GW00372695

IN ISADORA'S STEPS

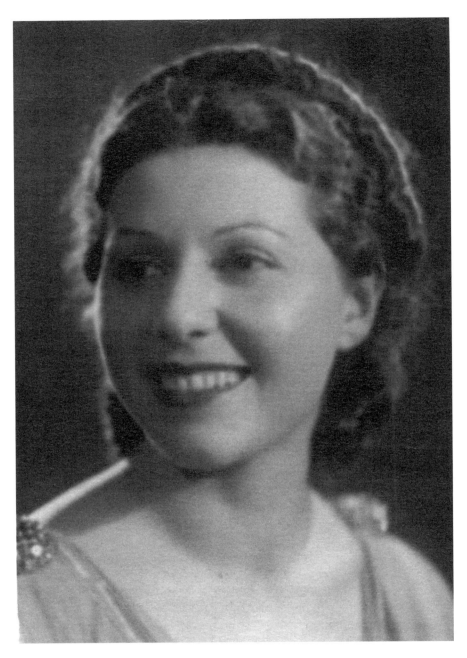

In Isadora's Grecian style, with hair braided and a tunic like a classical Greek *chiton*, fastened at each shoulder by a brooch, this is Lily ready to dance, aged 26.

IN ISADORA'S STEPS

*The Story of Isadora Duncan's School in
Moscow, Told by her Favourite Pupil*

Lily Dikovskaya
as told to Gerard M-F Hill

Book Guild Publishing
Sussex, England

First published in Great Britain in 2008 by
The Book Guild Ltd
Pavilion View
19 New Road
Brighton, BN1 1UF

Copyright © Lily Dikovskaya 2008

The right of Lily Dikovskaya to be identified as the author of this work has been
asserted by her in accordance with the Copyright, Designs and Patents Act 1988.

All rights reserved. No part of this publication may be reproduced, transmitted, or
stored in a retrieval system, in any form or by any means, without permission in writing
from the publisher, nor be otherwise circulated in any form of binding or cover other
than that in which it is published and without a similar condition being imposed on
the subsequent purchaser.

Typesetting in Garamond by
YHT Ltd, Hillingdon, Middlesex

Printed in Great Britain by
CPI Antony Rowe

A catalogue record for this book is available from
The British Library.

ISBN 978 1 84624 186 4

Contents

Acknowledgement

I would like to thank Keirsten Clark and Gerard Hill for their encouragement and support. Without them, this book could not have been written.

Lily Dikovskaya
2007

1

Prologue, 1905–21

Making friends with Grandma

The first time I met my grandmother, I was 8 years old. I was terrified of her, because she was wearing a scarf over her head. I had never seen people wearing scarves on their head, except witches in storybooks, so I thought she must belong to a witches' coven and I hid behind my mother. My grandmother never forgave me for that, never. She had expected me to come running to her.

Soon after that, my grandma came to live with us. I was at boarding school, but whenever I came home she would prepare a nice meal – she was an excellent cook and she kept everything spotlessly clean. Both those things pleased me very much, so I really tried to be friendly, to make up for our first encounter, when I thought she was a witch. I tried to make friends with her, and she responded, though it took time.

She was a very proud woman, who demanded respect from any-one who knew her. Even when she went downstairs and sat outside to get some fresh air, everybody who passed by greeted her – ''Madam Dikovskaya, how are you?'' – and she would be very pleased. After a while, I broke through to her and then I began to ask questions.

What my grandmother told me

My mother had never told me much about herself, but I knew that she came from a place in the Ukraine called Nikolaev. Funnily enough, I saw that town later on, when I was on tour with the group and we danced there. It was a lovely place: the streets were all adorned with acacia.

Whatever my mother told me was all very sketchy. Hungry to know more, I turned to my grandmother. She too told me that she came from Nikolaev - quite a large town, 70 miles east of Odessa - or, to be exact, she came from a place not far from Nikolaev. She started telling me about when she was young: she had a brother and a sister, and they lived with their father in a big house, which I think they rented. She never mentioned her mother, but that was because her father was always in the front of her mind: he ruled the family.

I don't have to tell you that the Jews had a very difficult time in Russia, but my grandmother's father rented land and he grew wheat and kept cows on it. They had a kind of farm, big enough that they employed farmhands. Actually, my grandmother's family were all rather educated people. She told me that her brother - who was tall and rather handsome - used to ride and he joined the dragoons.

When she came of age, my grandmother was lucky enough to have two suitors and to be allowed to choose the one she preferred. He was well educated and earned a lot of money. They married and were happy, I would think, until a great misfortune occurred. One day at the bank where he worked, a case of fraud was discovered - a forged cheque or something - and he was made the scapegoat. He was the only Jewish person there, so it was easy to pick on him. He told his wife he was very worried: he felt they would not be satisfied with his resignation and he would have to leave Russia completely, or they would pursue him.

When this happened, her husband - strangely enough, I never knew his surname - decided to go to America and asked her to come with him, but she said she was terrified of her father. What it had to do with her father, I have no idea, but she just let him go. He went to America by himself and she was left. She was never divorced - it was as if she was a widow.

So she got married again, to a man called Dzhikovski - a widower with a son. When I heard all this, I was incensed.

"How could you do a thing like that? Why didn't you go to America? We would all have been born there, and not here."

She laughed and said she was frightened of her father.

"What could he do, if you went?" I wanted to know. And how did her husband feel about all this?

Nevertheless, she settled down with this man Dzhikovski and they

2

had five children who survived infancy. The eldest was Isaac; the second was a girl who died of diphtheria. Then she had three more daughters – Liza (my mother), Luba, who was the beauty of the family, and Clara, whom I stayed with one summer.

"But then something happened I could never forget," said my grandmother.

"What did happen?" I asked.

Well, she told me that her children were engaged in politics. I didn't understand what that meant. She explained to me they were fighting for equality – they wanted to be recognised as people. The eldest son was in charge; I think he knew Trotsky.

It was 1905 and the start of all the revolutionary ideas. Being Jewish, this particular group always thought that one day they would be free, if they only had some idea how to make freedom for themselves. The irony of it was that it never worked out that way, but that's what they thought.

The elder son used to organise meetings where they lived, in a small house in Nikolaev. His sister, Luba, was very beautiful and she had been married only about six or seven months at this time. Auntie Luba was part of the movement, though she wasn't sure about it, but the rest of the family were not, apart from another uncle – the youngest, Uncle Peter. Now this episode my mother did tell me about.

It was all very quiet in the cellar, the meeting had finished and they were all chatting. A young chap stood up. There was a revolver lying on the table and he picked it up, pointed it at my aunt Luba and said, "I will kill you". Before anyone could do anything, he shot her. She was killed outright, on the spot. Why did he do it? Was it a joke? Did he really not know that the pistol was loaded?

They couldn't get over it. I know they hushed it up because at that time in Russia, as a group with socialistic ideas, they had to be very discreet. So they couldn't do anything. My mother never knew what happened to the man afterwards; all she knew was that her sister was dead. My grandmother nearly lost her senses: to lose her daughter, such a lovely girl, so full of life and just married, it was such a terrible tragedy. When I heard this story, I was horrified too.

Liza Dikovskaya flees Russia

And that's how my mother's wanderings started. After that dreadful tragedy, the authorities found out about the activities of this group – I don't know what they called themselves – and my uncle Isaac, who had arranged the meeting, decided it was time to leave Russia. He ran away to Belgium.

My mother wasn't there at the time – she was studying couture in Odessa – but when she came home she heard all about it. Her brother had left by himself and she felt very sorry for him. How would he manage? She decided to follow him. How they got out of Russia I will never know, because I learnt afterwards that the younger brother, Uncle Peter, tried twice, but was caught on the border and sent back. He was lucky they never put him in prison; instead, they put him in the army.

So my mother followed and was reunited with her brother. They found they did not like Belgium, so they decided to go to France. They settled in Paris, and Uncle Isaac found a job as an engineer – he could adapt to circumstances and he was a very intelligent, clever man.

Paris suited my mother very well, and not just because it was the home of *haute couture*. She was very arty and went to see any concert or show that was going; that was her, though she had no musical talent herself. That I inherited from my father. She never missed Enrico Caruso or Sarah Bernhardt, and Paris was where my mother first saw Isadora Duncan dancing. She loved the way Isadora danced and she said to herself, *This definitely is the dance for the future*.

Although she was a couture dressmaker, who had finished her apprenticeship in Odessa and trained a bit in Paris, yet she couldn't get work readily and never had a regular job. So after about three years she decided to move on. She heard that you could earn a very good salary in London and that on bank holidays there was no passport control at English ports. I don't think my mother had a passport, judging by the way she ran away from Russia. Of course, I wasn't even thought of at this time. She wasn't married.

So she went to London, took a room in the East End and settled there. She taught herself new skills and it didn't take her long to find a very good position. She worked for a couturier, earning £6, £7 or £8 a week, which was a lot of money when average earnings were

4

less than £2 a week, even for men. She could afford to go out; there were social clubs locally and dozens of theatres and concert halls in the West End.

Then Liza Dikovskaya met a young man, like her an immigrant in the clothes trade, and he lived close by. He was an Austrian tailor; she was a Russian dressmaker. His name was Joseph Lotterbach and soon afterwards she married him. Perhaps this explains why I am good at doing things, especially sewing, which I enjoy. In this I take after my parents.

When she discovered she was pregnant, my mother was very surprised. She had no desire to have children: that was the last thing she wanted. She tried various things to avoid having the child: she used to lift heavy things and did various strange exercises to get rid of me, but no, she couldn't do anything about it – I was very firm. I was born in the London Hospital in Whitechapel on 2 March 1913.

My mother told me often that she wanted to call me Shulamith, but they couldn't spell it in the hospital. She was in the Lily Ward and apparently the women who gave birth to girls on that ward usually called them Lily, so that's how I got my name.

Even though my mother never wanted me in the first place – she told me that – and even though she tried to get rid of me, nevertheless, when I was born she really loved me very much. Not that she accepted me, but she really loved me, and she loved to do things for me, things she thought would benefit me.

I still have a photograph of myself at six months and anyone can see I was cared for. She used to take me to Hyde Park. She dressed me beautifully; again, you can see that on photographs. I remember very vaguely one visit to the studio with her, when the photographer gave me a gold ball to hold. She looked after me very well and we lived quite nicely, until I was three.

My mother does things *her* way

My mother never talked about how she uprooted me at the age of three. She was very strong-minded, in her own particular way, and that is something I regret really. I know women always think they know best, so they have should have a very big say in all matters; but, when they get their way, it doesn't always work out for the best.

After all, people have to live together and that means they have to accept that other people will do things differently.

Meanwhile, my mother liked London and she had made many friends – one in particular, Annie Isaacs, remained a very good friend for many years – and she wanted to go out and meet people at these social clubs in the East End. She longed to go to plays and concerts, opera and ballet, as she had before. Time passed and my mother became more and more disappointed with my father, because he still had an independent life and she didn't.

She thought: *He doesn't understand the problem. He can go out with his friends and I have to stay in with the child, but I am working and I need a break too*. She didn't like it and one day she decided she had had enough of it – she walked out on him, with me. I was three years old.

When I was bigger, I used to ask her: "Why did you leave my father?" I always wanted to know what was the reason, but she would always say, "It is of no importance." She never understood that children need both parents; she just never understood that. She didn't think that she had done anything wrong. She thought a mother was sufficient.

But I thought: *Why did she take on all that responsibility, all by herself?* In fact, she wasn't quite by herself, because she had her friend Annie. I knew her as Auntie Annie – she was like family to me, though she was no relation.

Staying with Auntie Annie

When my mother walked out, she went straight to Annie. It wasn't so much because Annie had a house of her own – at that time she lived in Stepney Green – but much more because she was a lovely woman and a good friend. Annie had four children: her eldest was a daughter and then she had three sons, Barney, Moss and Freddy. Of course, when I arrived, the two younger boys were very interested in me. Afterwards I found out that, when my mother was bathing me, they used to stand and watch. I think that was so sweet, really.

Speaking of baths reminds me of the smell of soap, and that brings back memories of hospital not long after my fourth birthday. I had mumps, but as I got better the weather seemed to improve too, so the nurse said we children could play in the garden if we liked. We all ran outside, but by the door there were some sharp stones, which I hadn't noticed. I fell on them and very badly damaged my right knee. The nurse was very concerned and held me in her arms while she bathed my knee with Sunlight soap - I know it was Sunlight, because the smell has stuck in my memory. It must have hurt, because I still have the mark on the lower part of my knee.

I don't know how long we stayed with Auntie Annie, but it was coming close to my fourth birthday when my mother got her own place and we moved out. She had this independent nature and she could earn good money.

She kept in touch with my uncle Isaac - I have some postcards from him in Paris. She was still in touch with Annie too, because once she took me once to a club somewhere in the East End - I was just 4 - and she held me and danced with me, and there, amongst a crowd of people, was Auntie Annie. To me she seemed most beautiful, and she was. I stretched out my hand to touch her, and they both laughed.

Now that she was on her own, my mother had to take on more work to live and she couldn't cope with looking after me as well. I was a hindrance to her and she became desperate to settle me in a suitable boarding school. By chance she was recommended to a couple - Mr and Mrs Shapiro - who were thinking of starting a small boarding school, but not in London: they were moving to Lincoln, and they were going to open a school there.

At boarding school in Lincoln

I must have been a little over 4 years old when the Shapiros said they were ready to take the first boarders. My mother took me on the train to Lincoln and left me at their house. They took five boys and five girls, and they had two children of their own as well, Basil and Kitty. I was very friendly with Kitty. They had a big dog - Prince, his name was - and we used to sit on him and ride, because he was so huge.

I was very happy there: the house was lovely and its owners were charming people. The wife played the piano and her husband played the violin, and that was where my musical abilities started to grow. They were always playing us music of various kinds and he used to take us to concerts. Every Sunday we went to a cinema; they were all silent films then, so there was an orchestra. I think Mr Shapiro perhaps played in that orchestra.

We had music lessons, and after a while I started to tinkle the piano and play some tunes I had learnt. Soon I was learning how to play the piano. I used to sing too – I was told I had quite a nice voice – and my favourite song was the one about the little girl who had a little curl, right in the middle of her forehead.

I have such wonderful memories of Lincoln. We used to go on outings and once we were taken to the seaside. I looked recently at my collection of postcards and amongst them there was a postcard from the seaside in Lincolnshire. I signed my name on it.

We used to go to Lincoln Cathedral – a very beautiful building – though we never went inside. There was a little square park surrounding it and we used to go there quite often. It's funny, but I remember we never used to sit: we used to run about. I liked skipping and Mrs Shapiro noticed that – that I liked music, I liked to skip around and I could never keep still.

My mother used to come to visit me, and the last time she came Mrs Shapiro told her: "You had better take note of your daughter: she is very musical. She is going to be either a pianist or a dancer" – and that is where my mother got her idea.

A vitriolic attack

While I was in Lincoln, my mother was still in touch with Auntie Annie, who had been having a very difficult time. I didn't realise at the time, of course, but even when my mother and I were staying with her she was having terrible trouble with her husband. He was a gambler and it was difficult for her to pay the household bills, so she took two lodgers in.

By now Annie and her husband had moved to Finsbury Park, a pleasant district but more expensive than Stepney. When she discovered that Annie never had enough money to live on, my mother encouraged her friend to do something about it.

"Why do you stay with him? You have two lodgers. One of them is very handsome and he's very keen on you."

Indeed, this man *was* rather keen on her – she was very good-looking as well as capable – and he liked the boys as well. They were very intelligent boys and adaptable by nature. Funnily enough, at the time I thought this man was their real father.

Her husband used to gamble all his wages and Annie had three boys and a girl to care for and no money to feed them, so she was in despair. She told him so.

"I can't live like this any more; I have let two rooms and it is still not enough to live on. I think we had better part."

By this time my Auntie Annie had had enough of her husband and was determined to separate from him, but she had also got very close to this other man - Muscat, his name was - who was tall and handsome. He had money too, though where it came from and what he did were both a mystery.

It didn't take long for her husband to find out what was going on. It didn't worry him that the poor woman hadn't enough money to keep their children; but it did worry him that someone else might have her. He came home one day unexpectedly and threw acid in her face. He meant to damage her beauty for ever.

It gave her a terrible shock, but luckily my mother was there and managed to get her to hospital and saved her. Her face did heal up, but the case ended up in court; he went to gaol and afterwards Annie divorced him.

The middle son, Moss, could never forgive his father for doing such a terrible thing, because his mother was so beautiful. After that he refused to use his father's name, Isaacs. As I say, it was lucky my mother was there, and this episode made the ties between our two families even stronger.

The revolution reaches Highgate

Muscat was rather an attractive man; he proposed, and Annie married him. Despite the part my mother played in bringing this about, she was always doubtful about who he was and why he was in London. I think even Annie never knew where he worked or what he did, but he spoke fluent Russian.

Eventually we learn that this lodger was a big organiser in Russian revolutionary circles and was constantly in touch with Lenin; they belonged to the same Communist group. In fact, it was while Lenin was staying in Highgate that he first saw Isadora Duncan dance. Well, when the revolution was successful, Muscat was summoned to St

Petersburg and he asked Auntie Annie if she and her children would come with him.

Her daughter refused. She said she wasn't going to Russia, it wasn't the country she wanted to live in and she would stay with her father when he was released. He must have had some relations in London that she stayed with before that. I don't think he was very long in prison and when he was released they went to America. I know for a fact he was in New York.

Annie agreed to go with Muscat to Russia, with the three boys. That was in late 1917, when the revolution really hadn't come to an end; in fact it started again when Lenin arrived. Nonetheless, Muscat went to St Petersburg with Annie and the three boys, and they stayed in Smolny, the place where they made the glass. One of her sons, Barney, was sent to guard Lenin, where he was living, in a kind of office building.

Preparing to go to Russia

My mother kept in touch with Annie, so she knew when the revolution was over and the Bolsheviks seemed to be established. For a long time there was something like civil war there, as well as other wars, but eventually in late 1920 – though she didn't tell me that straightaway – my mother decided it was time to return to Russia.

Later on, when I asked her why, she said her family was still in Russia; when I pointed out that one uncle was still in Paris, she said he too was planning to go back to Russia, because he also was one of these socialists, and that decided it.

I was 7 when my mother came to take me away from the school in Lincoln, where I had been so happy. I felt very sad to say goodbye to my best friends, Kitty and Basil – I knew I would miss them a lot. They came to the station to see me off – in fact everybody came – and my mother and I set off back to London on the train. I had my things in a little basket.

When we reached London, we went to a new address in Russell Street, where my mother had rented one room, with a little landing where she did the cooking. It was very primitive, with hardly any furniture – just the necessities – and what we had was most unattractive. I was very disappointed. Then I discovered we were to go to

Moscow. Well, I was interested in a way, though I had no idea where Moscow was.

The owner of the house, Mrs Ostrovskay, was very kind and nice to me. She had three children - all grown up - two sons, who had just come back from the army, and Sally, who was a secretary. My mother always told me she didn't want me to be a secretary - but then I don't think I would have made a very good secretary anyway.

My mother had been in touch with the rest of her family, as well as with Auntie Annie, and as a result she had decided to go. I'm not sure why, but it seemed time was pressing. As soon as she got back to Russell Street, my mother started preparing. She and Mrs Ostrovskay talked a great deal about going to Moscow; they discussed what clothes we would need and then we went to buy them.

Amongst the people my mother knew from the social club in the East End there was a family - I have a photo of them - a taxi driver, his wife and their two children. We became very friendly with them in that short time. It was coming towards Christmas and we went with them to see two pantomimes, *Peter Pan* and *Babes in the Wood* - at which I cried. After that we used to spend a little time with the family. I remember sleeping with her daughter, who was about a year older than me - we had so much fun. We laughed all night! She was called Hetty and her little brother was Ben.

Those three months before we went to Moscow, they were hectic. There were formalities too. We needed passports, but the British Government didn't want us to go. They said that Russia was not fit to take children at present; grown-ups could go if they liked, but they were not to take children. My mother had to sign a declaration that we would never come back.

Fairyland

Of course, we visited all my mother's many friends; we went to see various stage shows; we went shopping; then one afternoon she turned her attention to me.

"Is there anything you would like?"

"Yes, I would like a nice doll."

So she took me off to buy a doll. We went down Oxford Street on the top deck of a double-decker bus and it was already dark, because what struck me were all the lights.

11

Coming towards Marble Arch, we got off on the left-hand side; we stayed on that pavement, turned our backs on Marble Arch and walked back along Oxford Street. The shops were glittering with toys and presents, there were Christmas lights and it looked just like Fairyland to me.

We came to a beautiful toy shop and stood looking in the window until my mother said, "Well, you can choose any one you like. Which do you like best?" As I liked fairy tales, I chose a fairy doll with a wand. We went in, she bought me that beautiful doll and we went straight back home.

Since our landlady was very nice to me, the first thing I did when we got back was to go downstairs to show her my doll. She had her two sons back from the army, her daughter had come home from work and they were all gathered in the kitchen – well, a big room that served the landlady's family as kitchen and sitting room combined. When I had showed my doll, they all stayed there talking.

I went upstairs to our room and I found four little candles. After that wonderful ride down Oxford Street, I decided I liked glitter, so I lit all the candles and stood them up on the floor, still alight. I put one in each corner and then I went down to tell them all to come up and look – and a good job I did, because otherwise I could have burnt the place down!

I never interfered with my mother's packing, but I know she took that lovely fairy doll with us.

An interview for stepfather

One day when I was at home, an odd thing happened. I must have been playing out and I came back home to find my mother had a gentleman with her. I was very surprised: I had never seen him before. My mother got up from her chair and came across the room to me – our sitting room was quite big – and she whispered to me: "Would you like to have a father? Do you want a new father?"

I looked at her and then I answered: "No, I want my own father."

At the time I could only say what I thought: I missed my father. I always knew there was something odd. I had noticed that other children had a mother and a father, but I had just a mother. I didn't know even my father's name.

My mother told me long afterwards that he was a friend of hers who came to propose to her. I was astonished at her. "Why on earth did you ask a child about it? What can a child say?" Anyway, my mother refused him – I always told her, "That was very foolish of you" – but nevertheless that's what she did.

Journey to Moscow

Then the time came when we were all ready to go. Early in 1921 we said goodbye to Mrs Ostrovskay and set off. I don't know how we got to the boat, but I certainly remember crossing the Channel. It was February, the seas were rough and there were people lying all over the decks.

I was walking about on deck and there was another girl walking about too. Her name was Cecilia Viviurka. I was 7½ and she was a bit older. I liked her, and she took to me too. I was always a serious child; I liked a laugh, but I was serious in other ways. She loved reading and I found out that her father was a writer, and she and her mother were travelling to Moscow to meet up with him.

Then we landed, we boarded the train and I lost touch with Cecilia for the time being. The journey was tedious and the train was awful. There were no bunks, nowhere you could really sleep. I couldn't get to sleep, so my mother found a little pillow for me to rest my head on. While I was lying there, all I could see was sausages hanging from God knows where, a kind of a stove in the centre of the train. The whole journey was so odd. Eventually I wanted to know how much longer this would last.

"How long will it take to get to Russia?"

"Oh, it won't be very long" she said. She was always very, very optimistic, but for once she was right: shortly after that, we arrived.

Moscow 1921

Now we were not the only immigrants – I heard there were about three hundred of us – and we had arrived in a country that was devastated, but they had tried to make at least some preparations for us. They took us to a large building that had previously been a hospital, but it hadn't even been disinfected and the whole place smelt of cabbage – it was awful. They had beds ready for us, but the men were placed separately from the women and children.

There were loads of children – Germans, Americans, Britons, all sorts – but they were dying like flies. I remember, the first night, we were given a bed next to a young German woman and she had such a gorgeous little boy and a girl with big, blue eyes. The girl was called Erica, and I remember her sitting on the bed, such a sweet child, and the next morning she wasn't there. She had died.

And then I noticed there were rats running about, there were rats on the tables by our beds. I felt it was unbearable; the place was infested with rats. I remember, when I was sleeping with my mother on the bed, I opened my eyes and saw a rat sitting there. I was horrified; this image has never left my mind.

Words cannot describe the terrible place where they put all the immigrants; the whole atmosphere there was so degrading and so ghastly. Half the English women went back immediately. I don't know how they arranged it, but they left their husbands and went back; they said they were never going to stay there.

Later on, I often asked my mother what possessed her to take me to such a place.

"What on earth made you move me from England, where I was healthy and happy, and take me through such devastating conditions? I will never forget my first impression of Russia as long as I live. It was so awful."

She had been in touch with her family, and with Auntie Annie, so she must have had some idea what conditions were like in Moscow at that time.

"Well, my family was there, and I felt a bit lonely, and in any event now you were with people who, if they made up their minds to do something, they did it. And now it's done, so there's no point in arguing about it."

My mother was immune to anything, because her idea was that the revolution was the important thing and there was a wonderful future coming. Well, you cannot argue about the future; and, after all, freedom is a wonderful thing and they all wanted it.

The Jewish people were so naïve: they thought that they would change the Russian attitude towards them – which they never did, as they found out eventually, but you couldn't argue with them then. The only thing that did change was that now they could live in the big towns. They could even live in Moscow, and nobody would stop them just because they were Jewish.

On the streets

We didn't stay at the hospital very long because it was so terrible and obviously dangerous. A few days passed and my mother took me out. The sights we saw, walking along the streets, were incredible. It was winter and there was snow on the ground; dead horses lay where they had fallen; there were people sitting on the pavement who were clearly dying. I thought it was a nightmare, as if I had come from another world.

I was dressed up, in a fur coat with a little fur wrapper, hat, boots and warm gaiters. We saw other children, but they were dressed very differently: they looked like urchins. I was well protected from the weather; they were not. They stopped to look at me: they thought I was a phenomenon.

Wherever we went, they crowded round us like beggars, pointing at us and calling, "Bourgeois, bourgeois!" I asked my mother what was going on.

"What do they want? Why are they so angry and calling us names? Why are they being so rude and pointing at us?"

"Oh, don't take any notice. It's because you are wearing such nice clothes, and they haven't any nice clothes."

"Why did you bring me here? Can we go home?"

"No – there is a big future here."

She spoke to me as if I were a grown-up. When I look back, I cannot understand my mother telling me simply to take no notice. Even then, at the age of 7, I could see this adventure was turning into something awful.

I didn't know how much money she had, but I knew I was hungry, because the food they gave us was not fit for the rats, never mind for us.

"Mum, I am starving."

My mother managed to buy me a kind of flaky pastry with meat inside – *pirozhky*, the Russians call them – and I tried to eat it very slowly, to make it last. That was all the solid food I got that day.

A room of our own

Not long after that, my mother found a room, not too bad, and rented it. The government helped, of course; they helped the immigrants as much as they could, because these people had come to help build a new country. The immigrants were so naïve: they thought it would be like going to America to build a new country. But in America there were different attitudes.

Very soon my mother got in touch with Auntie Annie. Until then I hadn't realised she was in Moscow, but now she used to send one of her sons to me with food every day. He used to bring me soup or whatever she could get, which was quite a lot, because after all she was married to this important official, Muscat.

One day I came home and found I had a grandmother. I was afraid and hid behind my mother; and from that moment my granny never liked me. She called me a foreigner and that's how we were to each other.

My mother was really desperate to get me a place in a dance academy. She hoped to get me taken on by the Grand Theatre, the Bolshoi, and I think we went there one day, to find out how to get started. She wanted me to be a ballet dancer, and I believe I could have succeeded in that.

Shortly afterwards I asked my mother when we were going to go somewhere better. She said, "Don't worry: I'm looking out for you, I'm arranging things. I've brought you here because I want you to dance."

We didn't stay in that small room long. My mother got a much bigger room and we moved in, together with my grandmother. Nobody had a whole flat then; it was one room, one household. The government had confiscated all the flats from their owners and split them up. This was a nice room in a pleasant road, a peaceful place, and we settled down there. My grandmother was never very loving, but I did try to make friends with her.

Off to the country

Summer was coming now and the authorities arranged a holiday for us. They found us a place somewhere in the country and took us there, all the immigrant families. The parents looked after the food and cooked for us. We had the same soup every day, and we didn't get much, but we didn't go hungry. It was usually made of beans, or whatever they could find, as long as it wasn't cabbage. We didn't like the smell of cabbage soup, especially since it brought back memories of that hospital.

There were many Jewish people and I was Jewish, but I remember eating all sorts of things. Facing me at the table was a boy called Michael. I had a pimple on my face as a result of malnutrition, and one of the other children said, "Lili, you have a pimple," whereupon Michael said, "Yes, that's where I kissed her." I thought to myself, *What a nasty thing to say*. I so disliked him then and, when I met him later, I found I still couldn't stand him.

In Moscow and on our summer camp, I had all my immigrant friends round me, which I preferred. We spoke English because it was easier. Up to that time I had always thought that everyone in the world spoke English when they were born, and then they learned different languages later. Now I discovered it wasn't like that – which was funny.

I first hear of Isadora Duncan

Meanwhile, my mother learnt that Isadora Duncan had arrived in Moscow in late July. She had seen Isadora dance in Paris and afterwards in London. Later they happened to meet – they knew each other by sight from visiting mutual friends in Paris – and my mother found out that Isadora was planning to open a school in Moscow. After that, there was no argument as far as she was concerned: Isadora's was the dance of the future and Isadora's school was where she was going to enter me.

All my mother said to me at the time was, "I want you to dance, because I have been told you have talent. Of course, we will have to see if they take you on or not, but I have seen Isadora Duncan dance, and her type of dancing I much prefer to ballet."

At last, one day my mother read an announcement in the *Moscow Worker* that the State School of Dancing was to open at Prechistenka 20 under the direction of Isadora Duncan, who would hold auditions there for promising young dancers, starting in early September 1921.

My mother was good at arranging things: she found out all about the school and made sure I was one of the very first children whose name was put down. She told her friends about it and they put down their children's names as well. So a whole group of us from among the new arrivals applied to join Isadora Duncan's school.

2

The Duncan School: its First Year, 1921-2

The commissar in charge of the arts, Anatoliy Lunacharsky, was a prominent figure and a very intelligent man who understood theatre and dance. He went to Paris to meet Isadora and invited her to start a school in Moscow; she was delighted. Yet no one in the Kremlin really supposed she would come. So, when she did arrive in July 1921, there wasn't even anyone at the station to meet her.

Prechistenka 20

Since the Russian authorities had not expected Isadora Duncan to take up their invitation, they had made no plans to accommodate her school. After a month or so, the Ministry of Culture allocated her a mansion on Prechistenka street, a very fashionable address. It had previously belonged to a millionaire called A. K. Ushakov and his wife, Alexandra Balashova, a leading ballerina. He was the owner of the Gubkin & Kuznetsov tea company, with tea plantations from Russia to Ceylon.

After the couple fled to Paris in 1917, the house was taken over by the Soviets, who granted it in 1921 to Isadora Duncan, newly arrived from Paris, where the Ushakovs had moved into a house previously owned by their new 'tenant'. Isadora, amused, called this stately international exchange of quarters "a quadrille".

Prechistenka 20 was beautiful and very spacious, with huge rooms. I remember on that first day entering what seemed to me like a palace. What struck me first was the great vestibule, with a statue – the Venus of Melos – and marble benches against the right-hand wall, which had a very large door in the middle, flanked by windows

19

looking onto the summer garden. On either side of the benches there were statues of satyrs playing flutes.

In front of you, on the left-hand side, was the most magnificent marble staircase supported by a huge pillar. I love staircases! This one was extraordinarily lovely. The school was laid out with the main rooms upstairs, on the first floor: our bedrooms, the two dance studios, Isadora's apartment and Irma's (Irma had been one of the pupils at her first school).

My first lesson with Isadora

Not long after she put my name down, my mother got a letter telling her when to bring me to Prechistenka 20. All the children had to go on the first day and register – over two hundred of them, not all Russian – and then Isadora would sort out the ones she wanted.

My mother had told other immigrant families about Isadora Duncan's school, so a little group of us walked there together on our first day. One girl, Yetta, was younger than me, so I was asked to take charge of her. In those first two or three months, I was usually paired with Yetta and I wouldn't leave her.

A maid met us, we said goodbye to our parents, and she took us up that beautiful marble staircase, across the upper vestibule to the Oak Room. There, a woman who spoke English – her name was Rosalin, I found out later – helped us to undress and put us into simple Grecian tunics.

Then, barefooted, we were paired off and taken across that broad landing at the head of the stairs, through open double doors into a huge studio draped with curtains – pale blue, with matching pale blue carpet. We called it the Blue Room, and our tunics were blue as well, to match; later, we had red ones.

There she was, standing, waiting to greet us, and next to her was Irma. They wore tunics like ours, but with drapes on top, and their feet were bare too. Isadora was tall for a dancer – about 5' 6" – whereas Irma was about 5' 2" or 5' 3".

When I first saw them, I thought Isadora was Irma, and Irma was Isadora. That was because Irma looked older, though she wasn't of course. But she was so pale, so drawn and very serious; she wasn't smiling. In fact she never smiled. Isadora looked younger, with gentle eyes set in a calm face. She moved gracefully and effortlessly, almost as if she was floating.

When we entered that big room, Isadora separated us and put us all in order in a line and then she said to us, "We will play music now, and I want you to listen. Put your two hands just here and listen to the music." There was no novelty for me in music; I loved it. The pianist played Schumann - I remember that, because I knew the piece. It was lovely.

Isadora said, "Follow me - just lift your arms, just lift them slowly, slowly up and make a wide movement." That was the very first movement. Then she said, "Follow!" and started moving her arms, up and down, and showing us these ordinary but beautiful movements - and I loved this, I really did. I didn't think about whether I was doing it well or not - I just followed what she showed us - and the time just flew.

We learn to move

After that, we were asked to come back at a certain time - some of us each day, in groups - because she couldn't see everyone at once. Each time we arrived at school, it struck us again how beautiful it was: we liked it so much, even just walking up the steps.

Isadora was looking for a sense of rhythm, a good ear, timing and of course the ability to move easily. Each day Irma would show us some new movements: first how to stand, but she made even that beautiful. After that she said, "Lift your hands up, then look down at the ground, then back up again." Everything was simple and I liked that very much.

Next Isadora asked Irma to show us how to walk - that was interesting, learning how to walk gracefully. "Walk always forward with your body, and not backwards. When you put your foot down, you put your toe down first and hold your arms." That's how she started us off, to make it easier for us. Isadora said, "Put your arms up as if you are carrying something, and then walk."

Irma showed us how to skip, but I always did skip. So I was very good - I was so light, as light as a feather. When Irma and Isadora saw that, they took great interest in me, in fact from the very first day I came. After skipping, we learned the polka and then the waltz, and every day we were given two of Gurdjieff's *Mouvements variés* to practise, and lots of other things to do.

When you are young, certain things stick in your head. The second or third time we went, there was a man sitting, watching. Yetta and I were paired; she had long blonde hair and I had long dark hair. As we came in, he evidently thought Yetta and I made a charming couple, and he stopped us and stroked our hair.

After that, he used to look out for Yetta and me as we walked into class. This was Anatoliy Lunacharsky, the minister who had asked Isadora to come and start a school. He had made all the arrangements for her, so he was at the school regularly, especially at the beginning when Isadora was choosing her pupils. He chose Ilya Schneider, a journalist who wrote about the arts, and especially dance, to be the director of the school.

In those first months, I also noticed a young man watching our classes. Lunacharsky, I knew, had reason to be there, but I wondered to myself, *What on earth is this young man doing here?* When the school opened, I found out why: apparently he was a well-known poet called Yesenin, and Isadora had invited him.

One famous writer who knew Yesenin used to say he was like a rough diamond, but I never saw him sparkle. He came from a village and had extraordinary ways with him. I disliked him from the start and I never did come to like him – and I was right not to. I didn't like his attitude, his over-familiarity when he came and watched our classes.

Lenin at the Bolshoi

Meanwhile, Lenin and Lunacharsky arranged for us to give a concert in the Grand Theatre – 'Bolshoi' just means 'big' or 'grand' – on 7 November, the fourth anniversary of the revolution, and Isadora thought she would teach us youngsters to sing and dance the Internationale. We didn't really know what Isadora was going to do, because we were too busy learning our parts.

We were beginners – for example, we had just learned how to waltz – and there wasn't much time to prepare, so she taught us a few movements that we could perform. Beforehand, we had a rehearsal in the big theatre – with the drapes brought from school, the blue drapes and the carpet – though the stage itself had to be made smaller because it was too large for us to occupy all of it. But the stage was arranged very well.

We had our little tunics on, and I remember walking across the stage wearing boots I had brought from London. They were buttoned boots, and the blue and red lights that shone from below the stage - the footlights - shone on my boots. It went through my mind that they looked very attractive. We couldn't dance barefoot in rehearsal, because they hadn't yet laid the carpet.

There were about 75 of us youngsters. We were not really needed until the last part of the concert, so we could watch Isadora. The theatre was packed with dancers who had come to see her. She danced the Internationale and then Tchaikovsky's 6th Symphony, which made a tremendous impression on me. I saw her dance it more than once, so I shall say more about it later. Her final solo item was Tchaikovsky's *Marche Slav*.

At the end of the concert, we all had to dance the Internationale. Isadora danced again, in front, but we girls - the whole school, and there were plenty of us! - all went in a row, holding hands over our heads. Irma led us like a snake until the end of the song, and we sang as well as danced, and even the audience sang it with us.

It was remarkable - and near the end, at the line 'Bring all the working people of the world together', we heard somebody shout several times, from the place in the balcony where the tsar had previously sat, "Brava Isadora! Brava Duncan! Brava Miss Duncan!" It was Lenin, who had arrived towards the end of the concert. That was really interesting for us girls, and Isadora was very pleased about it. The resident company perhaps weren't so pleased, though.

That first success didn't last very long, because the Grand Theatre - the Bolshoi - fought to prevent us spreading our art. It was nothing but a fight from the beginning to the end. It was a terrible thing, very bad, because they took everything from her that they could. Even the Bolshoi took all the beautiful movements and the freedom of moving that she had shown them, but they never acknowledged Isadora's ideas or talent. The spotlight remained on them.

The pink ticket

In our dancing classes we did marching and skipping first; then we learnt the polka, first on our own, then in pairs and finally in circles;

23

after that we practised running and big leaps; and only then did we dance the waltz. This went on for two months.

Then there came the day when Isadora sorted us out: some people got blue tickets and some got pink tickets. I had a pink one. It turned out that the ones with pink tickets were being taken on; the blues weren't. So I was among the ones who were taken on. I was 8 years old.

I nearly said 'I was one of the lucky ones', but there was no luck in it. Either you were good enough for Isadora or you weren't. It didn't even matter whether you'd had dancing lessons, because I hadn't.

Those of us with a pink ticket were told that, the next time we came to school, we should come prepared to stay. We couldn't enter straightaway because things weren't ready. They had to arrange everything – the kitchens, the staff, the bedrooms. While they were doing that, for a short period we came every day to train with Isadora and Irma.

Aunt Clara

Having only recently discovered that I had a grandmother, now I found that my mother had a sister as well. She never lived anywhere very near us, but she came to see us. Since Moscow was full up, it was difficult for my aunt to find anywhere to stay, so she rented a *dacha*, a cottage in the countryside near Moscow.

My mother decided that it would do me good to go to the country for a while, until the school opened. To be honest, I didn't enjoy it. For one thing, it was November, but in any case I didn't like the house and I wasn't much enamoured of my auntie Clara or her five children – to me they were all strange.

So far I hadn't spoken Russian and I didn't know how to get going with my new cousins, but it's funny how children manage. One of my cousins was a boy and he made me swear I would be his wife. I didn't say yes and I didn't say no; I was cautious, but also diplomatic. I said, "Let's wait and see – who knows?"

The facilities there were primitive and rather unpleasant. Unlike the room my mother was renting in Moscow, which had access to a proper bath, here my aunt had only a tub and that's where she bathed us. When my mother first told me to get into the tub, I

24

refused and that was the first time my mother had ever hit me. I cried bitterly – I was terribly unhappy there.

Malaria

I have photos from the first year of the school and several of them don't show me, because I was at home with a terrible fever. This was malaria. It begins with you shivering, yet with a high temperature. After a while, you seem to be recovering, but the illness comes and goes. My mother was very upset.

There had been mosquitoes around this *dacha* where we stayed with my aunt, and one must have bitten me. I didn't know then that I had caught malaria; that came out only when I got back from Aunt Clara's to our rented room.

However, in the block where we lived, there was a very good doctor. My mother contacted this Professor Frischkop, who gave her some drops for me, and they, rather surprisingly, cleared the malaria. For a while it kept coming and going – malaria is a very strange complaint: you feel cold and stop eating – but eventually I began to recover.

While I was getting better, my grandma looked after me. I used to be fascinated by a very big painting on the wall of our room, showing a synagogue and people praying. I didn't know what it was about: I had no idea about religion. All my mother ever told me was that we Jewish people were persecuted. And I knew there were some differences between us and the Russians. The painting didn't hang there for long, and I soon forgot about it when I entered Isadora's school.

Christmas!

Isadora opened her school officially on 3 December 1921. I had been going to Prechistenka 20 through the day since September, at first for assessment by Isadora and Irma, and then each day for classes in movement and dance, but now I became a boarder again. Straightaway we set to work, not just ordinary lessons, but also making paper chains, toys and ornaments for the Christmas Tree. They used to bring us all sorts of pieces of paper and glitter, and we would make whatever we could, whatever we were told. Our director produced many lovely things - he put up coloured lights in our dancing hall, he got hold of little baubles and things, and he arranged for the tree to be lit up. But what we could make ourselves, we did.

When Christmas came that first year, they put us all in little red velvet tunics - for best, but also to keep us warm - and my mother brought me some beautiful high boots. They were decorated all over with thin leather, like the ones Ukrainians used to wear. Isadora noticed them and said to our director, "You see what Lili is wearing? I would like all the girls to wear those. Can you get them?" I don't think he was able to get them, but I remember her taking note! And we were dancing round the Christmas tree and singing songs and Isadora was with us - she organised that.

On Christmas Eve, we all went to bed early but then Isadora used to come to wake us up at midnight. Yes, that brings back memories, especially since Christmas is coming as I'm writing this. We had nannies, but Isadora herself used to come into our bedrooms and wake us. "Children!" - and this was at twelve o'clock at night - "Up, up! Get up and put on your little red tunics and shoes, and follow me." We would follow Isadora and, when we got there, the tree was ready there in our big hall where we used to dance: we had a huge tree.

I remember so well that first Christmas, when I was 8 years old: we were woken up, dressed and taken to see the tree. I don't think there was any food, because I would remember if there had been: we were always hungry and food was so scarce. But we did have plenty of scenery and plenty of dancing at Christmastime.

Isadora used to make wings for us too; she would say, "Hold on to them" and then she would walk round the tree, with us following in a line, singing a pretty German song, 'O Tannenbaum'. We used to sing that with her, and then Christmas carols. All in all, we used to have a jolly good time. Isadora would then have a party in her own apartment, not with the children.

We would stay in the dancing hall to sing carols, and just look at the tree and enjoy ourselves, until about one o'clock in the morning, when we would be put back to bed. This was arranged just by Isadora and our nannies. I don't remember Irma being amongst us then, but I do remember Isadora. However, she was preparing to go to Paris after Christmas.

The ground floor

Let me tell you how the school was arranged. When parents came to the school, they sat on the marble benches in the great entrance hall while they waited to see their children or to see the director, whose office was on the left, by the foot of the marble stair. If, when you came in the front entrance, you walked to the back of the vestibule and turned left, there was a corridor running parallel to the street. On the left of this were some magnificent rooms.

First there was the dining room, which was large and quite grand. We used to have our breakfast and dinner there, because of course they made meals for us, but we also had lessons in that room. It had a very big black table, which had been taken out of the Japanese Room, next door.

The Japanese Room was a lovely, big room, very elaborate: everything was ebony, decorated with mother-of-pearl. It was marvellous, and that was where we did our gymnastics. At the top of the walls, at an angle and touching the ceiling, it had mirrors about two feet deep, going right round the room – the effect was most unusual. It was very strange because, when you did exercises, you could see your reflection as you did them. The mirrors had been installed for the ballerina Alexandra Balashova, when she used this as her practice room.

To make space for our gymnastics, they moved most of the furniture out of the Japanese Room. For a while they left a big sideboard there, but then it was taken upstairs to our bedroom. Valya told me that she slept in the Japanese Room at the beginning, and I have read that Yulia said the same, but I don't recall that.

Beyond that we had an 'isolator' – a sanatorium, particularly for infectious diseases – and next to that was the doctor's room. On the right-hand side of that corridor were smaller rooms, looking onto the big coach yard at the back of the house. One of these was a practice room for our pianist, and I used to hear music coming from this room at all times of the day. Our two nannies and the nurse had rooms there too.

At the back of the entrance hall was a door opening onto a long corridor. On the left were the food store and then the kitchens. Also down this corridor were rooms where all our washing was done: a laundry for our clothes and showers for ourselves. Yes, there were showers, which we used every day; and once a week we had baths, but not in a bath-tub: it was a kind of Turkish bath. That same passage took you to the dance room upstairs.

We had a summer garden and a winter garden. When you walked into the entrance hall, the summer garden was through the door on your right – that was where we would go when the weather was nice. It was a very fair size and, as well as playing in the garden, we used to plant little things. I remember we were taught how to put a seed in and we each had our own small container where we grew summer flowers. It was fun to watch them grow. The winter garden was indoors, beyond the 'isolator' at the opposite end of the corridor that ran from one side of the building to the other. We never went there; even in winter, it never attracted us. Behind the house was a great courtyard, big enough for a carriage-and-pair to turn in. We often played there in winter.

The first floor

I mentioned that, when you came in the front door, the main staircase faced you. If you walked up the great marble steps, the staircase ran straight up to the first-floor landing. Actually it was more like a great hallway, with a parquet floor, a high, painted ceiling and the walls hung with tapestries and large paintings in elaborate frames. Where it overlooked the entrance hall, the landing had an ornate stone balustrade. The pillars were of green marble.

At the top of the stair, on the left, was a large room that the school always used as a bedroom, with windows looking out onto the courtyard. The yard was very big and looked very nice, because it was meant to be seen. The main part of the house was L-shaped, but the building had been extended so that it was more or less like a square, with an opening where the carriages used to come in.

Upstairs was arranged much like downstairs, except that above the right-hand half of the vestibule there was another big room. When the school first opened, this was the bedroom where I slept. It had a musicians' gallery, so it must have been designed as a ballroom.

It was a lovely room because the windows faced the summer garden. It had an oak door and oak panelling, which made it rather sombre; I suppose they were inspired by the great oak tree in the summer garden. This tree had been left when the house was built, and it was surrounded on three sides by a huge balcony. In summer, the oak tree's foliage cast a dappled light across the room.

Later, Isadora made this into the Burgundy Room; it was the dance studio where she taught us. After her death, the Burgundy Room was dismantled and it became a bedroom again. Only then did we learn that it was really called the Oak Room. As you entered, to one side there was a little door to a staircase, which led up to the musicians' gallery and down to the cellar. Next to that, on the same wall on the left-hand side, there was a big door – glazed, I think – that led to the very big balcony above the summer garden.

When Isadora was away, Irma taught us in the blue studio. If you turned left at the head of the main staircase, this was the first room on your left. We called it the Blue Room because it had pale blue curtains and a matching pale blue carpet.

Its proper name was the Napoleon Room: the mansion had once been the home of General Alexei Yermolov, a hero of 1812. In the Battle of Borodino, he recovered General Raevsky's artillery from the French under Napoleon. The letter N in gold was repeated right across the ceiling and there was a huge painting, hanging in the middle of the wall on the right-hand side as you walked in. It showed Napoleon and it was labelled 'Vorobyoviy Goury'. That was the place, a few miles outside Moscow, where he stopped and commented he had at last reached "that Asiatic town with cupolas".

This was the room Isadora and Irma used that first autumn, when they were teaching and observing everyone who applied. After a while it became our bedroom – they took down the huge painting and the blue drapes, and then the room was much brighter – and it had a balcony overlooking the street. We each had a little bed, except for a short time when there weren't enough beds to go round. At about the same time they moved a big sideboard – it was beautifully made – out of the Japanese Room and brought it upstairs to our bedroom. We were told we could put our little belongings there. It was a huge thing and everybody had an allotted space. Of course we used to climb on it and jump down.

Next door was the Pink Room, so called because it had pink silk wallpaper. It had been called the East Room, and it was opposite Isadora's bedroom. At the beginning, we went through the Pink Room to enter the Blue Room for our dance classes. It also had an entrance to the winter garden, though that didn't interest us.

Opposite the Blue Room, across the corridor, there was a huge mirror, which ran from floor to ceiling. The door beside it led to Irma's room, which was very elaborate. I imagine it was originally the owner's bedroom. We went in there a few times, when Irma called us for something or other. Next to that – with a connecting door between them – was Isadora's room, which was perhaps used by the mistress of the house originally. She and Irma had one really big bathroom between them. The famous bathroom – famous because it was the only private bathroom in the house – was at the end of the corridor.

Between these two bedrooms was a small staircase. We only discovered this when our bedroom was changed from the Oak Room to the Blue Room. It was much more convenient for us, because it came out more or less opposite the dining room, where we also had some lessons, and the Japanese Room, where we started each day.

Meanwhile, our training? We loved it. The movements that Isadora had shown us at the beginning, they were so natural and at the same time so beautiful. And even at that simple stage she could somehow get us to use our imaginations to put the scene into good music, which is so very important, and put it into dance – but with time our routines developed.

Isadora could express the heart of music, which is so very important. We never did anything spectacular, but gradually we spent less and less time on the exercises we used to do when we entered the school. Eventually, we never did them at all: we only danced.

Beethoven

We had a second concert at the Bolshoi, in which Isadora danced the 7th Symphony of Beethoven. The music of that symphony dances; even Wagner called it "the apotheosis of dance". Speaking of him, Isadora also had a wonderful dance that she created for the Overture to *Tannhauser*. The older girls danced parts of the Beethoven, but in the second half there was a very vivacious part of the symphony, where we younger girls had to fly out from the side of the stage holding hands, and then fly back again, still holding hands, while Isadora danced downstage.

For the finale, Isadora danced on her own. I stood there in the wings and watched her dance the last movement of Beethoven's 7th.

I remember to this day the movements – skipping, and pointing, always pointing – and how extraordinary and light she was, and wonderful on her feet. The movements suited the music so well. I don't know whether any of the other girls watched her as I did, but I have always had such an interest in dancing and I remember that performance vividly.

After that of course I went to other performances. I am not sure how many girls went, because Isadora did some concerts of her own, quite separate from the school. This was in the early days of the school, but they took us to see her dance.

I remember sitting in the stalls at an evening concert, watching her dance a Chopin waltz, and I thought at the time – young as I was – I thought: *That doesn't suit her*. There were other views, of course, but that is what I felt. In fact, she didn't dance many waltzes – the majority of her dances were much more explicit. That was one of the things I liked about her, and not just the light movements. Her dances were so direct. They were good for young people. I realised that long ago.

The school day

There were about forty children taken on at the start – though I cannot remember the exact number – out of the two or three hundred who applied. Even though some of us had homes in Moscow, they made bedrooms for all of us, which wasn't difficult because it was a huge place.

The heating was difficult, because the central heating didn't work, but they got it going as time went by. Until they got it to work, they fixed big stoves in the main rooms and these were fed with logs. There was a lot of make-do-and-mend, and things were always changing.

After Christmas, we settled into our school routine. We never led an idle life, but I should perhaps explain our routine – it was rather a good one, actually. It was the same every day and it began early. The two nannies used to come and wake us each morning at seven o'clock.

Gym and breakfast

Before we did anything else, every morning we went downstairs to do exercise, or 'gym' as they called it. We had a special teacher for this - Irma and Isadora had nothing to do with teaching it - a young woman who taught only gym. We did it in the Japanese Room.

Isadora took a lot of advice from Anna Pavlova, when she met her abroad, and one thing she picked up from her was how to exercise - how to warm up - and how important that was. Our gym teacher showed us drill exercises and then we used to do all the rail movements, whatever was needed, with real gymnastic training, and then we practised all our dance movements.

After gym we were thrown under a cold shower, which was very, very cold, but then we were wrapped up, and dried and made comfortable. We put clothes on - the two nannies would help us dress. We were still shivering, but it did us a world of good, and we sat down very ready for breakfast, if you can call it that.

Our dining room was next to the Japanese Room and it had a very large black dining table. I think it was ebony; if so, it must have been brought in from the Japanese Room, because all the furniture there was made of ebony.

For breakfast we had just plain nothing; at least it tasted of nothing and it never filled us up. In the beginning it was always *kasha* (oatmeal), which we could not tolerate. All our school time, in the early days at least, there was nothing but hunger.

Lessons

After breakfast we went upstairs and had classes - ordinary classes with arithmetic and so on - with a special teacher for each subject. From time to time teachers used to leave and new ones came. One teacher used to teach geography, one used to teach Russian and we had two other teachers for languages, an English teacher and a French teacher. So we had four teachers and it was simple.

Our first lesson was arithmetic and astronomy. Of course we did sums every day, but I also remember the teacher telling us how the moon circles the world, while the world rotates around the sun and we had to make drawings of that. We learnt about the planets and the universe, and our place in it. Then we had geography. That took about two hours – or perhaps it just seemed like two hours.

Next we had an English teacher, Mrs Farrick, who didn't live far from our school. Some of the girls used to say to her, "Well, let's skip the lesson. Tell us about yourself." We were more interested in her life than her lessons and she was very willing to tell us about it. She was English-born, but married to a Russian – that's why she was in Moscow – so she used to tell us how she looked after herself, what she did when they had guests coming, all sorts of things. She used to lift her hands up and make very wide gestures as she told us how she lived. We were very charmed, and it's a good job we were because, if Schneider, the director, had known what was going on, he would really have given us what for.

Then we had a French teacher and she was rather strict – when we used to sit and wait for her round the table, she expected us to be 'at attention'. She used to say "Girls – backs straight!" and she had a little kind of stick to put at your back, to make you sit upright.

Then we had a teacher who used to do some drawing with us. The other day, I looked through one of my cupboards and I found there some of my drawings from school – and I see I was quite good.

Of course we had dancing classes during the day too, and I mentioned that Lunacharsky, the government minister, sometimes watched us dancing and stroked our hair as we passed. But that didn't last long – they cut our hair off short. There were so many children and no bath, so once a week we had a sort of Turkish bath, a sweat bath. Apart from that, there was only the one bathroom, which Isadora and Irma shared.

Afternoons

After our classes, we used to wash our hands and prepare ourselves for lunch – well, they used to call it *obiat* ('dinner'), so that was what we called it. We never called it lunch. Dinner was always cabbage soup, nearly every day, and *kasha* again. There were no other vegetables apart from what went into the soup.

After we had eaten our meal, which wasn't very nice, they would say, "You must lie down and rest now." We used to have an hour's rest in our bedrooms. If you wanted to sleep, you could, but whatever you did, you had to rest. Sometimes we slept and sometimes we didn't and after that we were taken for a walk for an hour or so, in pairs, right down Prechistenka. We lived in a very attractive part of Moscow, very near the big cathedral - that was very impressive and had little gardens, four of them. We used to like going there: it was near the river and you could see the Kremlin in the distance. We went there every day, and the routine was always the same.

We used to go to this beautiful church that they had, the biggest in Moscow. It was called Khrista Spasitela, meaning Christ the Saviour, and it was built in memory of 1812, when Russia was saved from defeat. They took it down afterwards. Actually, they destroyed it, blew it up. Stalin wanted to build a new campus for the university in its place, because they never had enough room to put up new buildings for the university, so the authorities said they had to take down this fantastic cathedral. Round it there were lovely gardens, and we used to walk there nearly every day.

We used to go inside the church sometimes, for various reasons, to have a look at paintings and other things, but not to pray. In any event, personally, I always found the church depressing. Did I like it inside? No, because it was so dark; but the outside I did like, because it was beautifully built and it had those lovely gardens. It was the nearest you could get to the woods in Moscow. It was a lovely spot there, and Auntie Annie used to live nearby. She was as good as a mother to me.

I should also mention the boulevards. There were two of them - one called 'A', which circled the city centre, and a bigger one on the outskirts, called 'B'. For our afternoon walk, we usually went to Boulevard A - it wasn't far from school, nor from where I lived, and it was very pleasant - and sometimes we walked to Boulevard B. Of course there was very little traffic; Moscow was so different then.

Free time and another lesson

After we had come back from our walk, we would have tea; after tea, we were given time for our own pursuits - reading or whatever one wished. We had that freedom of choice.

Then we had another session of study, and this time it was with our teacher of Russian language and literature. Although she was little in stature, she was the only teacher that we really listened to or respected. In fact, I think we feared her, because she was rather strict. Her name was Victoria Vakirovna and I remember her so well. She was the best teacher we ever had.

This evening class was downstairs in our dining room, so we would be sitting there waiting for her. Then we would hear her walking down the corridor and giving us instructions as she came along. We were ready to meet her of course, but she used to say, "Girls, girls, is everything ready? Have you got chalk? Are the dusters there?" – all this before she walked in. We didn't have monitors in charge of these things, but we made sure everything was in place ready for her.

With this teacher we learnt how to read and write Russian properly. She was very hot on spelling and we had to do Russian compositions too. I wouldn't say I was very good at composition, but I did my best! She was fantastic and we worked hard in Russian, which was very important for me. But I used to read a great deal, so I was interested in language generally and in Russian literature. I liked the history very much too. This teacher even talked about the economy. She was an excellent teacher, but quite adamant and she kept our class in check. We did respect her very much. That lesson lasted about an hour and a half and then, after she had gone, we had our supper.

Dancing in the evenings

After supper there used to be dancing, and our group was divided into the big girls and the younger ones. In the early years I was one of the youngest. One evening it would be the big girls; the next evening it would be the little ones. It was only when we had a combined dance that we would have a dance together. After the big girls had had their lesson, we younger ones would go through to find out all about it.

The big girls were equally interested in what *we* had been doing. They would run in to the bedroom after we had finished our class and say, "Girls, girls, show us! What did you do, what did Irma show you?" And we would all dance, to show them the steps and the movements – or sometimes just one of us would dance. Once, when we were doing a programme of Chopin, I was showing them the steps and one of them said to me, "Lilya, you do it the best."

So that is how the time passed, vigorously. It was so wonderful. I

35

couldn't wait to go back to school because it was so beautiful, being at school. You made your own life there.

Tsarskoye Selo and St Petersburg

From the start, we travelled to give performances. In the very early days of the school, when we were still learning basic skills and Isadora was there all the time, she started teaching us a polka by Rachmaninov, in preparation for a visit to Petersburg. Before we went, Isadora was vigorously training us. There were rumours that the composer himself would join us, but of course he went to America – we found that out later on.

Although Rachmaninov never came, a very good pianist did come with us, so it went very well. He was Lubovich, one of the best the Moscow Conservatory had. Isadora used to phone to find out who was their best pianist and then make sure they sent that person.

It must have been in the spring of 1922 when they took quite a few of us on that first short tour to Petersburg. We stayed in the countryside at Tsarskoye Selo, in the tsar's summer palace. They arranged beds for us in – the Alexander Palace, I think it was – the palace, anyway, where each summer from 1905 to 1917 Tsar Nicholas II lived with his family, 15 miles from Petersburg. We slept in the same beautiful beds they had slept in, because the royal family had many children. I remember that the bedclothes had embroidered designs in the corners: the tsar's monogram, I think.

A couple of boys came with us. Certainly I recall one of them by name, an American called Victor Kadovsky, whose sister Maria had joined the school too. I don't know where he slept, but I remember seeing him at breakfast at Peterhof. It was marvellous to have a good breakfast, and then a proper meal in the evening as well.

From Tsarskoye Selo we went to Petersburg, where we danced in a big theatre – I am not sure if it was the Mariinsky, but I know it was a big concert and we children danced the Rachmaninov Polka. It was charming music and a very lovely dance, the way Isadora choreographed it. It was she who made sure that everything worked well, with us showing the best of our abilities, but Irma also danced with us at the end of the dance and she took us out on the stage.

One morning at breakfast – funnily enough, I don't know how I did it, but I was always so careless – I managed to cut my finger, not for the last time. That night we gave a performance in Smolny. As we were dancing the polka, the wound opened up again and I had blood running down my fingers. I gave everyone a bit of blood, because we had to hold hands – you know, first in single file holding hands in a long line, then in pairs and then all of us side by side, facing the audience.

Isadora dances Tchaikovsky's 6th

After that visit to St Petersburg, we went back to school and Isadora started preparing her choreography for Tchaikovsky's 6th Symphony. She had danced it in that first concert, the one where Lenin applauded her, but now she included parts for the older girls. The girls in the dance were the best at that time: Shura, Tamara, Valya, Liza and two more. They were three years older than I.

We little girls didn't join the group – we were much too young then, though I danced this later – but we watched from the comfort of a box at the Grand Theatre (the Bolshoi) and we thought the dances were absolutely lovely. After the Tchaikovsky symphony, Isadora danced the *Marche Slav* – the 'Slaviansky March'.

How Isadora arranged a symphony was most interesting. Her idea was that the beginning of the symphony was the birth of a child; the second movement was youth, and the six girls were charming. Irma was out in front, but otherwise the six girls performed this section. In the third movement, the heroic part, Isadora danced with them – she portrayed the general and the rest were the warriors. She was in the centre and Irma led the other six – they had changed their costumes, so that their cloaks now were fixed in the Grecian style, with a clasp on one shoulder.

They did this part beautifully, but even more so the heroic last movement, where Isadora was so magnificent. I was there in the Bolshoi Theatre, sitting in one of the boxes, and I could see so plainly what it all meant. The last part of the symphony Isadora interpreted as death. Since she had endured such sorrow in her life, especially losing her two children so poignantly, she was expressing in movement the tragedy and grief she had already experienced. Yet she was absolutely in her glory in portraying them.

I never will forget the way she danced on that stage. Much of the time she was really expressing what you can hear in the music: the last movement of that symphony is pure desperation. So, when she took some earth and threw it in the grave, you could hear that plainly. Even more awful was when the music goes calm, the world is turning and she collects some earth and throws it down, only to find that the grave has gone. There are many things that Isadora put into her performances that people miss now. Irma was the only one who knew the last part of the 6th Symphony.

But I remember Isadora dancing it. She is in despair, then she begins twisting and she falls down on the floor. As if at a funeral, she takes some earth and throws it down. When the music rises to a climax and the cymbals clash, that's when that happens. In the very last part she is on her knees: she goes down, down, down. And that is the end. But she never makes any movement, just goes down with the music.

I have never experienced anything like the way Isadora danced the whole of the last movement; I was so young, but it impressed me so much. Whether it affected the rest of the girls in the same way, I don't know – we never discussed the matter – but something in me, even as a little girl, made me want to watch everything she did. I think I was the only one who was so interested in dance itself. I never missed any chance I got to watch Isadora and I could not take my eyes off her when she danced.

What was she like?

People now don't know what Isadora Duncan was like. She was very intelligent, charming and beautiful, and she had a certain way with her. When she walked, she never hurried – somehow, she seemed to glide. Even at her liveliest, she was always unhurried – serene, I would say.

Nor was there any sense of striving for effect when she portrayed things in dance. She made them real, and this was even more remarkable when she was in her mature years, because she had lost the advantage of youth. I mean, we met her when she was in her forties and even the older girls in her school were so young – 14, 15 or 16 – when they danced the 6th Symphony with her. They were so lovely and light, but she made it look even more effortless. The movements Isadora created were so light and easy to do.

She did some ballet dancing too, but not particularly well. She found it difficult, yet she moved beautifully. She wondered where she could learn more about movement and she found what she was looking for in the art of ancient Greece: the vase paintings and statuary. At the school, we children were taken to museums and picture galleries – I saw a Picasso, a real one, when he was still normal – and we looked at classical sculpture. It was all part of our education.

Isadora was extraordinary in many ways – in the way she dressed, for instance: she always looked different from other people. First of all she had such wonderful height, and then too she was very beautiful, but most of all it was her personality – that tremendous charm combined with knowledge.

Isadora Duncan was energetic and got on with organising things; it was quite something to set up a new kind of school, with little money of her own, in a country where she did not speak the language; and she did that more than once. She would have achieved even more, except that in some respects she was not worldly-wise. It would be an exaggeration to say she had her head in the clouds, but certainly her mind was focused on higher things. She wasn't always practical, and she wasn't businesslike or even astute in money matters.

Also she was naïve about politics. For example, I know she agreed with the revolution of 1917 in Russia: she said of herself that she was a very great revolutionist. She was, but from the sidelines. She never liked to be in the middle of any conflict; she just liked the idea of revolution.

Tragedy made real

When Isadora came to Russia for the very first time, it was just after the 1905 rising. She asked about all the fresh graves she saw and learnt that these were people who had died in the rising and its aftermath. This inspired her to create a dance to Chopin's Funeral March, and she was magnificent in this dance.

It was the one with the cape, where she uncovers her head and then shrouds herself again, until she is invisible, covered up. At the very end she lies down, becoming still, and a gentle rain of petals or flowers falls on her. When all seems over, she sits up, her hands rise up and she seems to float.

I remember seeing Isadora dance that: she was so magnificent and she still had a wonderful figure. We saw some of her concerts, especially in the first year or two of the school, which never had any money unless she earned some. Isadora used to travel a lot to Paris, partly for that reason, but also because she missed her French friends.

She was very popular in Paris: they all knew her, or thought they did. Everyone thought Isadora was so revolutionary, but she wasn't of course. She just liked the idea of revolution and change, nothing else. What she did revolutionise was the world of dance. She was an extraordinary person and her professional life was, in the main, triumphantly successful. She achieved such a lot and ballet would not be as popular as it is today, had it not been for her, yet hardly anybody seems to know that. What she created was a revolution in art.

Her personal life, though, was very, very unhappy: her parents separated, her children died young, her relationships ended prematurely. Her tragic life had left terrible emotional scars, yet she never allowed them to show. All that most people saw was a woman of great poise and personality, intelligent and lively, but also kind and sensitive, with a smile playing about her lips.

An incident

Sometimes we were allowed to go home and once during the week somebody ran up to me and said, "Lili, there's your mother downstairs." I said "Really?!"

I was so happy that I ran all the way down. I had been feeling miserable that day – I must have had a quarrel with some of the other girls – and I remember putting my face in my mother's fur wrap – it was wintertime. I was so pleased to see her. We sat down on the bench there and my mother said "Are you happy or unhappy?" I said "I am not very happy and I would like to go home."

As we sat there talking, facing the wonderful marble staircase that I talked about, Isadora came down the stairs – that was coincidence, but my mother knew her personally because, when my mother had had friends visiting from Paris, she had introduced them to Isadora, who was very pleased to meet them.

She came down and went up to my mother, who said, "Well, how is Lili doing?" Isadora said, "She is doing very well." Then my mother said, "She doesn't seem to be very happy: she says she would like to go home" - I remember this so well. Isadora lifted me up and said, "No, no, no! Never would I let Lili go: she is one of my best pupils - no!" and of course that soothed me very well.

Learning Russian

Many of the children that Isadora chose were, like me, recent immigrants and we had to start adapting ourselves. Most of our classes were taught in Russian, but of course some of us had first to learn the language. By this time I spoke some Russian, though not well. Our director, he was terrible: he would make me say things in front of the others and for a long time I never understood why. It was because of the way I used to talk, my appalling accent, and there would be little bits of laughter all the time. Once I realised what was going on, I refused to speak in class and I thought, *I am not going to; I am not going to be caught like that*. I was also adamant that I had to learn to read the language. In fact, long before I spoke it properly, I could read Russian easily.

I always loved reading anyway, but then on the boat crossing the Channel I met a lovely girl, Cecilia. She too was going to Moscow with her mother and we became very friendly. Funnily enough, when we did arrive, she also entered the Isadora Duncan School, so we were friends there. Cecilia and I spoke English together, not Russian. She wasn't the only English girl who entered the school, and she didn't stay long, but she was special. Cecilia was reading *She* by Rider Haggard. That struck me very much. We used to find a little corner somewhere and she would read aloud to me. I was so enchanted that I thought, *The first thing I'm going to do is learn Russian so I can start reading books.*

I found Russian very difficult to learn. It was often difficult to make the effort to practise it: I had always spoken English and there were lots of British and American girls at the school, so I used English with them; in addition, I always spoke English with Isadora, who never got very far with Russian, and with Irma, who did eventually become fluent. Isadora sometimes explained what she wanted in German to Schneider and he would translate it into Russian for the girls; or she would explain it to me and I would demonstrate it.

It took me three years before I really learned the language. Funnily enough, in the end I could speak it better than many Russians. I still speak it fluently now. I made up my mind to learn the language, and I think people should always remember that, wherever they live, they should speak the language properly. Many English people are not very good even at their own language. Some of them, I just cannot understand what they say.

Sport for all

Isadora was very keen to spread her ideas to youngsters beyond the school. She became friendly with the person in charge of youth and sport, a prominent man called Padvoyski, and asked him if it was possible to get together groups of young people, especially the Pioneers (the boy and girl scouts), in a stadium to learn about movement. He promised to arrange it and gave us permission to use a sports arena. On certain days in the week, he made a point of getting youngsters there, and we used to march out to meet them.

We marched in pairs, just as we did when we went for walks – we used to turn right, up the hill – and to march we needed drummers. So they gave two of us a drum: one to me and one to Yulia. Now don't ask me why, but they gave Yulia, who was older and taller than me, the small drum and they gave me the big drum. Still, I managed: I learnt how to play a drum to march to.

When we were ready to march off, Isadora used to come onto the balcony of our bedroom, the Blue Room. She used to come out to wave to us and wish us a very prominent walk, and then we would march off, with two girls carrying a banner in front of us. I think that is so funny.

I have a photo in front of me that shows us with the banner and it strikes me as very amusing. It doesn't show Isadora, because it was taken at the stadium, and it doesn't show me. I was missing that day, for a funny reason I shall tell shortly. You can read the inscription on the banner, in big letters – "The spirit can be free only when the body is free" – and, underneath, "from the Duncan School". On the other side it had some slogan to do with beauty, but you can't see that side on the photograph.

The people holding the banner are Shura on the left and Liza on the right. In the front row you can see Marisha Borisova and Natasha Nekrasova. The whole thing seems extraordinarily funny now, but

42

funnier things happened. We would intermingle, youngsters with the big girls. After all, they were young too and they still liked to have a game. That particular day, just before we marched off to the sports arena, we were all in high spirits, giddy with some wild chasing game.

Running past Irma's bedroom, I was the last one in our group. I heard the door open, and someone caught me by my hair: it was Irma. The other girls disappeared.

"What on earth are you doing?" she said in English; I was the only one in the group who spoke English.

"Irma, please do forgive me." But she would have none of it.

"Come along." She let go of my hair, but she took me by the shoulder and led me to the Pink Room. At that time it was an empty room, but there was a board on the wall, so we must have had some kind of lessons there.

"Now you sit here until somebody releases you."

You see how obedient we were: I sat there and waited for a while, for quite a long while, until they all came back. All the girls came to find me and they told me that, in the end, they had marched off with only one drummer. They wanted to know what had happened to me.

While I was explaining, Irma walked in. She had clearly forgotten all about the incident, but she could see all the girls were gathered there, so she got straight on with what she wanted to do. She came up to me and said, "Lili, can you do a Russian national dance?"

"Yes, Irma."

"Go, please, and show me."

So I did. She thought it very good and made a note of it. When Irma was putting together a programme for our American tour, she fitted the revolutionary song 'One, two, three, Pioneers are we' to that Russian dance that I showed her, and it became a great hit with audiences.

Now I think it was odd that she made me sit in a room when I was meant to be playing the drum and marching to the stadium, and even odder that she then forgot about me, but extraordinarily strange that she picked on me again. Why was it always me? I have no idea.

There was a board on the wall of that room and it was used as a classroom. Later, Irma used to gather us in that room every so often and try to teach us how to speak English. I think she had a very difficult time making any progress with most of the girls.

She came once wearing a very beautiful chiffon dress, with a pattern that you couldn't understand at first. She was always very well dressed; she used to get a carriage to take her into the city, to buy clothes. I would say she must have gone to one of the beautiful stores on Petrovska to buy materials, and then had that dress made for her. She knew some good dressmakers.

Well, she could see we were all looking at her and she didn't mind.

"Girls, I can see you have noticed my dress. Come closer, so you can see it."

We came closer to get a better look at the material, and she explained the design to us.

"You see, it is like a chrysanthemum."

We said 'yes' but, as a matter of fact, it was more like a box of matches with red heads, but with all the matches scattered round the back, because the tips were red. Still, I suppose it did look like a chrysanthemum. She was wearing little red shoes, and the whole effect was absolutely lovely.

High jinks

We certainly did have fun and we played games when no one was looking. We were fond of doing various little things that we weren't supposed to. One night, when we knew Schneider and Irma – and, I think, Isadora too – were going out to a concert or the opera, we decided to play hide and seek.

I am not sure if Isadora was still at school, but anyway she was out. I think one teacher lived in at school, whoever we had the first lesson with, but we waited until they were asleep and the others had gone out, and the nannies were in bed, and then we began. We got out of bed – we had our nighties on – and we divided ourselves: some were hiding and some were seeking. We played and played, until we heard the carriage returning. At that we quickly decided we had better disappear and go to bed, in case we were caught.

But one of the girls, Ulya, was downstairs in the big vestibule, and I suppose she hadn't time to get up the stairs without being seen, so she hid herself in one of those big empty baskets, like hampers, which were used to carry our curtains and carpets to the theatre when we had concerts. Of course she couldn't see if anyone had arrived, so she had to wait until she heard the door opening and they all came in.

They sat down, some on the benches, but some of them sat on the basket. Ulya held her breath. She was frightened she would be stuck there forever, but nevertheless she waited until they stopped talking, got up and went upstairs. When they had gone, she quietly got out and managed to get to our bedroom, the one that had been the Napoleon Room, the blue studio where we danced when the school first started.

That is how the evening passed and we all finished up quite comfortable, in bed. At that age it doesn't matter much where you sleep and what time you go to bed. We fell asleep and nobody ever knew what we had been doing.

Some visitors

During the week we were busy, but we had spare time in the evenings and especially at weekends, since we were all boarders. Our director Schneider must have thought about how we might use this spare time and, in the spirit of communism, he felt that we ought to mix with other people. Once we were settled at school, he used to organise things for us in the evenings and at weekends.

On one occasion he invited people from an orphan place to come and see us – they had many youngsters there. He thought it would be nice for us to meet people who lived very differently from us and he made an evening out of it. There were boys as well as girls and, though they were a bit strange to us at first, we became friendly. A girl there took a fancy to me and asked if she could correspond with me. I said, "Yes, of course" – and we started writing to one another.

Sometimes we had plays put on: they were done in our blue studio, the Napoleon Room, before that was changed to our bedroom. The bigger girls took the leading roles in these plays and I remember vaguely that Schneider was good at organising that – it was made like a theatre. I forget what plays they put on; I was so young, but also I missed part of that first year because they found I had malaria and I was off school for a while.

Our director also used to invite people to come and talk to us or demonstrate things. Some of them seemed to us strange people. There was a man called Evon 'Biesmiertny' – that was his nickname, meaning 'immortal'. We thought he would never die because he was like a Spartan – he used to walk around summer and winter in the same outfit – a Grecian tunic and sandals. Even in wintertime in this dreadful temperature, he used to come to the school in the evenings and show us how he used to move his muscles. We were interested in that because, if he could walk around in the wintertime like this, he must be a very remarkable person indeed.

From time to time our director used to invite an orchestra consisting entirely of wind instruments: there was no piano and there were no strings, just brass. The conductor was a little man who was something to do with the army, because he had a very strange title before his name. I told you before about the school when you used to walk up the marble staircase and we had balustrades – we had a very big vestibule there and we used to sit around in places listening to them. The conductor struck me as being so funny – he used to conduct in a military uniform and they used to play various types of music. I never really liked that band very much, but they still came to entertain us and it was all interesting.

Evening classes

Isadora also organised things for us. Amongst these were the special evenings when Grechaninov came to see us with his folk group; he didn't sing, but the group did. They were all from the peasantry and they had lovely voices; the songs were very sweet. They used to come and sing folk songs for Isadora. Then they would translate the words and explain what the song was about and, if she liked it, she would make a dance sequence with it, and it would be put into our repertoire. We youngsters used to have a separate children's programme.

This aspect of Isadora's work created great interest in the school. I remember all of these lovely songs – there was a very funny one about a crow, and another one was a lullaby that Grechaninov's group sang, in which they thanked her. All the peasants sing and dance in Russia and they all have lovely voices, so it was no novelty that they did this so well. But, even though we had been picked for our dancing, we children also had good voices.

There were other evenings with Isadora when we danced, but they were not lessons and sometimes they were not dancing at all. She would ask us to come to the hall – the Burgundy Hall – another room she had refurbished for evening dancing. It was draped in burgundy curtains, matched by a carpet in the same colour.

Sometimes Isadora would show us some movements or do some dancing herself, so if she was dressed in a tunic we knew we were going to have a very interesting evening. There was something of interest coming and she was going to dance. Whenever she had finished creating a dance, she wanted to show it to us. One performance in particular I remember, because she prepared the whole thing while I watched. I remember that: it was so very simple, and very easy for her to do, and the wonder has stuck in my memory. She was extraordinary, very, very extraordinary.

Schubert's *Moment musicale*

I remember once she did a lovely dance to the *Moment musicale* of Schubert - very nice, I did like it, and I always took notice of exactly what she did and how she did it. I don't know about the rest of the girls. I know they all watched whenever Isadora danced, but they still had to be taught the steps afterwards, whereas I took notice of her every movement and remembered the steps.

We were there, dressed in tunics as well - there were quite a few of us: not just the group of fourteen, maybe about twenty - and when she had finished she said to us, as we were sitting there, "Who could do that?" And I said - I don't know where I got the audacity from, to be so brave - I said, "I can!" So she said, "Go ahead - don't be afraid. Do what you can."

I was very observant, I remember, and though I didn't do it all correctly, I caught the first movement very well - she was amazed. The rest of the dance I managed and at the end of it she laughed and said, "Very good, Lili; you have done very, very well!" I was pleased with myself that I could follow what Isadora asked me to do.

She was very taken by that. After that episode she really counted me one of the best pupils. I kind of caught on to what she was doing, followed her very well, and so we continued. From then on, she spent a bit more time on my dancing and she really sorted me out, though she was never a natural teacher. Of her pupils, Irma was much the best teacher.

All the same, if Isadora was there in the tunic and with the drapes round her, we knew she was going to show us something. She used to dance for us and we used to sit and watch her. She never really taught us – she had no patience – but she would show you once and, if you were able to remember and grasp what she was doing, and if you said yes, you thought you could follow her, she would let you do it.

Isadora used to get bored in Moscow and she would go to Paris a lot. She very seldom stayed for any length of time with us, but nonetheless we did have many lessons with her, sometimes because she wanted to prepare a special performance with us. She used to invite the elite, because at the time they still had some very talented people in Russia, and she was especially interested in the revolutionary poets (Yesenin was one) and writers. She would put on a whole concert especially for an invited audience. But Isadora went to France very, very often; and in between, to make money to support the school, she went touring.

Yesenin

When she travelled, she took Sergei Yesenin with her. As he became more intimate with Isadora, he took liberties with her. He used to get terribly angry that she had such deep feelings for her lost children. The fact is, his morals were bad, whereas Isadora always had high morals, in the sense that she would never do anything unkind – she would never insult anybody or say anything nasty.

Once she had a party and Yesenin was there. He used to drink excessively, which was very unpleasant, and this night he got lost. I don't know how nobody noticed, but he started wandering about the school. He came into our bedroom and sat on one of the beds – poor Ulya's. She woke up, saw a man and screamed. She was terrified and of course he got really alarmed. Someone came and took him away, and we told the teacher that Isadora could do what she liked – we didn't mind – but her guests should not disturb us. After that Isadora never had any more parties at the school.

Unfortunately, Isadora didn't speak Russian so she never understood half the things Yesenin said; she thought he was a genius. Well, I doubt he was that. I know he was popular amongst the Russians – at least, they liked his poetry, which I didn't. I liked only one Russian poet and that was Pushkin: his poetry was just beauty itself – the very language of Russia.

Before her new school was a year old, and she had been married to Yesenin only half that long, things once again looked bleak for Isadora. She had to get rid of Yesenin: he had such unpleasant habits – drinking far too much and being very abusive to her. He was not to be trusted in a school and he made life awful for everyone around him – Isadora got tired of it. Let's just say that it came to her mind: she had had enough.

Sundays

We were often taken to museums on Sundays, particularly to look at the statues. I was very interested in these, especially when I discovered that they gave Isadora some of her ideas about movement. We also went to see paintings – but they were in different places, in picture galleries.

On Sundays they also used to take us to the Bolshoi Theatre to listen to the orchestra. They didn't have matinées, but there were rehearsals at that time each week and we were allowed to go. We enjoyed that very much – we always sat in one of the boxes – and paid great attention to the music. Well, I did, in any event, no matter what they played. I liked the orchestra very much, so it was never dull.

Our parents could come to visit us on Sundays. My mother always used to come, and I was very pleased to see her, but I was rather sad to see that all the other girls had visits from their fathers, whereas I never did. We had a daily routine and it was very strict, but every three weeks we were allowed to go home. At first, I think my mother came for me, but later I walked there and back by myself. I used to enjoy that walk very much indeed.

A year has gone by

All in all, the school was very well run. We were brought up in a sort of austerity, yet the school was beautiful. We never had enough clothes to wear or enough food to eat, but we had plenty of music and dancing. We all used to read a great deal and talk to one another about what we had read. We were given very good books at an early

49

age and we learned to reflect on them and express what we thought. It was a wonderful school: I loved it.

In the summer at the end of the first school year, Schneider arranged that we should all go to the countryside to enjoy the season, and perhaps to build us up a bit. He rented a small country estate, but I couldn't go straightaway because I still had a little of the malaria I had caught the previous summer. One of the nannies was left with me and, as soon I got a little better, she took me to join the other girls.

We were there nearly four months and we had a wonderful time. Each month was like a separate season with a different thing for us to pick: first came the violets and lilies of the valley; next the raspberries; then the strawberries; and finally the mushrooms. One day when we were picking raspberries, we met a bear! They are particularly fond of raspberries. We planted vegetables by the house, as food was so scarce, and we used to tend and water them. We helped as much as we could.

A year in a child's life makes a big difference. I was 9 then, nearly grown up, I felt. When we got back home to Moscow, I still had a slight touch of malaria, until my mother got rid of it completely with the help of a doctor who lived in the same building. He was called Professor Frischkop and he gave me some drops, a strange way to cure malaria, but indeed I soon recovered completely.

3

The Duncan School:
at Home and Abroad, 1922–5

Home and school

When I started school, my mother lived at Byshmitrika 23, Maly
Dmetrovka, near the centre of Moscow, in a very good district not far
from the school. The government gave her a room there, in an
apartment block. It had been part of a six-room flat, which also had a
big kitchen and a bathroom with a real bath in it.

The flat had belonged to a married couple, not even a family, so of
course the authorities confiscated it. The couple, who were allowed
to choose one room for themselves, chose a very big room with a
balcony. The rest of the flat was allocated to two families from
London, but then the wives went back and one husband got a flat
with his son.

There were four other households, two in the same family –
mother and grandmother in one, daughter and granddaughter in the
other – and one consisting of a young woman with her future husband (they soon got married); the other one was us. Everybody had a
room, nobody ever had two rooms. That is how it was, even though
the block was quite prestigious and the people who lived there were
very well-to-do.

I used to come home one, two or three times a month, less often
when I was very busy learning something in dancing. In any case, life
in that one room at home was very, very drab. Every three weeks we
could go home, but I used to get rather bored: I missed my school
friends and the fun.

I did know some children where we lived and I would look out of the window to see if anyone was running about. One family had three daughters – I think one of them entered our school at the start – so I used to pop in there and play with the middle girl, Esther. There was a boy called Michael, too, who lived in the same block, but he was the one who said the reason I once had a pimple was because he kissed me. I used to see him around, but I refused to be friends with him because I could never forgive him for what he had said.

Sometimes I slept at our flat overnight and went back to school – I nearly said 'went back home'! – next morning. My mother would give me the bus fare, but I preferred to walk down Maly Dmetrovka, left onto Boulevard A and so to school. It wasn't far – a half-hour's walk – and I knew my way. I used the bus fare to buy myself a toffee; that kept me going up the hill on Prechistenka. We had to be at school quite early, but that was no hardship: I would meet all my friends and get back to my normal life. I wasn't the only girl who occasionally went home during the week.

Comings and goings

While we were in training at the start, I was put in charge of a little group of immigrants, since I was the eldest amongst them. They were such sweet little children. One girl particularly stood out, called Yetta. She and her parents came over with us from England and they were very friendly with my mother. Yetta had straight blonde hair, with beautiful blue eyes; and I was just the reverse, with dark eyes and long, slightly curly black hair. We were always to-gether at the beginning.

There were quite a few boys at first, some of them – like Victor Kadovsky, who came with us to Petersburg – from America. One particular boy I remember because very often Isadora used to put me with him to dance; she would say, "Go on, pair yourself up with Tether." That was his name. But one by one all the boys left.

When we were being examined by Isadora, I met Cecilia Viviurka again, for the first time since the Channel crossing. I was pleased to see her, but she didn't stay long. She wasn't really very good at dancing and her father took her away from the school.

Many other girls left too, sometimes because their parents were not pleased, sometimes because the girl wasn't good enough. Even my Yetta never stayed. I don't think she had that much talent or the same interest in music that I did. She wasn't there long, but it was her parents who took her away.

We all moved in – the ones chosen by Isadora, that is – and settled down, but every so often new girls would appear. Someone would recommend the school to their parents, or the girl to Isadora, and they would come to audition. Isadora didn't want to see what they had learnt at ballet classes; she wanted to see them doing *her* movements, so someone had to teach them a few basic movements first.

Isadora always asked me to show them the movements before the audition itself.

"Lili, show her our movements – how to skip and how to run – and let us see how she does it."

Shura Aksimova

One of the new girls I showed our movements to was Shura Aksimova, even though she was about two and a half years older than me. I taught her how to move and how to hold her body, or at least I tried to. She had grace, but she couldn't do the movements properly. They were quite pleased with her, though her movements were not wonderful at first, but all came in time – as the saying goes, Rome wasn't built in a day.

Shura was not exactly a beauty, but she was beautifully built, even as a child, with a figure like Diana the huntress. As a dancer she was neither too light nor too heavy. She was not very lyrical, as I was; I did intricate things. She was not a brilliant dancer, but she was certainly the best all-rounder.

How she got to the school was through my mother, who, at the time, was at a sanatorium where she met Shura's elder sister. They had lost their parents during the revolution, even though the family came from peasant stock – well, half-peasantry, anyway. Tanya was an intelligent woman, quite a lot older than Shura, and she told my mother that she had this younger sister and she didn't know what to do with her or how to manage. When my mother discovered that Shura liked dancing, she suggested sending her to Isadora Duncan – and that was how Shura came to audition.

I think Shura may have been the only person who danced the solo that Isadora created for the Chopin Funeral March. I don't recall even Irma ever dancing that. But when we were in China, I think we girls suggested that Shura ought to dance that solo. It had so much of Isadora's spirit in it; I remember that especially.

Natasha and Lolya

I auditioned Shura, and I auditioned Natasha Nekrasova. This was after the blue hall became our bedroom – it was a very bright room once they took all those curtains away – and then we used the burgundy hall for dancing. Now I remember that Shura, when I first showed her the movements and she tried to copy them, she wasn't doing so well, but I could see she had some talent. Natasha had no talent whatsoever, and yet they took her on. Isadora took her on for her looks – she was very dark, very extraordinary – though she couldn't dance at all. Nevertheless she tried and she did manage various movements, but she never became a dancer.

This Natasha Nekrasova was an orphan and lived with her grandma and her aunt. She used to make up poetry and she had a gift for it. Funnily enough, there was a well-known Russian poet called Nekrasov. Now whenever any of us did something outstanding, we had a special board in our schoolroom where we could write congratulations or commendations. She was praised there and ever after we called her 'the poet'.

Natasha's bed was next to mine; Mooshya's was on the other side. Natasha was extraordinarily funny. She would wake me up in the middle of the night.

"Lilya, I was thinking. It just came to me..."

"But look at the time!"

"It doesn't matter; don't take any notice of that."

Then she would read me some poetry she had just written.

"Natasha, that is very nice, but please let me sleep."

It would take me quite a while to get back to sleep again, but that was Natasha.

We girls knew that Natasha kept a diary and it was bound to be very funny. Now we used to get that orchestra coming to play for us and the conductor was a little man and quite funny-looking. His name was Kapududkin, which sounds funny enough in English, but it sounds far funnier in Russian. Well, like any youngsters, we could be naughty and we found her diary. When we read what Natasha had written about the conductor – she had fallen completely for him – well, we were in fits, especially when we got to the bit about the piercing look she was getting from him.

One day Natasha was standing by the window in our bedroom when Manya came in with her notebook.

"Natasha, I want you to listen to my poetry."

"Right, I am ready."

Manya began reading her poem and Natasha was saying, "Very good, very good" and pulling the curtains as she said it. Over the windows we had very big pelmets made of mahogany – all the rooms had them, even where the central heating didn't work (though they tried to put it right) – along with very heavy curtains.

Natasha kept on saying, "Very good, very good" and pulling the curtains in a kind of rhythm as she said it, and then the whole thing collapsed on her head, this very heavy pelmet with big brass ends in the shape of horses with wings. Natasha fell down under it; Manya was horrified and all of us in the room were alarmed.

Natasha managed to open her eyes and lift herself up on one elbow to speak to Manya: "Quickly, go and tell my aunt, and tell her that I have concussion, and don't forget to tell her to bring me lots of pastries with plenty of cream." It seemed she wasn't too badly injured to seize such an opportunity. Even awful events can have their funny side. She soon recovered: she had only slight concussion, which was lucky because it could have easily split her head open. It must have caught her just a glancing blow.

Like Manya, most girls go through a stage when they think they can write poetry, but it wasn't like that with Natasha or me. I had no interest in writing poetry. As I said before, I liked only one poet and that was Pushkin. I liked reading his verse, but I had no inclination to sit and write any of my own. Natasha liked making up verses and she was very good at it.

Very shortly afterwards, another girl applied to join the school, called Lolya Terentieva. She was the same age as me, and her elder sister, like Shura's sister, met my mother at the sanatorium. The upshot was that Lolya too came to audition and Isadora again said, "Where is Lili, to give her the examination?" I showed Lolya the basic movements, she did them for Isadora and she was taken on as well. She turned out to be a really fine dancer later on.

Marisha

Towards the end of the school's first year, a new girl came – a big, tall girl – and her name was Marisha Borisova. As a newcomer, she didn't know anybody; and she found that nobody much wanted to know her. So I befriended her. At the time, I was recovering from malaria and my mother, wondering if I was eating enough, had brought me some nice little cakes. I got these out of the cupboard in the dining room where we kept our own food, and asked her if she was hungry and would she like one. She said, "No, thank you" but my gesture had its effect.

Marisha came from a working-class family. They lived in Dresden, a factory town named after the one in Germany. She was sent to us by Mikhail Fokine, the ballet master. I don't know how it happened – I suppose he saw her dancing in a show of some kind there – but he must have got in touch with this girl. Isadora took her on his recommendation and she did have talent. She was rather impressive, a heroic type, never lyrical like most of us.

She was about three years older than me and seemed quite mature. When she entered the school, people cold-shouldered her – partly, I think, because of her plebeian background – and I felt sorry to see her all by herself. Then, as she became familiar with everybody, she began to get a bit bossy. I couldn't understand why she did that. It took her a little time, but eventually all the other girls were a little bit frightened of her. I never was. She never bothered me. In fact, she was always very friendly with me, but she reigned over the other girls.

As time went by, she started to be envious of Shura, who was a lovely dancer and very much admired by the rest of us. Marisha felt jealous of her and after a rehearsal of some sort she punched her in her ribs. She really hurt Shura. We were horrified and she was punished for that. Nevertheless, she kept on being bossy and later on she caused us a lot of trouble.

Winter 1922–3

By now we didn't need help from Auntie Annie and I lost touch with her. My mother and I had been in Russia nearly two years; I had grown, of course, and my clothes were getting very scanty. I had boots, but the weather turned bitterly cold and I began to notice my clothes were no longer warm enough. I don't think my mother had noticed.

Our routine never changed, summer or winter: we used to go out for a walk each day, after we had rested. This day I wasn't dressed very warmly for the time of year and I wondered why. When I got back, I must have caught a cold and I began to cough very badly. Nobody usually took any notice when this happened and I just carried on, until I developed a very high fever. After that I don't recall anything. It turned out to be pneumonia and, when Auntie Annie heard about it, she said to my mother, "Lizzie, please bring her here: I will nurse her", and she did.

The next thing I knew, I was waking up and Auntie Annie was standing in front of me. I was so surprised, and it must have showed. She reassured me.

"Don't worry, Lili dear, you were very ill and I have been looking after you."

"How did I get here? I have no idea. I don't know why it is, but I don't remember."

"That's because you were very ill, and you're still not well. You have pneumonia."

Two doctors came to see me and Auntie Annie arranged everything. She had a very spacious flat, since her husband was an official – a three-bedroom flat with a lounge and dining area. She had made a bed for me out of a settee in the lounge. The doctors used to cup me: they would put those glass containers on my back and use them to suck out whatever it was. The only trouble was that it felt unpleasant and it left round marks, like the marks you get when you hurt yourself – not exactly like that, but marks all the same. Still, eventually they went.

I soon became very friendly with my aunt Annie and, of course, her sons too. The younger ones, Moss and Freddy, were delighted to see me. We hadn't seen each other for a long time, not since Freddy used to bring us food just after we arrived in Moscow. I was busy at school and my mother never mentioned Auntie Annie, but their friendship continued and my mother told her when I fell ill. I spent six weeks convalescing with Auntie Annie and I was very happy there.

I was very comfortable and I was getting better, so one of the boys went to school and brought home my doll, the one my mother had bought in London, and I began to make little clothes for it. I had a way of making up clothes, with very neat little stitches. I was fortunate that I was very good at sewing; I think I inherited that from my parents, since my mother was a tailoress and my father was a tailor.

Although I didn't see it at the time, I think the middle son was in his childish way trying to court me. Every time the two younger ones passed me they would stop to play with me. Auntie Annie would say, "Leave her alone: she's not well", but I didn't mind – I liked fun. Eventually it was, "Lili, would you like a piggyback?"

Of course, through the day the boys were out at school. I know they had to learn to read, write and speak Russian, just as I did. They didn't go to boarding school; there was no need. I was at boarding school for my dancing, and no other reason.

The school begins to change

Dance pupils were not enough to keep the school going. I was only dimly aware of it at first, but the government had stopped paying the school's bills and we had to support ourselves. Our director had to have other paying pupils, so they started taking day pupils. They weren't there to dance; they came because our school was so very much talked about. Their parents liked the way we were brought up – the system of teaching and the routine – and you could do exercise and dancing if you wished. The majority of day pupils came from very good families, so they had to pay.

I was off for a good while with pneumonia. I came back to school to find my bed had been taken, so I was given a bed beside a new girl. This was Lucy Flaxman, an American girl about three years older than me. I am not sure when Lucy arrived, but she stayed quite a while. Her mother was friendly with my mother, and she took me in for two weeks to feed me up when I was recovering from malaria, because they had a bigger place.

Another new arrival was Mooshya, who came in spring 1923. Her mother, Elzbieta, was a trained nurse who looked after our health and took care of Irma – after a while we found out that Irma was suffering from TB when she arrived in Russia with Isadora.

The core group

As the school was thinning out, somehow only the very talented were left and we had to learn to support ourselves. Now that we were getting older and becoming better dancers, we were divided. Irma took on the six best of the older girls, amongst them Shura, who had started to come of age; later she turned out to be absolutely wonderful as a dancer.

Irma did most of the teaching. Whenever a new girl joined us, she would call for me to demonstrate the movements. From an early age I was very light, so dancing came easily to me. Despite that, Irma would say, "You can do better." I loved to dance, whether or not I had an audience.

Before we had our supper, we had a dancing class, but now the core group was taught separately from the other girls, because we were to form a dance group. We were chosen as the best, and with Irma we trained, practised, learnt new repertoire and rehearsed. When we had achieved a professional standard, we went touring. We first danced on the stage about two years after the school opened and then we travelled a great deal, all over Russia. We needed money, because the school had no money at all.

Let them eat cake

Now that I had made friends with Auntie Annie - after she had nursed me when I had pneumonia - well, of course she found out where we girls went each afternoon when we marched off for our walk. We were friendly with Freddy, her youngest son, and he used to come home by way of the cathedral and those little gardens where we played. Freddy would call out, "Lili!" and I was so pleased to see him. He gave me a nickname - 'Monkey-face' - which looks bad when I write it down, but it was affectionate really.

"Do you want a piggy-back?"

"Oh, yes!"

I would run up to him and he would carry me about for a while. Then he had to leave me and go home, but we kept that friendship going, on and off.

It was a lovely spot, those gardens near the cathedral. Auntie Annie lived nearby, so I very often used to say to the other girls,

"Who would like to run and say hello to my auntie? She is very kind and she will definitely give us something nice." Lolya and Mooshya would come with me. We used to run there very quietly, I would ring the bell and Annie would open the door.

"Lili, what on earth are you doing here?"

"Auntie Annie, we haven't got much time. Is there anything nice going?"

"Yes, hold on, hold on! I will give you a few pieces of cake each."

We were always so hungry. Although we had teachers with us, they never realised what we were doing, because it was really just round the corner. Even so, we only did it every so often. We felt it wasn't right to keep doing that to her. Later, I used to be invited to stay with Auntie Annie at the weekends, but that was when I grew up a bit.

As time went by, things got better. Thanks to the Americans, we began to get food. It was still a struggle, but our parents managed to help a bit too: my mother used to bring eggs, because she felt I needed them, and apples. They made us take cod-liver oil too. I remember that. (Well, you can't forget cod-liver oil!) We had to queue up for it. We were so undernourished: meat was scarce, so they used to make us cabbage soup every day, but it was like water. Sometimes I used to go very, very hungry.

The housekeeper

Now I must say a word about our housekeeper, who did an excellent job in very difficult circumstances. She was in charge of the kitchen, but food was in short supply and cash was scarce. That wasn't why she used to make cabbage soup every day, though. She explained to me that this was because Isadora had insisted that cabbage was very good for you. I liked the way she put it: 'She had been told that cabbage was good for you.' We were given many things that we didn't really want, from cabbage soup to cold showers, because they were good for us – and probably they were.

The housekeeper, whose name was Alexandra Edmundrovna, was always very kind and, strangely enough, I was her favourite girl. I don't know why exactly. I think she liked me because I was very lively, and perhaps also she liked the way I did things. At any rate, she would never refuse me anything.

One day she told me that my mother had brought some eggs for me and I could have one every morning. I thought, *Well, that's very nice*. Now we were always hungry and one day not long after this we were gathered, when the talk turned to food.

"How can we get hold of some food?"

"I wonder if Lilya could help us there. The housekeeper is especially kind to her."

"Lilya, could you arrange to get some eggs and sugar? Then we can make a very special dish. Oh, and make sure you get some little containers and little cups."

There were a couple of new girls who could cook and knew how to make this dish, which has a very funny name, *gogyelmogyel*. It is rather like the Italian *zabaglione*. You take the eggs, separate them, add some sugar to the yolks, then mix the two parts separately, mixing the whites until they are fluffy and mixing the yolks with the sugar.

So I went downstairs and found our housekeeper. She was in charge of laundry too, and very organised, because every week our beds were changed. We had nannies who helped to do that, but our housekeeper made sure everything was spotlessly clean. I remember watching her putting sheets away, because I always noticed what was going on. Everything she did was done so beautifully, and I liked that.

So I went and found our housekeeper in the kitchen, and told her our predicament.

"The girls begged me to come and ask you something, if it is possible, because we are all so hungry."

"Yes, dear. What is it you would like?"

"We need at least two eggs, and a bowl, and some cups, and some sugar, because we want to make *gogyelmogyel*."

"Right," she said, and smiled. She always smiled whenever I asked her anything.

She took me to a little pantry where she kept food, including whatever our parents brought for us; she had it all under control, what was bought and for whom. So she gave me all the things I had asked for and I took it upstairs, where the others were all anxiously waiting for me. I gave them all the containers, the eggs and sugar, a fork to beat the eggs and spoons to eat with, and we did it. When it was ready, the girls were very fair. They thought I deserved my full share after all that.

Speaking of the housekeeper, who liked to keep things 'just so', reminds me that sometimes they had a little raid, to inspect the little baskets under our beds where we kept our belongings. They wanted to know what we kept there. After one such raid, our director and one of the teachers called us all together.

"We raided all your little baskets. Why is it that Lili always has everything so neat and tidy, while the rest of you just push things in any old how?"

In the same way, Irma very often used to stop us in the corridor and inspect us.

"How is it that Lili's socks are always nice and pulled up straight, and you girls – just look at you!" Well, I'm just tidy; that's the way I am. Other people are different.

'Varshavianka'

Sometimes Isadora wanted to put on something a little different. She was interested in the revolutionary songs and I remember her inviting a composer and lyricist, who translated the words for her and explained the ideas behind them. One of these was a very vivid song called 'Varshavianka', which was used in the film *Dr Zhivago* – the part where they march off singing the Russian song.

She listened while they sang it, and took in the words as they translated them. When they had finished, she asked for the music again and then she went dancing, and I was there to see her. Unplanned, without any rehearsals or anything of the sort, she began at once to dance, portraying the spontaneous movement that began when the starving poor – they were asking just for bread – marched to the palace, and how in the end they were shot. That was the episode from which the song originated.

It was extraordinary, wonderful in creation. I have never experienced anything like it. She didn't have to stop and think, and start arranging how the dance would go: she just went. She took a red scarf and made it look like a flag. She leaped with her scarf – she was wearing a red tunic as well – and then she backed down.

The idea was that she leaped out from one side of the stage and, in crossing to the other side, she portrayed the advance of the revolution. She could see they were going to kill her, but she struggled on and kept marching until she was shot. When she was shot and fell

62

down, that is what stuck in my memory so much. She tried to get up, only to be shot again and wounded. She still tried to get up and go forward, but at last she fell to the ground.

After that, she started creating the rest of the dance. She wanted us to be the crowd, to continue the push forward, and she started telling us how she would like it done. After she fell down, she wanted others to come up, and more and more to go forward, only to be shot. When the music repeated itself, Isadora would repeat the dance steps - always, regardless.

After that, we were taught two by two how to do our steps. It was a very impressive dance. In fact, that is the reason I remember it, out of all of the revolutionary dances she created, because I thought this one much the most impressive. Almost immediately Isadora put the dance on as part of one of our stage performances.

After that, she wanted to learn other revolutionary songs and she did create dances with some of them, but they never appealed to me personally as this one did. For the last item in the programme, she wrote a song for us. The words are very difficult to translate from Russian to English, but roughly they said:

One, two, three
Pioneers are we –
We're not afraid of fascists:
We'll round them up. You'll see!

The music was very vivacious and she made a dance with it for the younger girls. When we went to America, that dance was immensely successful.

Isadora and Anna Pavlova

I must stress that Isadora did not think she knew all the answers and she was willing to look, listen and learn from other people, but the only classical dancer she really liked was Anna Pavlova, both for her dancing – "She feels it!" – and for herself. On one of her visits to Paris, Isadora saw Pavlova dance 'The Swan' of Saint-Saëns and made a point of meeting her afterwards. She liked her very much, both as a dancer and as a person, so she went to see her quite often.

Isadora got the idea of exercising from her. One day, she called on

Anna and found her doing her exercises. Isadora was interested, and Anna explained that you could never make a good dancer if you didn't loosen up your body beforehand, to prepare it for dancing. She said, "You can't dance without doing exercises." She taught Isadora how to warm up, and told her never to dance until she had thoroughly loosened up first.

In the light of this advice, Isadora went several times just to watch her warm up, to learn about that, and after that she changed the way her pupils were taught. As a result, we danced quite differently from the pupils at her previous school. When Isadora came to see how we had progressed, she said to Irma, "You know, they dance better than the first school did." When she said 'the first school' I think she included even the six girls who took her name – Irma, who agreed to come and help her in Moscow, and Anna, Teresa, Lisa, Erica and Margot, who didn't – but she meant the way they danced when they were our age.

Isadora and Irma

Over the course of the school's first year we saw more and more of Yesenin; and then we discovered that he and Isadora had married. Despite that, Yesenin seemed to get more unpleasant than ever and he was often drunk, so Isadora would go away to avoid him. She also went away because she got bored in Moscow – inevitably, since she never learnt the language. The result was that Irma had to work harder and she didn't hide her feelings about it.

Everyone said Irma had been adopted by Isadora; that was why her surname was Duncan. What we didn't know was that Irma's own mother was still alive then. We found that out only later. In fact we knew very little about Irma, though we knew she wasn't well and had to have different food.

What I did know was that Irma was in some ways unfair to Isadora. After all, everything Irma achieved was thanks to Isadora, who had trained her. Without Isadora there would have been no school, and she worked hard to arrange everything, especially with all the party and government officials, the events, tours, visits and concerts. But teach? No. In her first school she had managed it, but gradually she had realised that teaching wasn't for her. She left it to Irma.

Isadora was vague: she would show us a dance, but she couldn't really be bothered to teach us the details. And she used to get bored. I remember she went on tour in Russia to raise money for the school, because the touring group wasn't yet ready, and not long after her return she went to France with Irma. I don't know if Isadora came back from France when Irma did, but I remember Irma coming back. She was a wonderful teacher.

Out of the whole school, Isadora and Irma had selected the very best dancers, and there were fourteen of us. We kept training and rehearsing, and then we began to go on tours, giving concerts. We did very well and we kept the school going, with Irma teaching us.

Irma Duncan was married to Ilya Schneider and one year they went to Paris. They came back with a tremendous amount of gifts, because Schneider by nature was very kind. They brought us many things, which were unpacked on the big table in our bedroom – the room that had been our dancing hall. I remember our director emptying out suitcases and boxes, filled with so many things, while we girls stood around watching.

Touring

We became very used to touring. We travelled the length and breadth of Russia, and we discovered what a beautiful country it is. It is no good me telling you, of course: you have to see for yourself the beauty of Russia, from the Caucasus to the Urals, from St Petersburg to Samarkand, from the Caspian Sea to Lake Baikal. It is a lovely country.

We had to tour to help the school, because we had no longer had any subsidy from the government. We had only the building and nothing else, so it was pretty difficult for Isadora and for us. But it was also good for us to travel. It was an education, and so was the discipline of public performance, though we never thought of our art as being so important. We liked it, we enjoyed doing it and we used to show each other how well we could do things, but still it wasn't the most important thing.

No, what we really liked about touring was the food. That was the big attraction. Really and truly our main thing was to make sure we got a good square lunch.

The Caucasus

We went to the Caucasus several times and it was always an interesting trip. We travelled most of the way by train and it took three days, but what I recall plainly is the last part of the journey. For that, we had to get in an open car and there was a road specially built (though not for us!) through the mountains, called the Caucasus Military Road. It was a very long road, but lovely; so, even when we had done that journey a few times, we always looked forward to it.

Part of the road ran alongside a mountain river, the Tierek. Near Beslan it left the river, and the car had to climb up to a pass, then down the other side until we stopped at Grozny. Well, there has been a lot said about Grozny and Beslan since then, and the Russians had trouble with the Chechens even then. That's why they built the road. However, we never met any problems.

Grozny was a beautiful town and we had boat trips there. I still have a photograph of myself on the boat. We gave concerts, of course, and once we had a visit from some young people during the day. They were pioneers – so were we – and they made friends with us. They brought me an owl! I was thrilled with it and put it on the window sill next to my bed. I had to tie it up so it wouldn't go away or bother the other girls in my room.

From there we went to Tiflis, the capital of Georgia – it is called Tbilisi nowadays – and we put on concerts there. For myself, I liked to notice everything around me, what was what, and I liked Tiflis very much. Along the streets there were green trees growing, the whole atmosphere was charming and I liked the people. The men were so light on their feet and the women were so slim and graceful; they really caught my eye, especially if they were wearing their colourful traditional clothes.

On one of our visits, there was quite a big group of us: besides the girls of the main dance group, there were quite a few little girls, and our director had his sister and her daughter with him as well. It was summer and so very hot that we had to sleep on the first-floor balcony. This stretched all way round the hotel and it was more like a big veranda. They put out beds for us, but they had to separate off the beds with mesh curtains because of the mosquitoes. The beds were quite comfortable and we never slept in our rooms at all.

Tiflis itself was most interesting and we had great success there, but of course what mattered most to us was the food – and the food was lovely there, better than in Russia. That was perhaps because it was divided off from Russia and far away from Moscow. We followed the same itinerary more than once; I recall recognising the hotel in Tiflis when we arrived the next time.

At least once we went on to Azerbaijan and stayed in Baku, which was more of an industrial town because they had oil rigs there on the Caspian Sea. I liked Tiflis better. We used to go the same way back by the military road and then by train. By now we were doing very well indeed.

Crimean holiday

One year we had a seaside holiday. For once we didn't have to give any concerts: it really was a holiday. The place was Yevpatoriya – it was on the Black Sea, in the Crimea – and we stayed there quite a while, a month I think. It was well known as a resort for children, because it had a sandy beach. It was a lovely place.

We used to go out in the sunshine, but we couldn't get away from our nurse or a nanny. We could sunbathe, but they timed it to make sure we didn't get sunburnt. It got really hot there. Schneider, our director, said "It's about time I bought you some hats" – and he did. The hats were not made of straw, as we had expected, but of felt; they looked rather nice.

He also bought us some very beautiful embroidered dresses, in one of the traditional styles of the Caucasus, with very high necks, but-toned across the shoulders. I remember, when I went to put the clothes on in the hotel, I laughed for sheer delight when I looked at myself in the mirror.

Irma never ate with us – she always kept herself separate, which is why I don't recall where she was – but the rest of us had our dinner in the garden, at a big table. All the girls were there, younger girls mingling with the older ones – they were only three years older, but they looked like grown-ups to us.

It was suppertime, and Schneider had administrators with him. When grown-ups were talking, I always listened. I don't know why, but on this occasion I was particularly intrigued to know what they were talking about. Our director was asking one of the people who was sitting there about somebody they all knew.

"Do you remember So-and-so?"

"Oh, he got married."

"Oh, yes? Well, how did it work out?"

"Well, he had a heart attack and he died."

From that point on, I thought there must be something not quite right about this marriage business, if a person could die of it.

Volga boat-girls

Another tour that we did more than once was down the River Volga. We gave concerts at places on the river and we were taken between them on the Volga boats. They still had the old Russian *lilos* – they had survived from before the revolution – and these old boats were wonderfully equipped.

We slept on board and we might travel two or three days before we came to a reasonably sized place where we could perform. The cabins were lovely, quite luxurious in fact, and the cooks were excellent. In fact, as soon as we got back from one of these trips, we would start thinking about when we could go again, because we were always very hungry. We really had a marvellous time.

The food was still the old pre-revolution *cuisine*, with various types of fish – sturgeon, caviar, salmon and others – and fish soups, wonderful *bouillons*, as well as *kulibaki*, which were pastries with fish inside. It was all so delicious!

I can't describe the reaction of the people when we arrived in the town. All I know is what happened on stage. Very often we did a matinée for young people, for children, and Irma always used to get me on stage to show the movements.

Our first Volga cruise was a big success and after that we went touring regularly. Of course we went wherever they took us, but we were very comfortable on the boats, so we always looked forward to going down the Volga. The last time we went on those boats to give concerts along the way, we went all the way to Astrakhan, on the Volga delta. We used to like travelling and we brought in money, which helped the school a great deal. In term-time we gave concerts in and around Moscow.

Summer garden concerts

When spring comes in Russia, there is such a difference in the air. In Russia they have real seasons: the weather changes completely, from bitter winter to refreshing spring. Summer is something lovely and then we used the summer garden for concerts, since we always needed extra money. Our director, Schneider, used to organise our concerts; he was very efficient, he started advertising and many people came – cultured people and not just our parents – in fact, so many people wanted to come that the concerts were always sold out.

He organised a number of these summer evenings each year from then on. He went to a lot of trouble, with curtains and backdrop, everything just as if it were in the theatre, with a stage and even the big lights from the side and overhead. He was able to make a replica of the theatre, because the garden was so spacious. Meanwhile, Isadora would get in touch with the conservatoire and ask them to send us the very best pianist they had. And, of course, they had to get the piano outside and set out chairs in the garden too.

One time, when we were getting changed into our costumes in the bedroom, Schneider happened to pass by the doorway as I was trying to pin up something. I must have looked very awkward, because he laughed and said, "What are you trying to do?" and I said, "I am trying to arrange my tunic." Well, no doubt I was making some strange shapes and it was rather funny.

Not far from the school, there was a chap who sold ice-cream at the corner of the street. He used to do wonderful ice-cream, so our director used to arrange for him to come to our summer evening concerts and sell ice-creams at the interval. The man would make sure he didn't run out, so at the end of the evening there would always be some left.

After the concert, our director would come to us and say, "Girls, upstairs!" We all ran upstairs to the Pink Room, the bigger girls' room, and finished off the leftovers. That was fun, because it was a very big container of ice-cream and we scraped it clean. Schneider saw to it that we all got a fair share and it was delicious!

These concerts were very enjoyable, they were good publicity for the school and they did help us to raise money. We also had four or five similar concerts during the summer term, for which people paid, so that was rather clever of Schneider.

Some more girls

I wasn't the only girl that went home during term-time. Marsha Toropchenova did too; she was one of the bigger girls and I liked her, because she was very vivacious as well as being a good dancer. She went with us to China and later to America. Her name was really Maria, but we called her Marsha for short.

Then there was a girl about two years older than me called Yulia, who went with us to China, but Irma never took her to America. She was rather naughty, though I was rather fond of her. Moura Babed was my age; she had auburn hair and some of the girls used to call her 'Ginger'. Now Moura was rather timid, and Yulia could be quite bad. She got hold of a worm in the garden and put it down Moura's back. I was horrified, the girl was screaming and I said to Yulia, "How could you do that to her? Get it out! Otherwise I will tell the teacher the way you have behaved." Well, she got it out and she never did it again; but, really and truly, Yulia could be very naughty.

There were a few girls that were very friendly with me, amongst them Mooshya and Marsha. Mooshya's bed was next to mine and Marsha slept at the back. Somehow, all the big girls slept all at the back and we youngsters in front. Marisha Borisova had one of the beds at the back, but she used to disturb the other girls with her peculiar behaviour. She evidently thought that, as she was the oldest, she could boss us about. Well she couldn't boss me about – I would never let that happen – but the other girls were a little bit timid and so they had to learn to cope with her behaviour. I told them, "Don't take any notice of her. Let her carry on in her own sweet way."

Stories

As the school began to shrink, Schneider let our Japanese Room to a prominent advocate and his wife, who was a very well-known actress from the Maly Theatre – the Bolshoi was for ballet and the Maly was for plays – and they used to come to our summer garden concerts. Her first name was Nidegda, she was very lovely and she had a beautiful voice. She used to come in the evenings to read us stories, and we absolutely loved them – especially Gogol, but other stories too.

Whatever I read as a child – and I read a lot – it was always

Western literature. As a girl, I never had much to do with Russian authors, though I read them later on. When I was getting a big girl, I used to read Andersen and Grimm. I liked fairy tales, but especially Andersen's wonderful stories.

When we travelled and stayed in hotels, we often slept many to a room. Amongst the girls I was sharing with on one occasion was Valya, a girl I was very fond of. I was fond of some girls more than others. We were all in bed when Valya piped up, "Lilya, you have read such a lot: you must know a nice short story to read us." Well, as I mentioned before, I like the great French writers and I was reading Prosper Mérimée at the time – his short stories, which were captivating me. One of them particularly was a most original story, called 'Venus Milovskay'.

So I started telling them that story, because it was a little bit scary. After a while, as I was telling the story – and, even with a short story, that takes time – it seemed to me that everything had gone very quiet. I thought had better check, so I asked quietly, "Valya?" There was no sign: they were all fast asleep. And I thought, *It's time I also turned in*.

4

Across Siberia to China, 1926-7

Isadora's plans

In 1926, our French lessons suddenly became very important and the teachers began desperately coaching us in speaking French, not just reading and writing it. We learnt that Isadora was in Nice and she wanted us to join her there. It sounded rather fun and we looked forward very much to that. Things had been pretty difficult for Isadora, and for us. Now we were to perform in France and then she was supposed to take us to America.

But instead of going to France and then America, we went to Siberia and then China. Yes, after all that work getting our French up to scratch, and looking forward to meeting up with Isadora, for some reason or other – I still really don't know why – Irma decided to take us over 5,000 miles in the opposite direction, to Vladivostok.

On the way through Siberia

In the late summer we set off. You could do the journey to Vladivostok in nine days, if you slept on the train, but we took quite a lot longer. The train was well equipped, so you could always get something to drink, and thankfully we could get food at many of the stops, even if they were just villages. Travelling with us we had our nanny and nurse, Mooshya's mother. She was also looking after Irma, who had been ill, and Irma appreciated that. It was a wonderful trip, because we stopped at such extraordinary places along the way. It was still old Russia that hadn't yet been destroyed. In the towns along the way we gave performances and then stayed there for the night.

One afternoon we stopped at a mining town in the Ural Mountains. I didn't feel very well so when they went off for a rehearsal, I stayed behind. I was only 13, and I was left alone in the place – you couldn't call it a hotel, I would say it was a kind of hostel – in my room. Now, although I didn't feel a hundred per cent, still after a while I was a little bit bored, so I opened the door to the corridor. Facing me, the door opened and a little boy came out. He looked at me and spoke.

"Do you speak English?"

Luckily enough, yes, I spoke English.

"Yes."

"What are you doing here?"

"Oh, I am waiting for the rest of our group to come back."

"Um. Would you like a cream cracker?"

"Yes, very much." I was always ready to have something nice. He went back into his room and came out again with a tin.

"Take as many as you want."

So I did – I took only a few of course, not many – after which he put the tin back, but then he came back out again. He wanted a chat with me because he also was bored. His father was an engineer. The government had introduced new rules about that time and there were many foreigners working on the mines in the Urals. I am not sure, but I think he was British, because cream crackers are English. After that, I walked down the corridor, and I met a Japanese or Chinese woman – Chinese, I think. She came out of her room, and to me she looked like absolute beauty itself.

Earlier I mentioned Marisha Borisova, the girl who was a bully. One day not long before we set off for Siberia, I was in the bedroom at school when Natasha Nekrovska came up to me.

"Lili, I want to tell you something. You know Marisha Borisova, the one everyone is afraid of?"

"Well, what about her?"

"So you don't know what's happened?"

"No, I have no idea."

"What's happened is that Irma has just found out that Schneider has been having an affair with Marisha."

"My God! Really?"

Later that same day, we heard the water running in Irma's

bathroom. When we went past the bathroom on our way down-stairs, we could hear the water running very fiercely. What Irma was doing was this: she had got all Schneider's things, all his clothes, and put them in the bath and soaked them. Then she threw him out and told him not to pester her any more. She told him to stick to his job and sort out this intimate relationship with Marisha.

When we were downstairs, Natasha said to me, "I don't think I like her any more."

I said, "I don't particularly like or dislike her."

That happened before we set off because, as we travelled through Siberia, Irma would have nothing to do with Schneider. Every time we stopped somewhere for a concert, she always had arguments with him - about arranging the lights or the stage, or the programme - because she wanted everything done her own way. In this she succeeded, which was just as well because she had more sense. She understood that side of things better than Schneider - he was a good organiser and administrator, but when it came to managing things on stage he wasn't as competent as Irma.

I had my own problems on our journey across Siberia. I think I mentioned before that the nurse gave me a difficult time and there were a lot of unpleasant incidents. Her name was Elzbieta Grigor-evnya Mysovskaya; I never got on with her and that was because she took advantage of me. Whenever we were staying at a hotel and she wanted something, she used to send me for it.

I got sick and tired of it and one day, when she asked me to go somewhere, I said, "Look, Elzbieta Grigorevnya, stop bullying me and sending me on your errands. If you want something, either you can do it yourself or you can send your daughter. Why should you send me?" Then I walked out of the room - this happened in a hotel - but that stopped her behaving towards me like that.

I disliked her, but only because she always disliked me, for whatever reason, and I have no idea why she did. What it was that so irritated her - especially when I was so friendly with her daughter - I don't know. I suppose she was probably a little bit jealous of me, perhaps when she saw that I got on with Irma very well. She thought Irma owed her a great deal because it was she who had cured Irma of TB. But what had that to do with me? Nothing at all. And why did she behave like that only to me and never to the other girls? I have no idea.

Performances *en route*

Each day the train took us hundreds of kilometres further east. At lots of places we stopped and gave concerts. We didn't have a class beforehand, but what we did do was gymnastics in the morning. Then, if we had to dance at night, Irma would put us to bed before the theatre: we had to sleep, and that we always did, to wake up fresh. But she would never make us go through our dance routines, oh no. It was not necessary: we already knew everything we had to do. Once we had warmed up, we were ready to dance straightaway.

En route, we used to give matinées and there were many children at these, of course. With Schneider's help, Irma used to invite people onto the stage and we used to show them movements. Many children would come up and we had little tunics prepared for them. We had nannies with us who would help them change, but we girls used to help too. We used to sit them in the corner while we put little red tunics on them.

When they were all ready, we started a slow march by Schubert and I showed them all the movements. Then we used to stand them up and they would repeat it – you know, follow me. That was a routine at matinées: we very often did that. However, Irma never told me beforehand when she wanted me on stage with her: when she was ready and everything was organised, she would simply call, "Lili!"

At one small town on our journey – and where it was, I have no idea – but by now it was cold, winter was coming on and this place had some Dutch-style heaters to warm it. They were used to warm up a few rooms at the back, but also at the side of the stage and centre stage. They burnt logs, I think, and they had vents, made of tin or something of the sort, that were opened to let the hot air come out. On this occasion, I suddenly heard Irma calling, "Lili! Lili, where are you? Come on!" and I dashed out onto the stage. I injured my arm because I caught it on that vent.

It was terribly painful; in fact, I still have the scar. I really hurt myself because when I went on stage to show my movements, the blood was running down my arm, but I never noticed that at the time: I just carried on marching. Irma noticed, but there was nothing she could do about it. She said later she couldn't believe her eyes, but then she added, "You should have been on stage. Where were you?" It is true that I always used to show the children what to do,

75

but she hadn't warned me to be there at that particular moment, when the children came onto the stage. She hadn't said, "You must be there and show them all the movements."

White Russians

At another place where we stopped – I think it may have been Sverdlovsk, the main town in Siberia – there were many, many White Russians, middle-class, from good families. They were called White Russians because they supported the White Party, rather than the Red Party; we used to call them bourgeois. They didn't all flee Soviet Russia, at least not immediately. They went to Siberia for one reason only, to get to China, and they were called *Bivshye* – which meant they were running away from Moscow.

Later they moved on to Vladivostok and eventually I believe they all went to Harbin, in Manchuria, and from there to China. Many of them went that way, to try to start a new life. It was so heartbreaking to see these people who had lost everything. Whatever they could put their hand to, they would do it, just to make a living. People are resilient on the whole; they try to keep afloat.

So for the time being they had settled in this town and some of them had opened little restaurants in order to make a living. The Russians always cooked well – I am speaking of their *haute cuisine* – and that came from French influence. I think it came about when Pushkin came on the scene – he really turned things over and made Russian culture much more important – that's when it changed. In those years after Waterloo, the French were forsaken, but they had great influence in Russia – at one time, Russian high society spoke only French – and especially in cookery, because French cuisine was so very good. As a result, the best Russian cooking was very, very good.

In this particular town where we stopped to give a concert – I think we were getting quite close to Vladivostok by this time – we went into one of these little restaurants run by a White Russian couple running away from Moscow. We enjoyed the meal so much that we thought we would like to thank them. Schneider was with us; I am not sure where Irma was. She never ate with us; she led a separate life, but we didn't mind. Anyway, we more or less filled the place. We praised them for the food. They were delighted to see us; we told them that we were dancers and we got talking.

In the midst of all this talk, one particular woman, one of the White Russians, said, "Who is that girl hiding back there?" and that was me. I was always at the back; I never used to go forward. She said, "What a pretty little girl she is. Can she come forward?" I was quite amazed, but I came forward and she started talking to me. After a little longer, we repeated all the nice things we had said about the food; then we said goodbye and walked off, in pairs.

As we went, Schneider came up to me and said, "Now, don't you be getting a swollen head. I hope you won't take any notice of what she said: it is nonsense. Just forget about it."

Well, I had been surprised, of course, to be picked out, but after that I had never even thought twice about it – so I said, "What on earth do you mean?"

I didn't know what he was talking about, so I didn't say anything more. I never took that much notice of what people said.

I was always at the back and I never used to go forward. Some girls used to push themselves forward, but not me, and I am still that way. I never liked to push myself, though I liked to give an opinion: oh yes, if I am asked I will tell people what I think. But to push myself on stage, I never did that. Irma used to get very cross with me and say, "Come on, Lili: you can do better than you are." Really and truly I always did the best I could, but she had the impression that I could do even better. She would say, "You lazy girl." I wasn't lazy; it was just that I danced without any effort. I still feel the same way now. You don't have to struggle to move beautifully. Even now when I watch dancers, they must move as easily as possible if they are going to be good to look at. That is how I like music too, played without any effort.

We saw some very lovely sights in our journey across Siberia, and I have very good memories of it, even though winter was coming on. One place we stopped at was Baikal; it was beautiful there. We went to see the lake and it was so clear you could see every stone at the bottom, though it must have been 100 feet deep or more. The scenery around was wonderful too, but my memory is that Baikal was something quite extraordinary.

Vladivostok

Then we continued our journey and we reached the sea at the port of Vladivostok. We had to get special permission to go abroad and China seemed impossibly distant to us. All the same, we were told that Schneider had been in touch with officials in Moscow to arrange for us to travel to China. While we were waiting for this to happen, we gave concerts in Vladivostok.

At that time, we knew that Russia had a very good relationship with China. What we didn't really know was that over the previous few months the Chinese Communists had been fighting alongside the Kuomintang to take control of much of China and they had set up a new government in Hankow. This was the Chinese Government that agreed to let us visit China, though most of the country was still ruled by various warlords. Even so, that is how we entered the country.

Manchuria

We were very excited at the prospect of entering China. I don't remember if we had to show passports or not, but our first stop was Harbin in Manchuria, and we felt the difference straightaway. It may seem funny to say it but, after we had travelled all those thousands of miles east from Moscow and had at last reached this famously oriental country, when we reached Harbin it was like coming into the West. I liked that: it was like my early upbringing. I could never forget that. In fact, Harbin seemed to me more Western than Moscow. The whole time I was in Russia, it was a strange thing with me: I always looked to the west.

Harbin itself impressed me very much, it was a very Western type of city, with boulevards and fine, modern buildings. It was still autumn there, and my favourite time is autumn. We used to go walking down the boulevards; they were lined with trees and the leaves were all golden-yellow. I was in delight; I used to kick the leaves up. Somehow, my mind was always at ease when I walked along the boulevards, and it's funny but I don't remember the other girls walking there with me.

Then we saw the shops. For us, the sight of these well-stocked shops was quite extraordinary, because there were hardly any shops in Russia where you could just walk in and buy what you wanted. Even in Moscow, my mother tried once to buy me something nice, and she just couldn't. I wanted some special shoes, and she had to go through the whole of Moscow to find anything. It was so difficult. They were very, very bad times.

As a result, on our journey through Siberia, we never even had decent sandals to wear. Mine had two holes underneath, and I still have hard skin on the sole of my foot that I got from wearing those worn-out sandals: it was as if I was walking about barefoot by the time we reached Vladivostok.

So, when we got to Harbin, the first thing Irma did was to take us to a clothes shop. We had new outfits, including nice little sweaters or cardigans and, I think, little skirts, but she bought us boots, stockings, scarves and hats too. We were transformed from looking like poor orphans to reasonably dressed young people. She bought us quite a number of nice things to wear, especially the four youngsters. I have pictures of us in Tientsin, wearing these clothes. We looked very nice and we were still wearing these outfits when we got back to Russia. I think the money came from the concerts we gave. Much later, after we returned from China, Irma bought us more clothes, lovely things; it made you feel better to wear them and we looked so nice.

We were at the back of the stage once, when the audience was coming in, and our director came over to a few girls – I was among them – and he said, "Girls, would you like to see a Chinese family?" Naturally we said, "Yes!" One by one we peeped through the curtains. We were astonished, because one family must have been about three to four hundred people. We said, "How on earth can that be?" He pointed to a very grand figure at the head of the crowd and said, "There's the cause of it. Mandarins used to marry several women, all of whom had dozens of children – and, I suppose, scores of grandchildren."

We could hardly believe him, but indeed, when they queued for tickets, just two families took up the whole place. The only reason I remember this particular performance is because it was the first time we had ever seen a family of that size. That was a very great novelty for us; we really found it fascinating. Of course, as visitors, we had to accept their customs and I suppose they had to accept us the way we were. We gave four concerts there, and our performances were really successful.

79

By then I was 13, and five and a half years had passed since I first entered Isadora's school. In that time I had learnt a great deal. We all had, and we danced very, very well. You can tell from the photos: we looked grown up. We were dancing almost every single day. From Harbin, we set off for Shanghai.

Shanghai

The people in China did not look at us in a strange way, and – even though so much that we saw was new to us – I don't think we looked at anybody there in a strange way either: we just accepted people as we found them. By that time, we were used to travelling: we had been all over Russia. Manchuria was only a step further, and China proper was just one step beyond that. In any event, Harbin, Tientsin and Shanghai were partly Westernised.

We didn't go to Shanghai by road, but I think we may have gone part of the way by train. What I do know is that we went most of the way along the Grand Canal on a little Russian steamboat – I know it was Russian, because I remember its name – the *Indigirka*. It was a long journey, and we slept one night on the boat.

When we reached Shanghai, we thought it was a very strangely organised place. It was a very mixed city, but the Westerners and the Chinese lived separately. It seemed that some quarters of the city were only for Chinese; these we only ever passed through. Also, there seemed to be something very strange going on, because we were always seeing people running down the street, waving some kind of placard. Only later did we guess what was happening.

I remember walking through the streets of Shanghai and noticing how some of the women, especially elderly women, not the young ones, walked oddly, as if their feet were crippled; really, they could hardly walk. They could only hobble and Schneider, our director, told us it was because their feet were still bandaged in the old way.

I also saw quite a number of people who were walking about with no noses; it was very odd. I pointed this out to the other girls and they said, "Isn't it strange?" They were just as amazed as I was. So again we asked our director: why was it they had no noses? They had only holes instead of noses. "Oh," he said, "it is because they have a terrible disease here called syphilis, and it makes their noses disappear."

It seemed there was an epidemic there and people suffered terribly; that is how we learned about that dreadful illness. Of course we were terrified of eating or drinking anything, because we were so afraid of catching the disease. We hadn't a clue how it comes and how you get it, and all our director would say was, "Girls, you must keep your hands very clean, and just be careful."

I remember we gave a number of concerts in Shanghai. At the time I wondered why we stayed in such poor lodgings there. It was because Irma was very short of money, and they wouldn't let her leave until she paid the hotel bills. Eventually the Soviet Government paid her debts and contacted the Chinese Nationalists. As a result Madam Sun Yat-sen, widow of Sun Yat-sen and a sister of Chiang Kai-shek, came to meet us: she was determined we should visit them, and she invited us to come and stay in her palace in Hankow – so it was arranged. As a result, we didn't stay in Shanghai very long that first time.

Madam Sun Yat-sen was rather beautiful and when we met her she was wearing a sable coat; we could not take our eyes off her. I thought to myself, "My dear, and you supposed to be a revolutionary!" We thought Sun Yat-sen was the beginning of socialism, but in fact the beginning of their revolution was really going on when we were there. They called themselves socialists, communists or whatever, so how was it that his widow was dressed in sables? Still, I thought she looked quite wonderful.

The palace of the People's Party

We travelled on a Japanese river steamer up the Yangtze-kiang to reach her palace. We travelled third class, even Irma on this occasion, because she was still very short of money. We couldn't even go and eat in the dining room on the boat; we lived on baked beans and bacon. We had some bread and butter too, but that was the main diet. Luckily enough I liked baked beans, so that didn't matter. Our nurse used to warm the beans and some bacon – she had a little food-warmer – and I think that was all we had for two days. It wasn't pleasant, but we didn't mind too much.

When we reached Hankow, Madam Sun Yat-sen was there to welcome us. She introduced herself and her brother, Mr Chiang Kai-shek, and they took us to the palace outside the town. We stayed there for a whole month and it was a very interesting experience. They gave us a limousine, with a driver, for the whole of our stay there. The palace itself was extraordinary, and very comfortable. I couldn't get over the luxury of it. We had two or three girls – no more than four – to a room, and the rooms were very spacious.

The dining area was so wonderful, and the breakfast! We were bowled over. We had porridge, we had juice drinks, we had toast, marmalade and – heaven, absolutely heaven – boiled eggs! We loved the food, because we had so little to eat in Russia. Long afterwards, my daughter used to say, "Mum, I bet it was because you were so underfed that you never grew your extra two inches that you wanted so much." I always did wish I was a little taller. At this breakfast, though, nearly every girl had a servant standing at the back of her chair, asking what she would like to eat and seeing that the food was served properly. Such luxury we had never experienced before. It was very pleasing.

After breakfast, we used to run about a bit and follow our own pursuits. The palace had beautiful gardens and, funnily enough, I still have a programme – I saved it from being thrown out, many years ago – and it includes pictures that show the palace gardens, with the gazebos; but of the palace itself, I haven't any photos.

The city of Hankow was very different from Shanghai. At that time, several Western countries had a foothold in China, small territories called 'concessions'. The further away from these you went, the less safe it became. In fact, much of the rest of China was ruled by warlords, who were like gangsters, only grander. So Shanghai was quite like a Western city, and near Hankow there was a small 'concession' where we danced a few times, but Hankow itself was more or less old China.

The Chinese theatres were not like European theatres at all: they were more or less like circuses, and they were cold too. When we arrived in Harbin, it was autumn, but now in Hankow the weather was changing to winter and we found it difficult to warm up properly, to be able to dance. I recall this theatre in Hankow: it was in an enormous building, like an amphitheatre or a circus ring, and around the 'circus ring' they had containers of some kind, four of them I think, with a fire burning in each. The audience sat in a circle: there were seats all the way round. There was only a small 'backstage' space for us, at the very back.

The audiences did not behave like Western audiences either. Most of them were men, sitting there with hot towels over them. What surprised me was they were drinking tea and throwing towels at one another, wiping the perspiration from them, and shouting, "Chin hor!" ('very good') – or there was another word – if they liked it. If they didn't like something, they would put their thumb down and say, "Mumandi!" or something like that. That was how they behaved, and it was so cold, it was awful. I remember being very, very cold.

Alone in the palace

Within a few days I had caught a very bad cold; in short, I had pneumonia again. So I spent about three weeks of my stay in bed, in that palace. I had to stay very quiet and be looked after. I couldn't dance or even go out any more. We had concerts galore, but they had to do them without me. The other girls went out nearly every night and I was left by myself in that very big palace.

I was terrified really. It wasn't just the palace: I was very frightened of this dreadful illness we had been told about and I didn't know how to get hold of anybody who could say more than a few words in Russian or English. I used to ring the bell and a servant would come in, bow to me and say, "What would the young lady like?" And I would say, "Can I have an orange?" or anything that came into my mind, just to make conversation, but at a distance because I was frightened of the Chinese servants.

I was so lonely lying there. I had books to read, because I used to love reading, and it's a good job I did. I was very, very frightened the whole time, until at last the girls came back. The funniest part was, they never walked in: they would only peep in at the door to ask how I felt.

"Lilya, how are you?"

"I think I am getting better. Why don't you come in to see me?"

"Oh no, no, we can't now. We are very, very busy, we can't."

They used to make any excuse; I couldn't understand it. When they learnt that I had pneumonia, they changed their attitude.

Later on, I brought this up and asked them, "Why didn't you come in and see me?" They told me, "Well, we were so frightened. We thought you had syphilis and we were scared of catching it." At that, we were all laughing our heads off. We had no idea how you got it;

all we knew was there was an awful illness called syphilis, and people caught it.

My mother's dream

My mother had always believed in dreams, as all Russians do. She said to me that she didn't hear from the school and in fact she didn't hear anything at all after we left for China – we didn't correspond, she didn't hear from Schneider and there was no news – so she became very worried.

Then she had a dream, a very bad dream, that she was in the market buying meat, and the meat was not very good. She was carrying me on her back and I was very heavy. Now, for the Russians, dreaming of a market with meat lying about definitely means an illness. That is how they translate it.

She told me afterwards that she had been so worried about me; she really felt something must have happened to me, so she wrote to Schneider and asked him, "Is there anything wrong with Lili? I haven't heard from her and I am concerned." He wrote back to say, "Yes, yes, she hasn't been very well, but now she is getting better."

Irma never visited me either. However, the food was very good and after a couple of weeks I was really well again. I still didn't start dancing again, though, because they wanted to make sure I had completely recovered.

At the court of Chiang Kai-shek

Once I was well again, I re-joined the others. We all used to meet each evening downstairs in the big hall. There would be Chiang Kai-shek sitting there, Madam Sun Yat-sen and a man called Ying Chen, who had been prime minister in the Philippines, with his family. Madam Chiang used to come over as well, to see Madam Sun.

They were all there in our palace and we had pleasant evenings, except that we girls used to have to go to bed earlier. We would rather have stayed up and listened to all the talk. In the meantime Irma stayed in the same palace and she behaved like a queen herself: she was dressed in an extraordinarily rich Chinese outfit and entertained the guests.

Chen's family were nice. They were grown up: he had two daughters, Sylvia, who was petite and very beautiful, and Yolanda, the youngest who was rather plain, and they had two brothers, Percy and Jack. Sylvia was the eldest and used to do a lot of riding. I still don't know why they were in Hankow. Apparently, although they were Filipino, they had been forced to flee from the Philippines. Were they thrown out? I have no idea. I know this, though: that when we went to Shanghai and later stayed at the embassy, the Chens turned up there; and, when we went back to Russia, they came too - not on the same boat, but they did come to Moscow - and they used to visit us at school.

If they were not performing in a concert, the other girls could go out into Hankow itself. When I was getting well again, I began to go with them, because there were cinemas in the town. After we had been to see *Peter Pan*, which we liked very much, I was left on my own again the next day. I got bored and found my way up onto the roof, where I skipped and jumped about, pretending to be Peter Pan. I always wanted to be him and I wished I could fly. He so appealed to me, that Peter Pan. We had all seen the stage play, but the film was wonderful: it was just for me.

We went to see two other films that I remember: one was a very nice film called *Midnight Sun* with Laura LaPlante, who was a big star just then. The other was *The Four Horsemen of the Apocalypse* with Rudolph Valentino. Of course we girls went potty over him; we all fell for him - he was so good-looking. After we had seen the film, we learnt he had just died - he had something wrong with his appendix - and we were so upset, we cried our eyes out. We couldn't get over it - such a handsome man to disappear at such an early age.

On the riverboat

We had a most interesting time in Hankow, but eventually we had to pack and set off again. We travelled on the steamer once more, down the Yangtze-kiang. On the way we had to pass Nanking; there was trouble there, so we stayed on board. I remember it very well. There were a few of us in each cabin and we were told not to step out of our cabins, but sometimes I used to peep out to see what the boat was like. I used to look out and see such funny people sitting there.

When you came out of the cabin, before you came on deck, there was a kind of big hallway and there would always be some Chinese sitting there, smoking – not tobacco, nor cocaine, nor marijuana, nor hash, but opium. There would always be five or six old men with long pipes, smoking. I have seldom seen anything so strange in all my lifetime.

Even after such a long time, certain things can sit in your memory. I can still picture those old men smoking their long pipes, long enough to reach right to the ground and up to their mouths. They were puffing away, in a kind of trance. It never occurred to us to try it. It never even entered our minds – in fact, we were a bit concerned about it, so we felt safer staying in our cabin for the two days and two nights. Nowadays I wonder why people do these strange things; I really do.

We were busy with our own things, busy thinking of our dancing and what the next day was going to bring. Where were we going? Would we be met there? And where were we going to stay? We were kept tucked away in these cabins, until we had passed Nanking. After that things were all right. I don't think we knew it at the time, but the revolution was beginning.

Tientsin: where East and West met

It was a longer journey than before. Below Nanking, instead of continuing downriver to Shanghai, we turned north to Tientsin. When we got there, we were very surprised to find that Tientsin was like a Western city, with beautiful streets and beautiful houses very like those of European capitals. The people we saw were all very, very well off, but they seemed to be all Westerners. I don't remember even seeing any Chinese people in Tientsin. I don't know who it belonged to. I don't think it was German or French, but I am not sure. There were many English people – and, I think, some Americans – but we saw mostly English people, so perhaps it was British.

It was not by the sea, but it was on an estuary and it had a big port. It was the most delightful place, Tientsin. I have some photos taken there. We gave a number of concerts – not very many – but we had great success because there were so many Europeans. We danced in proper theatres in Tientsin, not like in Hankow, which had been such a disaster for me.

Lots of families came to see us, of course. After one concert, a woman came backstage. She came up to our director and said she loved the dancing: it was so absolutely wonderful. Then she explained: "I have a daughter and we wondered - if you wouldn't mind - we wondered if we could invite one of the girls back to our home for a few days? There is one girl in particular that we would really like to invite: she looks so much like my daughter."

She meant me! Our director, Schneider, said he would ask. He came and explained all this to me, and then asked, "Lili, would you like to go?"

And I said, "Yes, very much. I would love to."

So I went and stayed for a few days with them - three days, I think - and they were a lovely family. They had a beautiful house and they were so kind to me. The mother said she liked me and I looked like her daughter. I don't know if I did, but she dressed me up in beautiful clothes and gave me many presents. She was certainly rather taken with me. I don't remember her name, but I remember the woman's face, and I remember the girl, who was just a little older than me. They were European, and I wouldn't be surprised if they were Jewish. I was the only Jewish girl there, so that could have been the connection. Her daughter and I had a lovely time together. Years afterwards, when we went to America, she came to New York to see us. I think she came specially to see me, because she came backstage to see if we still looked alike.

In Tientsin, the other girls said, "Lilya, aren't you lucky!" I never thought like that. If people were kind to me, that was fine. But even if they made a fuss of me, it never made me think more of them or myself. I cannot explain why exactly, but I suppose I wasn't easily swayed by other people's opinions.

We stayed a while in Tientsin and then we went on to Peking, which wasn't far away.

Peking: an imperial museum

I still have a couple of photos from our time in Peking. We gave concerts there, and I know I liked the theatre, though I don't remember it very well. What I do remember is Peking itself. It was fabulous, absolutely wonderful: the city itself was beautiful, the buildings were extraordinary. They took us all to these wonderful palaces, which were beautifully built and finely decorated - I don't think they exist today - and we looked at all the museums. We enjoyed Peking, because it was an old city and had such a lot of architectural interest. I always used to take particular notice of buildings, but some of the other girls did too.

The city then was a kind of wonderland, with beautiful gardens, wonderful palaces and all those marble statues. They were Buddhas, of course, but that didn't stop them being of great interest to us. I remember the city so well, because it did impress me: the city walls, the extraordinary buildings - especially the palaces, which we went to see - and most of all the gardens; they were wonderful. They are stronger in my memory than even the dancing.

Back in Shanghai

From Peking we returned to Shanghai. While we were in China, we naturally stayed most of the time in Shanghai: it was the biggest and richest city, and we gave many concerts there. Even so, I definitely preferred Peking.

When we had settled in a hotel, our director Schneider gave us something to read about syphilis. I'm not sure that we understood very much of it. We had to stay in a very small hotel, the second time we were in Shanghai. It was more like a guest house. It was so awful, the bedrooms were absolutely appalling, and the conveniences there - well, they were non-existent.

On the way upstairs to our room, we had to pass a landing where there was a big mirror on the wall. The owner of the place was a very strange little woman, who had a grown-up son living with her, and he by accident broke the mirror. There was such shouting and commotion; she was in tears with despair, crying, "Only the gods know what bad luck this is going to bring me!" I don't know if it ever did bring her bad luck, apart from losing the mirror. Well, perhaps it did bring bad luck in a way, because we didn't stay there long.

Shortly after that, much of Shanghai became very unsafe. We had to be very careful where we went: there were lots of streets you couldn't walk down. We managed to do a little shopping just here and there, because it was so dangerous to go out in Shanghai at that time – there was so much villainy going on.

I remember Lolya was out shopping, I don't know who with, but she took someone with her who knew the way, because she couldn't find it by herself. What I do know is she came back with her eyes bulging in horror; I thought they would come out of their sockets. We thought, *Gosh, what has she seen now?* It was some-thing extraordinary. She couldn't believe it; she had seen sticks with heads walking about, walking in the streets. When she had calmed down a bit, she started telling us what she had seen.

She had noticed some people who were dressed in a peculiar way, walking down the street in a procession and carrying things above their heads. As they came closer, she saw they were carrying long stems and on each stick was a severed head. My goodness me! She nearly collapsed in horror, and when she told us, we couldn't get over it either. At that point our director said, "We are going back to Russia." We gave no more concerts in China; it was now obviously very dangerous, even in the big cities.

It was certainly too dangerous to stay in this little *pension* in the heart of the town, so we were to move to the Russian embassy and stay there until we could set off home. Our move to the embassy took a few days to arrange. Meanwhile, the woman had no food in the place, so we went to a restaurant to eat. That was one good thing about this crisis, because we were always thinking of food: that was our number-one priority. We didn't mind the rest as long as we had a good square meal, and Schneider would always find a good place for us to eat.

Our director found a place where they made European food and it was very good. We had lovely fried fish and chips, salads and various tasty home-made meals; we liked it because it was wholesome and clean, and we would all eat there. The couple who ran it were Westerners and very kind. I don't know who they were, but some of the meals were Jewish, so I think perhaps they were too. We all liked Jewish food.

Over the sea to Russia

While we were staying at the Russian embassy in Shanghai, waiting for a boat to Vladivostok, Schneider told us that the liner he wanted to book us on was full, and he couldn't get any tickets. So we had to wait a little longer and then he booked our passage on a relatively small boat.

The weather was still bad, there were big waves and this small vessel was really tossed about. It pitched and plunged and rocked, so that everybody was lying as through dead. I was the only one walking. They said to me, "How do you manage it?" They were all ill. They couldn't move, but I never thought anything of it, though it was not very comfortable, I must say.

After we reached Vladivostok, the director told us, "You know the big liner we were going to go on? Apparently, the weather on their crossing was even worse. They met a storm and it went down." I don't know how true that was. He said it was sheer luck that we were not on it. I have a picture of us sitting on the boat to Vladivostok.

The sleeper

Irma and Ilya Schneider were anxious to get away from China, so we didn't stay long in Vladivostok. We set off again on the Trans-Siberian Railway, but 400 miles along the line we stopped at Khabarovsk, which is the furthest east on the railway. From western Europe, it is three-quarters of the way to the other side of the world. We spent about two weeks in Khabarovsk, giving concerts and making some money for school funds. After that I don't think we stopped to give any concerts, because we had danced a great deal in China, and Schneider was anxious to get us back to school.

Our director got tickets and there were to be no more stops; we slept on the train. Unfortunately, he couldn't get any tickets for second class, the way we usually travelled, so we didn't have bunks. We travelled third class, where you had to share a compartment. It had only couchettes, but all the same our director managed to make beds out of them. He got hold of some mats and sheets, and laid them for us so that we could sleep.

We had entered China with nothing, but we came back with tremendous amounts of beautiful things, lovely clothes, shoes and boots, which Irma and Schneider had bought for us, as well as some presents. All our things were in big baskets, stowed overhead in the compartment.

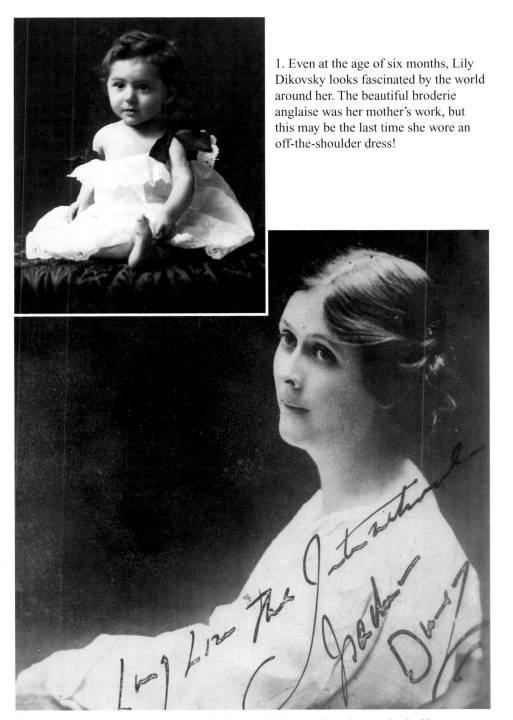

1. Even at the age of six months, Lily Dikovsky looks fascinated by the world around her. The beautiful broderie anglaise was her mother's work, but this may be the last time she wore an off-the-shoulder dress!

2. Isadora Duncan was more romantic than revolutionary, but she was both. She wrote 'Long live the Internationale' when she signed this photograph and then told the girls at her Moscow school to 'Make everybody dance'. Lily remembered her as funny, but quite delightful, with china-blue eyes and a gorgeous smile, which captivated all the men.

3. Right: Liza Dikovskaya *c*.1906, before her marriage. Lily's mother was a proud woman, always impeccably turned out. Her fashionable hairstyle is reminiscent of the style that took its name from Lehár's hugely successful 1905 operetta *The Merry Widow*, which could also have supplied the model for her independent lifestyle.

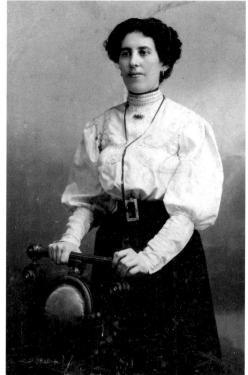

4. Below: A studio portrait of Lily's uncle Isaac, taken in Liège on 13 March 1911. After he fled Russia, his sister Liza followed him and they lived in Belgium for a while, before moving to Paris.

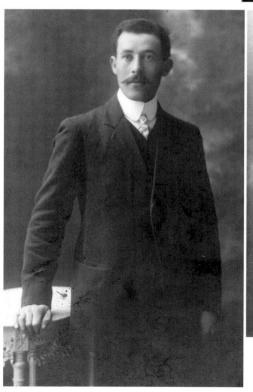

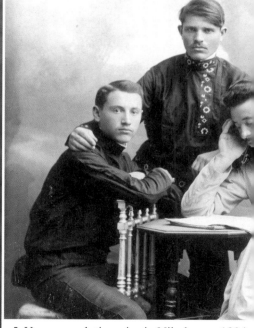

5. Young revolutionaries in Nikolaev, *c*.1904. The two in white are Liza's brothers – Peter facing the camera, Isaac leaning on

6. Right: Liza Lotterbach and Lily, aged about 2½. She can remember the photographer giving her that golden ball to hold, in a studio in London in 1915, just before Liza left Joseph Lotterbach for ever. Liza liked simple clothes, but they had to be of the highest quality.

Lily was quite happy as a small child, but those big eyes took in everything that went on. Once she began asking questions, she wasn't always satisfied with her mother's answers.

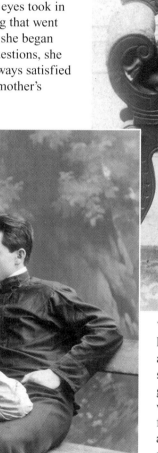

the table – before Luba's tragic death forced them to flee. The other three are unknown.

7. Nowhere: All her life Liza carried a picture of her husband, Joseph Lotterbach. Lily found it after her mother's death, but she was so upset that she forgot to take it with her. When Lily had gone, someone threw out whatever was left; she went back next day, but the photograph was never found. In the picture Joseph wore a velvet jacket and dress shirt, with a large black bow as a necktie. Lily said his face was the image of hers at the same age, his eyes were exactly like hers and he had a dimple in his chin. She liked the look of him very much.

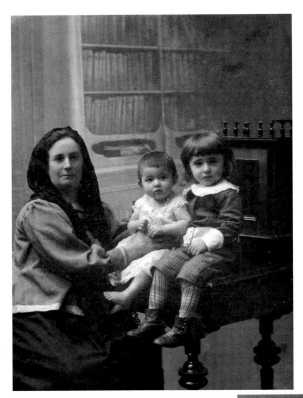

8. Liza's mother with Luba and Mark, her younger daughter Rosa's children, in January 1911. Lily didn't know she had a grandmother until she was 8, and at first sight was terrified of her. But later she found that Grandma was willing to answer all those questions that Lily's mother wouldn't. The inscription on the reverse is in someone else's hand; their mother spoke Russian, but never learnt to write it.

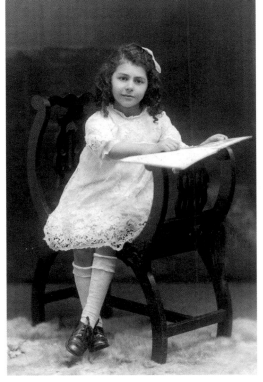

9. Lily boarded at a very small, family-run school in Lincoln, where she was very happy. This picture was taken in a studio in the town when Lily was 7, but within months her mother took her to Russia, where it was winter, the country was in chaos and people were dying in the streets of starvation and disease.

On the way, the train stopped somewhere – I think it was a big village, it wasn't even a town – and we were going to be there for a while. I was lying down at the time and I decided to stay on the train, but the other girls got off to buy something. Before they left the train, the director came up to me and said, "Lili, if you are staying here, stand guard. Keep an eye on those baskets and see that no one comes in." I said, "I'll try." Unluckily, I felt very sleepy and my eyes must have closed.

The next thing I knew, there was some commotion going on and I woke up to find Schneider standing next to me. He said, "You fell asleep and didn't notice, but someone has taken those hampers with all our clothes."

Now our director was very quick-witted; he ran down the platform and stopped the train moving. He told the driver, "Our goods have been stolen" and he could see at a little distance someone moving, alongside a horse and cart, which had big containers lying on top – these were surely our baskets.

He thought to himself, *How can I chase him?* He looked around and spotted some kind of vehicle. He ran across, jumped on board and told the person who drove it, "Hurry! Go after that man. He's making off with all our clothes!" This driver made chase as fast as he could, but Schneider wanted to stop the thief.

Again he was quick-thinking. He took out a very big key that he had in his pocket and started shouting to the driver in front, "If you don't stop, I will shoot you!" The thief saw that our director was holding something in his hand and the chap must have thought he was going to be shot, so he left the cart and ran away. And that is how Schneider got the cart and all our luggage back.

The director didn't scold me very much when he came back, but he kept saying, "Lili, you were a fine one, to fall asleep when I asked you to watch. I did ask you to keep an eye out."

I said, "I couldn't help it. That's why I was lying there, because I was ready to fall asleep."

In any case, I don't think any thief would have been afraid of little me; a fat lot I could have done to stop them, when I was the only one in the compartment.

5

The Death of Isadora
and What Followed, 1927-8

While we were in Khabarovsk, a letter reached Irma from her stepsister saying that her (real) mother had died in Germany. We had never even known that Irma's mother was still alive. We knew only that Isadora had adopted her, but we naturally assumed she was an orphan. While we still on our way back through Siberia to Moscow, Irma decided she would travel onward, first to Germany and then to Paris, where she was determined to get in touch with Isadora. When we reached Moscow, we went back to school and after that we were allowed to go and see our parents.

A tense interview

Irma went first to Germany, much too late to attend her mother's funeral, but at least she was able to find out where her mother was buried. Then she travelled on to Paris and went to see Isadora. They hadn't seen each other for nearly three years and they were glad to be reunited, though Isadora was still angry about what Irma had done, taking us to China instead of joining her in France.

Isadora had been in Nice, expecting us; when we didn't turn up, she got in touch with the government in Moscow and asked them where we were. They told her they knew all about us and that we had gone on a long tour to Siberia and China. When Isadora heard this, she was incensed – she was so angry, she called Irma a bandit – and she still wanted to know how Irma could do such a thing without her permission?

So at first Irma didn't get a very favourable reception. She had some explaining to do, but I don't think she was very apologetic.

"After all, be fair, Isadora. I have been doing everything at the school. You never did have the patience to teach. You were sitting in France somewhere" – even if Isadora did try to speak, Irma probably ploughed on – "well, in Nice, wherever you were, but who was organising the school? You were never there. And what were we supposed to live on? We couldn't sit and wait for you to come back with some money: we had to go on tour to earn some. Well, we can't go on like this any more: it won't work. From now on, unless you are going to be at the school all the time, you must allow me to take charge."

Isadora was at first very taken aback at this, but on reflection she agreed. They came to some arrangement, though I don't know exactly what. I think Isadora still wanted us to come to Nice and meet her, and then go to America and perform with her. She told Irma she had started writing her memoirs and, as soon as she was paid the advance and had done one last concert in Paris for which she was booked, she would come back to Russia. Irma said there was no reason to be angry; they parted as good friends, and Irma went back to Moscow.

My mother had some good friends in Paris, with whom she kept in touch. They had two daughters, one of them a dancer, and the mother decided that her daughter Marguerite must go to Isadora's school, the one at Bellevue. I met Marguerite in Paris in 1929.

Mme Bouquet wrote to say that she had been to see (what turned out to be) Isadora's last performance in Paris. "She was fabulous! She could portray emotion just by standing on the stage. At the end, the audience went wild, applauding and cheering; they wouldn't let her off the stage. Paris adored her."

We hear the news

Following the meeting with Isadora, Irma returned to Russia. At the end of the summer, we went on tour to the Ukraine. We performed in Nikolaev, the town my mother came from, and while we were there I heard there was someone asking for me. When I came down to see who it was, there was our pianist, Moise Borisovich Shane. He couldn't take his eyes off this very beautiful young woman, who turned out to be a relation of mine that I never knew about. We performed in Odessa, Kiev and all the cities of the Ukraine. Everywhere we had huge success, but most of our concerts were in the 'Donbas' region. The Donets Basin was mostly heavy industry, so we danced lots of concerts for the ironworkers and coal miners, who liked us very much.

We were on this tour of the Ukraine – far away from Moscow and twice as far from Paris – when we heard on the wireless the tragic news of Isadora's death. We were stunned. Irma said later that she fainted, but I was there with her and I don't remember her doing that. But we couldn't get over it and deep down we knew that half the school had died with her.

How on earth could it have happened? And what were we going to do now, without Isadora? It seemed to us it was all over. We were all very sad, the whole way home. The mood was just as sad when we got back to school, because they were all waiting for us with the bad news.

Now to me it will always be a mystery: why didn't we go to Nice, where Isadora was waiting for us? We were growing and we were now quite good dancers, good enough to be engaged for all sorts of concerts in and around Moscow. We had reached a professional standard, and Isadora clearly had something in mind for us. So why did Irma not listen to her?

I thought it was very wrong, the way Irma took us to China when Isadora was waiting for us. No one else ever mentioned it, so perhaps it didn't strike them – but then I always did have different ideas in my head from other people.

Mary Desti

Shortly after we came back from the Donbas tour, Irma set off for Paris. While there, she saw Raymond Duncan, who wanted to talk, and Augustin Duncan, who didn't. She visited Isadora's grave and she met Mary Desti, who gave Irma a piece of the scarf Isadora was wearing when she died.

This Mary Desti was a big designer in America. She was an artist, but an artist in textiles, especially in beautiful silks. I remember Irma wearing a most interesting dress by her. She had designed the material too – it wasn't embroidery – and the style of the dress was very simple. Isadora didn't wear any of her designs on stage, only the Grecian-style tunics.

Mary Desti came back to Moscow with Irma and told us all about how Isadora died. It was better for us to hear it from someone who was there at the time. We were all still in mourning, and Mary was still very upset, because she had been a very dear friend to Isadora and had been staying with her, keeping her company in Nice, where the tragedy happened.

She had tried to persuade Isadora not to drive that day. It was dull weather, with no wind. Mary told us how she tried to talk her out of going, but Isadora said she was so lonely and bored, she felt she had to do something and she loved riding in open cars. She also loved to wear a scarf – it was rather theatrical, I suppose.

Mary said that, when Isadora got in the car, there was hardly any wind, so that wasn't the cause. What happened was, the car set off very suddenly and threw her back in her seat. Her scarf got caught in the back wheel with such force that it threw her out of the car, and that was how she died. It was awful even to think about it.

Isadora had always believed in fate and she always felt that, if anything ever happened to her, it would be in a car. I remember hearing that from somebody who had heard her say it. She wouldn't have told us girls a thing like that. Nonetheless, that is what happened.

The Oak Room and the treasury

Irma picked up very quickly and took charge. There was a lot for her and Ilya Schneider to catch up with because, all that time we had been away in China, the rest of the school had carried on as before. Also, the school was a bit chaotic for a while after Isadora's death, because things were being altered or refurbished.

First of all, the Burgundy Room lost its red decor, all the carpets and curtains, and it became the Oak Room again. They made a bedroom out of it for the girls of my age. Five or six of the big girls, I don't know how many exactly, always slept in the Pink Room and that never changed. The Napoleon Room was the other dormitory.

Isadora's room, which was very large, became the Blue Studio and Irma now used it for teaching. As you entered it, in the corner on the right-hand side was a door to Irma's apartment. It was convenient for her: when we arrived for our class, she used to come through her bedroom. Sometimes she was in a tunic and we knew she was going to dance with us, and sometimes she wasn't. This room was as big as the Oak Room, even as big as the Napoleon Room. All our vigorous training, preparing for America, was in this room that had been Isadora's bedroom.

That room faced the yard, as Irma's did, so it was quiet. There was no traffic passing by. Actually we never took any notice of the traffic, because our bedrooms were always facing the street – except that our last bedroom, the Oak Room, also had windows facing the garden, which was lovely. I often used to lie there, reading or thinking, looking at the trees and wondering what the future would bring. From that great Oak Room we left Russia for America.

When you walked in, there was a little archway on the right-hand side, and we had a big stove there to help warm the room. We used to gather there and sit round it to talk. We had just got settled in our new bedroom when one morning someone reported seeing a ghost in the night.

A few mornings later, we woke up to find that the panel next to that archway was broken through and removed. Thieves had been in our bedroom! We learnt that the rumour was that there was a treasury somewhere in the house and the thieves had brought a plan that showed them where to look. They took quite a few panels out, but I don't think they found anything, because there was no treasury.

We couldn't get over it, because it was awful in a way that we had strangers coming in at night. How did they get in? Of course they climbed onto the balcony, but our garden had a very tall fence, very tall. They must have arranged beforehand how they would get in.

I had always admired the very big oak tree that stood right outside our windows. In fact it stood so close that they built the balcony round it on three sides, so the balcony was unusually broad. Those thieves weren't the only people to make use of the balcony and the oak tree.

After Isadora: the wheat and the chaff

We had a girl – she had entered the school quite a while before – who turned into a rebel, and we had such problems with her. I think she was an orphan and everybody felt sorry for her because she lived with her grandfather, not even with an aunt. Her name was Natasha Shlahtina. She used to get out at night, go out onto the balcony and climb that beautiful oak tree. She was like a tomboy. They really couldn't cope with her; eventually they had to discharge her.

Many wives came to Moscow without their husbands, to place their daughters at Isadora's school, but one by one they all went home again. I could understand that. I was very fond of my mother, but I could never forgive her for bringing me to Russia. I never took to it, to the harshness of the climate or to the Russian people, though I got to know many wonderful individuals. But I so liked the school: the building itself was a thing of beauty, and there was wonderful music and so much going on. That's how I remember the school. Yes, I was hungry and often cold, but I learnt from Isadora to rise above things like that.

She showed us how to move and dance, but she was also a model of the way beauty is not just on the surface. Without even moving, Isadora displayed another aspect to beauty, the beauty that comes from something fine at the heart, an inner strength. That spoke to me. I like to know why and where things come from. I don't like to live on the surface; I like to know what is underneath.

A new tour programme

After Mary Desti had left, Irma began a vigorous training programme with us. We knew that we had to work very hard now: the school depended on us. She decided to work separately with ten of us. There were six older girls and four of us younger ones, and we had extra classes on alternate evenings.

One night the older girls went, the next night we went. Each time, when we had finished our class, they used to come into our bedroom. We had enormous bedrooms. "Well, girls, well, what is happening? Show us! What did you do, what steps, what were the movements?" We were working at that time on a whole programme of Chopin. We had never danced that before. It was so exciting.

About twice a week we would all ten have a class together, to work on Schubert's 9th Symphony. Nonetheless, each group had its own part: we didn't dance together. We younger girls had the scherzo; the bigger girls danced the first movement until they scattered and then there was a section where the four of us younger girls danced, and so on. We worked very, very hard.

It was a long time since Irma had danced the 9th Symphony and I noticed she really had to put her thinking cap on to remember the movements. Now that Isadora wasn't there, it was difficult for her to remember even where to begin. At the beginning there is music but no dancing; it is only later on when the andante comes that the girls start to dance.

She had even forgotten the first movement. She had to ask the girls, six of them, to do that particular passage at the beginning. How would they respond? We had one girl who was so wonderful, Shura – she was really the best dancer in lyrics – and she came out and showed how she would dance it. Irma liked the movements, and that is how they started rehearsing the 9th Symphony.

With possibly the exception of that opening that Shura improvised, the 9th Symphony as we danced it was Isadora's choreography. I didn't realise it at the time, but Irma had never done any choreography; I found that out later. I thought some of what we did was Irma's idea – the parts based on folk dancing, I thought she did those – but no, she took it all from Isadora, and I never knew that at the time.

I remember very well how it was arranged. When I listen to the music now I recall the whole dance, especially the scherzo – which we younger girls danced – because I liked it so much. But everything Irma was teaching us was what Isadora had created – Isadora worked very hard and Irma had to remember everything.

She started learning some new Chopin too; the idea was to make a whole programme. We also had these very vigorous exercises with Irma and she worked us really hard for about six months, until we found out that an American impresario was coming to Moscow to have a good look at us, to see if he wanted to engage us.

Two kinds of contract

The impresario was called Sol Hurok and he knew about dancing. He had previously organised concerts with Isadora and Anna Pavlova. Well, he came over from New York and we showed him what we could do. We were well prepared by then and he liked what he saw. He went home to arrange bookings and draft contracts. Since we were still at school, we had to get permission from the government before we could go abroad. All this took time, but eventually the government agreed and in March 1928 Sol Hurok signed a contract with Irma and separate contracts with us girls – I still have my copy of the contract.

At that point we discovered what we were going to be paid and what Irma was to be paid. We were to get $60 a week! At that time it was an enormous amount of money, but that hardly entered our minds. We never dwelt on it or thought how wonderful it would be to have so much money. Instead, we were intrigued and fascinated by the idea of going to New York. It was the month of my fifteenth birthday.

Before that happened, though, the school got to know about the affair between Ilya Schneider and Marisha Borisova – they had been to bed, though with her consent, otherwise it wouldn't have happened – so a letter was sent, asking her parents to come to the school. When the parents came and they were told what had happened, they insisted that Schneider should marry their daughter. He was incensed. "How can you expect me to marry a girl from a working-class family?"

"Look, you had enough audacity to get intimate with her, so now you're going to have to marry her."

He argued, but they insisted. He must have divorced Irma, because he did marry Marisha.

When it came to signing the contracts – which is why I mention it here – we signed for a year, but she signed a contract for six months only, after which she would go back to her husband, Schneider, in Moscow. Irma never considered taking him to America. She was so angry with him and tired of his behaviour. Of course, there would be other girls still at school while we were away, so it made sense to leave him in Moscow.

So Irma signed a contract, and Marisha signed hers and she told Irma not to prevent her coming back after six months. We of course had no worries about going with Irma – we had no ideas of leaving or coming back, or whatever – but Marisha did. Only later I realised that both of them, Irma and Marisha, had been rather cunning.

Annie's boys

I must go back a bit now, to the early summer of 1927. Since I had a very close friendship with Auntie Annie and her sons, my mother thought she would take me round to see them one Sunday, because they would be very interested to hear about our trip to China. The eldest brother, Barney, was there; he was extremely handsome and had not long been married.

This was the first time I had met his wife, Tatiana, and I liked her at first sight – she had such a lovely face. She was very pleasant, but later on I learnt that this marriage had caused Barney some difficulties, because his wife came from a well-to-do family – the sort of people that would be called White Russians.

Auntie Annie had separated from her husband, Alexander Muscat. It seems he wanted her to go off with him, just the two of them, and she said she would not leave her sons. That was how the rift between them started. Now I discovered that they were making plans to return to England. A treaty had been signed by the Soviet Union and the United Kingdom; as a result, lots of people who had British passports were now leaving Russia. Barney and Tanya were going to London shortly, along with Moss, the middle son. Annie and her youngest son, Freddy, were to remain.

Polyanna and Grigori

We younger girls were growing up now and, between our return from China in spring 1927 and the exchange of contracts with Sol Hurok in spring 1928, we started to get a little bit more freedom. In this period, my mother took me to see some people who lived not very far from our flat in Maly Dmetrovka.

I thought they were friends of hers, but it turned out they were related to my mother in some way, though it seemed to me a very distant relationship. The family lived in a semi-basement – it wasn't too bad, just a few steps down – and they had a very big apartment, because there were quite a few of them.

Amongst them was a brother to the husband of my auntie Luba – the one who got shot – along with his wife. Now, he was a very pleasant man and I didn't dislike him, but his wife was absolutely lovely; her name was Pollyanna. I don't know where they met, but

100

Pollyanna told me afterwards that, wherever it was, she was playing the piano and he walked in. Somebody was going to introduce them, but there was no need: when he walked in, she told me, she looked at him and she liked him straightaway; he looked at her and he could not help but like her, she was so lovely. So they got married.

Pollyanna came from a big family, and a very different sort of family. They were from Samarkand, strangely enough, but they were Jewish people. I hadn't realised there were Jews amongst these people. My uncle brought her to Moscow, along with his father, his sister and her two children, and some other relations. One of these was Pollyanna's younger brother, because she wanted to give him a good education to start him in life. I met him too at this get-together, and lots of other people.

Pollyanna introduced me to her younger brother. I must confess Grigori was tall and very good-looking – in fact, I would call him handsome. He was one of a group and we were all sitting there, talking to one another. They were interested in me because I was a dancer and I was going to America. Suddenly Grigori stood up, came over to me and spoke. He really took me by surprise.

"Would you like to go with me for a walk?"

"What for?"

"Well, it would be nice. I would like to walk down Tverskay."

There were two main shopping streets in Moscow, Pietrovska and Tverskay, and I liked Tverskay, because it reminded me of St Petersburg and its prominent avenue Nievska, where they had the same shops as Tverskay. For instance, both cities had a branch of the same big grocery shop – with a wonderful delicatessen section and all sorts of beautiful things – called E. Ilyasevski's.

Grigori wanted me to take down that street. I knew it would be very busy, especially on a Sunday, so I said, "Well, I don't mind, if my mother can come with us." I was never keen to go on my own with someone I had just met; and at the time I was so young that I had never walked out with anyone. My mother agreed – "Why not?" she said – so we went out and walked a little bit up and down the street, which was busy with people. That was fine and I enjoyed it. After we got back, we sat for a little while and then I said to my mother, "I think we should go home now," because I knew that the next day I had to be at school early, working on our programme for America.

Golden Samarkand

After we signed the contracts for America in March 1928, we went on a short tour that took us to Samarkand, where Pollyanna came from. I can remember groups of buildings – all in blue and gold – and they were entirely different to the Western architecture I was used to. The people there weren't Arabs, but I didn't know what to call them. I know they used to drink a lot of tea and sit down in a circle to drink it – sit down on the floor, wherever they were – and I thought that such strange behaviour. They drank very pale tea; I don't know what herbs it was made of.

We were even taken to see one of the harems, where so many poor girls had to live, who had been captured by some potentate. In the garden of this harem near Samarkand was a fountain, called the Fountain of Tears. I recognised it as the name of a poem by Pushkin – 'The Bakhchisaray Fountain' – and we went especially to see it. It got its name from the way it was built. From the top to the bottom, each tier of the fountain had teardrop shapes around the rim, and every little teardrop had water dripping down in droplets. They represented the tears of the young girls in the harem who were locked up. We travelled a little bit further in Turkestan, before returning to Moscow.

A day in the country, and what followed

In this period we continued to give little concerts here and there, because we always had to earn some money. Irma also danced with us in these concerts, because it gave them added prestige. We were working very intensively on our preparation, but sometimes we could go home for the weekend. One Saturday, my mother said, "Would you like a day in the country?" and I said, "Oh yes! I would love that."

It turned out that Auntie Annie and Freddy were staying somewhere in the countryside, not very far from Moscow, and they wanted to say goodbye to us before they set off for England. Early on Sunday we set off to see Annie, Fred and various friends. Fred was so pleased to see me. I wished him *bon voyage* and said, "Enjoy the rest of your holiday!" and that evening we went back to Moscow. When I got back to our flat, my grandmother said, "Oh, there was a telephone call from school – 'Where is Lili? There is a rehearsal coming up' – they wanted you for various things and you were not there.'' The rehearsal was on the Sunday, but they had never warned me about it.

Anyway, I got back to school on the Monday and Irma was very angry with me, wanting to know why I hadn't stayed at school, ready for the rehearsal? But nobody had told me there was this very important exercise we had to do, to polish up our dancing. Apparently she wanted all of us.

Irma continued with the rehearsal on the Monday, when I got there. We were practising waltzes, which I was very good at – Chopin and Schubert – and there were some new dances that she had showed us, which I did very well. However, she took me off them and put our nurse's daughter, Mooshya, in instead. I was very upset and even Irma noticed. She commented, ''Lili is so quiet'' and I said, ''What do you expect? Why should I be happy about it?'' I was very upset because she took me off three dances, a mazurka and two waltzes, and she put Mooshya instead of me. I was terribly heart-broken. I was so upset, because all the other girls told me that I had been the best in those dances, but I had to resign myself to it and that was that.

I never said anything, but I knew that it must have been our nurse who did this to me, because it was the kind of thing she would do. Apart from that, Irma always seemed to think she owed the nurse a favour, so she had put her daughter in the leading roles instead – but I got over it.

Uncle, Valya and I

After some very vigorous rehearsals at school, we were unexpect-edly given some free time, with permission – and this seemed very strange – to go out in the evenings for a little while. One of the girls, Valya Boye – I was very friendly with her – said, ''Lili, would you like to go to the cinema?'' and I said, ''Yes, I would love to. But do you think we can?''

Her uncle was manager of a cinema not very far from school – you had to go by way of one of the boulevards, which I knew (we used to go there for walks anyway) – so Valya explained where it was. Another girl came too – either Manya or Lolya.

Anyway, there were three of us and we went to see a film with Conrad Veidt – a very good actor that we liked – and we couldn't tear ourselves away from the film, though it was getting late and we were getting nervous. Her uncle said, "Don't worry, I shall see you halfway back," so we sat there until it finished.

By then it was 11 o'clock at night. Gosh, how could we go back? Well, he took us halfway and after that we went on our own. The school was all locked up, but we got in, because we knew how; we all three of us were hushed and we went to bed as quiet as mice. The big girls were sleeping separately from us and they never heard a thing. And that was our last escapade before we went to America.

Saying farewell

When I was ready to set off for America, I had to say goodbye to my neighbours. My mother and I had one room in a big flat, but there were several other households besides ours. They were nice people, all quite friendly and interested to know how I was getting on. The (former) owners of the flat had the best room, the one with the balcony. Next to us was an elderly woman with her grand-daughter Cecilia, a lovely girl – but not the Cecilia I met on the boat. I think her parents lived there later.

A corridor divided the flat. Opposite us were a couple from England with their son and next to them was another family who, I think, were related to Cecilia's family. Cecilia, who was getting tall and nice-looking, was friendly with me, even though I was much younger than her.

Just before I left for America, she came with me to the cinema, along with my mother and some friends of hers. It was a very old film, I recall, but we all liked it and when we got home they all said goodbye to me. They were very interested in my going to America, especially New York. I said goodbye to everyone and went back to school.

Irma left Schneider in charge of the school, because there were many other pupils still there. Only eleven of us went with Irma, and one of the eleven was Schneider's new wife Marisha. She was going to stay only six months and then she would come back to her husband.

Form No. 257—CONSULAR
(See General Instruction No. 926, Sec. 3)

No. 52

DECLARATION OF NON-IMMIGRANT ALIEN
ABOUT TO DEPART FOR THE UNITED STATES
AMERICAN CONSULAR SERVICE

AMERICAN CONSULATE, _____ RIGA LATVIA _____ December 12, 1928
(Place) (Date)

I, Lilia DIKOVSKY, a {citizen / subject} of _____ Russia _____
(Country)

bearer of Passport / Laissez passer / (Other document) No. 183334, dated _____ November 28, 1928
33698

issued by _____ Soviet authorities Moscow Russia _____
(Nationality and title of issuing authority)

am about to go to the United States accompanied by _____
(Names of persons included in declarant's passport, photographs of

whom are attached thereto) _____ none _____

I was born _____ March 14, 1913 London _____ -- _____ Great Britain
(Date) (City) (Province) (Country)

My occupation for the last two years was _____ Dancer _____

and at present is _____ Dancer _____

I desire to proceed to the United States for the purpose of _____ fulfill contract with _____
Nurok Attractions Inc. New York N.Y.

to remain for _____ six _____ months, and my address in the United States will be _____
New York N.Y.

My references are _____ Nurok Attractions Inc. 55 West 42nd St. New York N.Y. _____
(In the United States)

_____ none _____
(Local)

I consider myself as a non-immigrant under the provisions of the Immigration Act of 1924 on the following grounds:

that I am proceeding to the United States for the purpose of temporary visit.

and offer for inspection the following documents in support of my claim: contract with Nurok Attractions Inc. New York dated March 1928

c1—1008

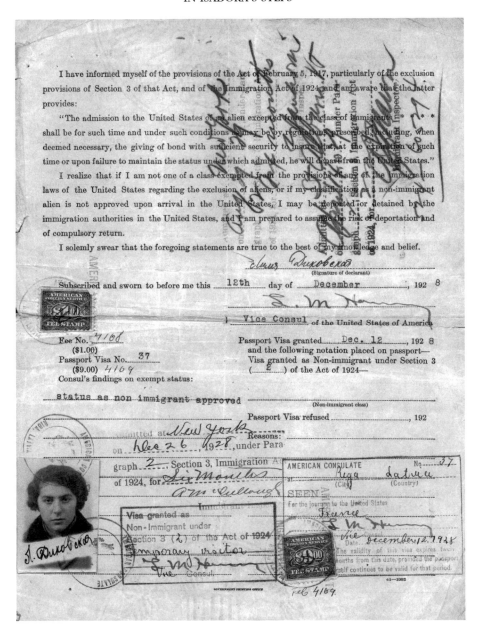

I have informed myself of the provisions of the Act of February 5, 1917, particularly of the exclusion provisions of Section 3 of that Act, and of the Immigration Act of 1924, and am aware that the latter provides:

"The admission to the United States of an alien excepted from the class of immigrants * * * shall be for such time and under such conditions as may be by regulations prescribed, including, when deemed necessary, the giving of bond with sufficient security to insure that, at the expiration of such time or upon failure to maintain the status under which admitted, he will depart from the United States."

I realize that if I am not one of a class exempted from the provisions of any of the immigration laws of the United States regarding the exclusion of aliens, or if my classification as a non-immigrant alien is not approved upon arrival in the United States, I may be deported or detained by the immigration authorities in the United States, and I am prepared to assume the risk of deportation and of compulsory return.

I solemnly swear that the foregoing statements are true to the best of my knowledge and belief.

Cluus Duxobexa
(Signature of declarant)

Subscribed and sworn to before me this ___12th___ day of ___December___, 192 8

_S. M. Ha___
) ___Vice Consul___ of the United States of America

Fee No. _7108_
($1.00)
Passport Visa No. _37_
($9.00) _4169_
Consul's findings on exempt status:

___status as non immigrant approved___
(Non-immigrant class)

Passport Visa granted ___Dec. 12___, 192 8
and the following notation placed on passport—
Visa granted as Non-immigrant under Section 3
(___2___) of the Act of 1924—

Passport Visa refused ___, 192

...mitted at _New York_ Reasons:
on _Dec 26_, 192 8, under Para
graph _2_, Section 3, Immigration A
of 1924, for _Six Months_
a. m. McCullough

Visa granted as
Non-Immigrant under
Section 3 (2) of the Act of 1924
Temporary visitor
_S. M. Ha___
Vice Consul

AMERICAN CONSULATE No. _37_
at _Riga_ _Latvia_
(City) (Country)
SEEN
for the journey to the United States
via _France_
_S. M. Ha___
Vice Consul
Date _December 12. 1928_
The validity of this visa expires twelve months from this date, provided the passport itself continues to be valid for that period.

c1—1093

GOVERNMENT PRINTING OFFICE

Feb 4169

First stop, Riga

At last the day came and off we went. We went by train, but there was no comparison with the journey seven and a half years earlier, when my mother brought me to Russia. This time it was well prepared and comfortable. Our first stop was in Riga, the capital of Latvia, a most beautiful place; we were very charmed by it.

We stopped there because Irma wanted to buy some clothes and dress us up, so we would look a bit more respectable when we arrived in America - not like poor orphans. She didn't buy all that much, just what she could afford. She bought us shoes, I remember, and matching berets, sweaters and skirts. We each had our own outfits and we looked quite nice. Our old coats were renovated, and my mother had even put a little fur on top of mine, because it was late in the year when we set off and the weather was already autumnal.

We didn't give concerts in Riga, but we went to the ballet and became very friendly with the *corps de ballet*. They seemed to like us, because they invited us backstage. Riga was delightful but still, after three days, we resumed our journey.

Köln

The next stop was Köln. Schneider had told his new wife, Marisha, that he had relations living there and they would come to meet our train. She was looking out for them and there they were. In fact we got off the train, because there was a long stop there. We saw the cathedral, a beautiful building, which was close to the station. I bought a card there, wrote it and posted it to my mother. I had done the same in Riga, and my mother never threw out cards - letters perhaps, but never postcards with views. Recently, when I was looking for photographs, I found these cards.

Amongst Marisha's relations by marriage who came to see her was a young woman of about 18, very good-looking - a very handsome girl. The others were older people and Marisha told us afterwards that they gave her a couple of diamonds, in case she ever needed money.

Her husband, Schneider, had wanted to come with us, but Irma absolutely refused, because they had had the most terrible row not long before and got divorced. She used to say, "No, I could never take a man like that with me. He's the kind that, if you show him the door, he will fly in through the window." She could be very fierce. They always used to be arguing backstage, how to arrange the lights, this and that, and he used bad language very often; on the other hand, he worked very hard and he was a very good manager. I wouldn't say he was a bad man, but his behaviour in the affair with Marisha was dreadful.

Schneider's family was in tailoring. They were Jewish, at least to the Russians, but they had converted to Christianity, the whole family. They considered themselves Russian, but other Russians never did; they were just Jews. He had seven sisters and he was the only boy. He made a poem out of it:

Seven sisters and
I the only brother;
Where the sisters went,
I went with them.

Lisel Duncan in Paris

In Paris, we got off because we had to change trains and we spent a few hours there. We got into taxis and I happened to get in the one with Irma and a young lady who sat next to her, chatting and chatting. I discovered this was Lisel, who lived in Paris and was one of Isadora's girls.

From her first school, Isadora had chosen the six most talented girls and 'adopted' them; they took the surname Duncan. Only one of them, Irma, had agreed to come to Moscow, to continue studying with her and to help teach in the school. Lisel broke away from Isadora when she was in Paris and set up her own dance group. Isadora went to see them perform and she was surprised. She told Irma afterwards: "If you could see what she is doing, you wouldn't believe it," and indeed I saw this for myself. After I had come to live in England, I went to Paris and met the group that Lisel founded – and what they did was something unbelievable.

Lisel was blonde and I remember noticing that she had very long legs. Irma was delighted to see her and they were very happy, chatting all the way. I don't know what language they used – it wasn't English or French; it could have been German. In the taxis going through Paris, we just couldn't take everything in. It was evening and we girls were enchanted with the lights, jumping from one window to another to see all we could of Paris; it was so extraordinary to us. But before long we had to catch the boat train. We didn't dance on our way to America, not even in Paris.

The liner *Caronia*

The train took us to Cherbourg, where we boarded the Cunard liner *Caronia*, outward bound from Southampton to New York. The boat trip itself was very interesting. Everything was like a dream: the boat, the people, the cabins. We were divided into couples, and I shared with Liza Belova, one of the big girls. When we first saw our cabins, I exclaimed: "Liza, just look at these blankets, look at the sheets! Aren't they absolutely wonderful? Isn't it marvellous to have such luxury?"

Every day it was the same routine: in the morning we had a shower, dressed and went down to breakfast. After that, we all met up with Irma and Elzbieta Grigorevnya, our nurse. She also travelled second class, I think; at any rate, she was never far away. She looked after our health constantly, but when we were performing, she was always at Irma's beck and call, mostly helping her backstage, doing whatever was needed.

We very seldom came across Irma except at mealtimes. After we had seen her, we did whatever we fancied, usually walking on the deck during the day. We girls always kept together and the time soon passed. We didn't mix with anyone; we didn't particularly like the way some of the young people behaved, and none of the other girls spoke much English. Most of the passengers were Americans, and many of the rest were British.

The school was always short of cash, so I suppose that's why we went second class. The food wasn't anything special – in fact, we didn't always like it – but I could not get over our beautiful cabin and the beds. They were absolutely wonderful! At least, that's how I felt. I don't know what the other girls thought, because they never used to talk about that sort of thing. I didn't talk about it either, but I thought about it a lot.

We brought our own pianist with us from Russia. His name was

Moise Borisovich Shane – 'Maurice Shane' in the American tour programmes – and he was a very good pianist. We often used to ask him, "Moise Borisovich, are you going to stay in New York?" and he would always answer us, "Oh no! I would never leave my family or my parents." Well, of course, that wasn't what happened; nevertheless, that's what he said at that time.

Our pianist and Irma travelled first class; we were in second class and we were very happy. It never occurred to us to think, *Why does Irma have more privileges than us?* It seemed natural, a matter of course, and in any event she deserved it: she taught us and organised everything for us.

Irma and Moise Borisovich sat with us at meals: we ate all together. I am not sure if we went to the first-class dining room or the second-class, but we always met to eat. The days were exactly the same: lunch was at 1 p.m., we had something at teatime and then in the evening, dinner – or, as we Russians used to call it, supper. After supper, Irma usually stayed with us until it was time for bed.

After dinner, there was fun and games and dancing, but we were not allowed to go. In any event we couldn't have gone, because it took place in the ballroom and you had to wear evening dress. It was extraordinary to watch them, though, the women in ballroom dresses and the men in tails, a scene we had only ever seen in films. We watched from the balcony by our cabins, which gave us a very good view. Our nurse would say, "You see that woman down there, glittering? You see, girls, that's because those are real diamonds." And we used to say, "Are they?" – that's all. We thought they looked so artificial.

The behaviour of some of the passengers was not very good, we thought. We girls were so strictly brought up that we never even dreamt of doing something that wasn't entirely proper. And some of their behaviour was bad. Even so, we had never seen such people in such gear. We couldn't get over it, we couldn't really. To us the whole spectacle was a novelty, and we watched it every night. They used to dance slow foxtrots, quick foxtrots and tangos – which I really liked – and it struck me for the first time, I think, that ballroom dancing is a rather graceful form of dance. I liked this kind of dancing and I liked some of the tunes the orchestra played.

Island Christmas

The Atlantic crossing took five days. The big girls were always by themselves; well, we four were a good bit smaller, after all. Lolya, Mooshya and I were 15, and Little Tamara was about a year and a half younger than us, which at that age does make a difference. So, we four youngsters were sitting together on deck when the Statue of Liberty came into sight and we got really interested. As we were sitting there, Big Tamara came by and saw us sitting there. She always wanted in some way to frighten us or make us a bit unhappy, and she could see how we eager we were, so she taunted us. "You know what? You little ones, they're not going to let you in."

We looked at her, astonished.

"Why? What is wrong with us? You must be joking."

She just walked away. But the funniest part of it is, that is exactly what happened.

When we arrived at New York, we all had to pass in front of a kind of examiner. That was before you entered, even before they checked who you were. They used to turn back your eyelids to see if your eyes were clear. They were looking for trachoma, an illness. Well, we had nothing wrong with our eyes, but nevertheless four of us were kept to one side.

We couldn't get over it: they let the other girls into New York, but they wouldn't let us in. It was very close to Christmas when we arrived. So they took us to Ellis Island, and we were stuck there. We were absolutely in despair, but there was nothing we could do. Of course, Irma wouldn't abandon us, I felt sure, and Mr Hurok, the impresario who invited us, would make sure we were released.

The accommodation wasn't bad and our nurse was with us too. She would never have just left us; after all, amongst the four of us was her daughter, Mooshya. But we were stuck there in torment, while the big girls were celebrating Christmas and enjoying themselves, for three days and three nights.

I don't know how many people – immigrants I suppose you would call us – there were then on Ellis Island, but when Christmas Day came they were so good in those days. I don't know if they do the same now, but they gave us gifts: they took an interest in everyone and gave them something nice.

There were little parcels of some sort, with various little knick-knacks and things. Each of us had a big bag and, when we opened it, there were various things. I know there was a sewing kit, with scissors, and besides that other nice things they gave us. That was kind of them, but nevertheless we wondered how long we were going to be there, and kept on talking to one another to keep up our spirits.

The reason why we were there, apparently, was because it was Christmas and they were all on holiday, so there was nobody to take action and release us. At last the rumour reached us that we were going to be let in. They knew we were dancers on tour, but we were under age, and that was why they wouldn't let us in. They had rules, but once everything was done and signed we were allowed to enter New York.

6

New York, New World, 1929

A La Marque

As soon as Christmas was over, we younger girls were released from
Ellis Island. We could hardly believe it. At last we could enter New
York and join the rest of our group. They were staying in a brand-
new hotel, a lovely place called the Hotel A La Marque. It was very
central, and that was rather pleasant. There were just two girls to a
room; it was like on the boat, absolute luxury. Altogether we were
enchanted with it.

They put us on the 14th floor and that seemed remarkable. The
heating was so hot that we had to turn it down. But what we
couldn't get over was that you could open a window whenever you
wanted, get fresh air and close it. We thought this was quite extraordinary: it was like going to the moon. In Russia, all the windows
were fastened shut for a good six months, because it was so terribly
cold and the heating couldn't cope. Irma stayed at the Astoria; she
never stayed in the same hotel as us.

Our hotel was on Ninth Avenue, which wasn't really finished. That
didn't bother us; what we didn't like was the hotel's food. It was
worse than on the liner, which we didn't like very much either. We
were used to a very different type of cooking. We used to ask our
nurse to take us somewhere else to eat, not in the hotel, and later we
found for ourselves a place where they served very good steaks. Even
then, the food never tasted the way it did in Russia. I think they must
have tampered with the food there, or perhaps it was our imagina-
tion – I don't know.

As we younger ones settled in, the bigger girls were bragging
about where they had been and what they had seen; but we four

were soon getting experiences of our own. While we were in America, people used to come and seek us out, and we thought some of them very odd, really. But they were often very kind to us.

A man called Jannett, who knew Isadora, took us under his wing and promised to show us New York. The bit I remember best was when he said, "Girls, I am going to take you, just the little ones now, to Woolworth's. I'll give you a dollar each, and you just buy whatever you fancy." And he did. At that time, everything in Woolworth's was 10 cents – whatever you chose – so that dollar went a long way. It seemed to us that for a dollar you could buy nearly the whole of Woolworth's, so we went berserk and bought stockings and all sorts, whatever we put our hands on. It was so exciting.

After that we went to Fifth Avenue, 47th Street, which must have made a great impression because I've never forgotten that address, and then we went back to the hotel, where Irma was preparing us for our first concert.

New Year, new audience

We began our tour with four concerts in New York. The first was just over a week after we younger girls had been released from Ellis Island, so we started work straightaway. We had to find our way to the theatre for rehearsals, first with our pianist and then with a full orchestra.

That first concert was in the Manhattan Opera House on Saturday, 5 January 1929. I can be sure of that because I still have the concert programme. First there were some waltzes, followed by our usual programme, including a few dances that Irma did. We had a symphony orchestra playing for us and the centrepiece was the 6th Symphony of Tchaikovsky. Finally we young ones danced our own little programme, with the revolutionary songs that Isadora had put on. That little dance – 'One, two, three, Pioneers are we' – was the last item.

In the audience there was a young girl, eleven years old, called Lilian Loewenthal. We impressed her so much that, thirty years later, she was inspired to write a book. She called it *Search for Isadora*. I'm not sure how hard she searched – even though it took her thirty years to get to the bottom of Isadora – or how she managed to write

Manhattan Opera House

5th Anniversary of

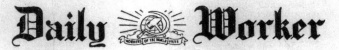

Daily Worker

The Only Communist English Daily in the World

SATURDAY, JANUARY 5th, 1929

Isadora Duncan Dancers

from Moscow

Supported by

SYMPHONY ORCHESTRA

Read THE DAILY WORKER Daily

Buy it at your Newsstand

Domestic and Foreign Labor News—Special Cable Service—

Begin Reading Bill Haywood's Book in The Daily Worker Today

THE DAILY WORKER

26-28 UNION SQUARE   NEW YORK CITY

No admittance into the hall during performance of musical numbers.

1—INTERNATIONAL
Orchestra

2—WALTZES . . . . Schubert
(a) Under the Scarf .... Irma Duncan and Tamara, Marie,
Alexandra, Manya, Maya, Vala, Vera
(b) Game with Ball .... Irma Duncan
(c) Three Graces .... Irma Duncan and Tamara, Alexandra
(d) Ecossaise .... Irma Duncan and Dancers
(e) Around the Linden Tree .... Irma Duncan and Dancers

3—SCENES FROM CHILDHOOD . . . . Schumann
(a) Blindman's Buff .... Maya, Lily, Tamara, Manya
Lisa, Lola
(b) Zizilienne .... Lisa, Manya, Lily, Lola, Maya, Tamara
(c) Soldier's March .... Lily, Lola, Lisa, Manya, Maya, Tamara

4—POLKA . . . . Rachmaninoff
Irma Duncan and Dancers
Maurice Sheyne at the Piano

5—MOMENT MUSICALE . . . . Schubert
Irma Duncan with Orchestra

6—MARCH MILITAIRE . . . . Schubert
Irma Duncan and Dancers with Orchestra

7—OPENING REMARKS BY BOB MINOR, Editor of The Daily Worker

8—GREETING BY JAY LOVESTONE, Executive Secretary of the Workers
(Communist) Party

9—GREETING BY WM. Z. FOSTER, Member of the Secretariat of the Workers
(Communist) Party

Intermission 5 minutes

10—IMPRESSIONS OF REVOLUTIONARY RUSSIA
(a) Varshavianka
(b) Dubinushka
Irma Duncan and Dancers with Orchestra

11—ADDRESS BY BOB MINOR

12—IMPRESSIONS OF REVOLUTIONARY RUSSIA
(a) Funeral Song
(b) Trilogy: 1. Workers and Peasants
2. Famine
3. Labor Triumphant
(c) Blacksmith
(d) Pioneer Song
Irma Duncan and Dancers
Maurice Sheyne at the Piano

Hardman Piano Used

LENIN MEMORIAL MEETING
MADISON SQUARE GARDEN
SATURDAY, JANUARY 19, 1929
Soviet Sports Spectacle and Pageant
JOIN THE WORKERS (COMMUNIST) PARTY

Tear off and send to District No. 2, Workers (Communist) Party of
America, 26-28 Union Square, New York City

NAME ....

ADDRESS ....

OCCUPATION ....

116

the book. She never got in touch with me, and of course she had never seen Isadora, only us.

Someone sent me a copy of her book a few years back, and I read it. I was surprised at how taken she was by our dancing, when she was a child of eleven. She said she couldn't get over it. So, a couple of years ago, I thought, *I'll find her address and write to her, if she is still around*.

She did reply, and her letterhead said: 'Professor of Dancing, especially Isadora Dance'. I have no idea how she became that, since she had never seen Isadora dance, had never even got in touch with me. In her letter, she wrote, "When I found out you were one of those lively girls, Lili, I had tears coming into my eyes." We corresponded for a short while, but I realised that she was interested only in the idea of Isadora, and she had no idea at all what Isadora was really like.

All in all, we had a very big success, right from that first concert in New York. It seemed that American audiences had never imagined they would see anything like the programme we put on, so extraordinarily different and so wonderful to look at. The press were very taken by us too. They used to surround us, firing questions. I couldn't get over that, how fascinated by us they seemed to be. I remember being interviewed by the American press. Their questions were nothing to do with dancing; they never even asked us about Russia or what life was like there. They did ask where we came from; and they wanted to know what we loved more than anything else, and what we liked doing best.

But the thing they were really concerned about was: Why did we have such lovely skin? What did we eat? Apparently this was the most important thing. They wrote about what we had for breakfast, but of course we never really thought about it; we just ate whatever we fancied. We never thought diet was something of great importance. Anyway, we were young: we were supposed to look lovely. I would like to know who doesn't look lovely at the age of 16 or 18?

Mr and Mrs Rice

Irma met a family, a prominent family who lived near Central Park, and soon became friendly with them. They used to arrange evenings at home and invite the dancing world; and they invited us, because they very much liked the way we danced. This was Mr and Mrs Rice. I remember them very well, because they were very friendly, lovely people and very kind to us.

They had a little girl; her name was Barbara, and she was such a sweet girl. We liked her, but we didn't often see her because she was either tucked up in bed or she wasn't around, even if we popped in during the daytime – because often Mrs Rice wanted to see us for something or other.

The Rices had two flats together, so they had plenty of space to entertain. We usually stayed next to Irma, since there were so many people and we didn't know anybody. These occasions were usually in the evenings, and the food was beautiful. We never sat down to eat, but you could help yourself from a buffet spread through two rooms. I always used to say it was like a delicatessen in two rooms. One room was filled with food; the other room was for drinks, but there were also lovely savouries.

We would help ourselves and then sit down near Irma; she liked that. Towards the end of these evenings, we used to return to sit by Irma before we went home, and she would ask us to sing something, because we sang so beautifully. We were never very keen on doing that, but we did as we were told.

Anna and Teresa Duncan, and Augustin

Once they made a special evening for us, and there for the first time we met Anna Duncan, as she called herself. Well, we called her Anna, and she never mentioned Duncan, but there she was, and most attractive. I remember the way she was dressed: she had a velvet outfit – not a dress, but a wrap of some sort, strangely made – and underneath she wore a kind of blouse, in cream. She certainly looked very attractive.

When Anna was there, she used to sit near Irma and they used to chat together. She never made any attempt to speak to us – though, of course, the other girls never spoke English, and she probably didn't realise that I did – but in any event I don't think she had any inclination to get to know us. She wasn't as friendly as she should have been, though she was very attractive and walked about as if she were royalty, I used to say. I never cared for her: that type of person never attracted me.

118

Mr and Mrs Rice were very friendly to us and quite often invited us. One afternoon Irma arranged for us to meet Teresa Duncan at their flat. Now Teresa was lovely: she was so friendly and equally so nice to all the girls, and she was married. Irma never got married again after her divorce from Schneider, but Teresa did and her husband was rather nice.

They had two little boys, still very young, and she was so pleased about them. She gave them Russian names, I remember: Serge was one, and I think Sasha was the other one. She insisted on showing us where they were, in their little cots, and she was so sweet, so motherly. We became very friendly, and she gave me a photograph of herself and wrote 'To Lily' on it; I was very pleased with that.

It was there we met Isadora's eldest brother, Augustin; I remember him vividly. He was there with his wife and a grown-up son – a very good-looking young man, blond and very handsome, I would say. Augustin had become blind, but he knew we were there and he was trying to communicate.

I remember him saying to Teresa, "Oh, Teresa, take off your shoes please, and just stand somewhere where I can reach your feet to touch them." He thought she had such beautiful feet. And I thought how very funny that was, but also very nice: it was done so spontaneously. I also thought: *What a difference between her and Anna.*

Detroit

We didn't stay in New York very long the first time, because we were preparing for performances in other cities, that were already booked. Shortly after those visits to the Rices, when we met Anna, Teresa and Augustin, we started preparing to go to Detroit, Michigan. Our first night there was a very strange affair. There was a very big stage, and we had brought our blue curtains and blue carpet with us, so the stage was always much the same from our point of view – except we were surprised to find we weren't in a theatre at all.

Where the audience should have been there were tables, and people sitting round them. I don't know if they were drinking something or not, but whatever they were doing, our concert went on: our pianist played and we danced. After that very strange performance, even the other girls commented, "What a strange affair!"

The audience somehow wasn't like a theatre audience; they were all relaxing at tables. I don't know what that place was, but it reminded me of China, where the audiences drank tea and threw towels. It could have been a club. Whatever it was, we found out after the performance that Henry Ford had been in the audience and he had invited us to see his factory.

Next morning he sent some wonderful cars for us. They were limousines and every car had a wireless. We were most impressed by the beautiful upholstery and the luxury. We had never experienced anything like it, though we took to it like ducks to water. That bit we found very, very easy.

The Ford factory was interesting in a way. We watched the production line and then they wanted to show us the end of the line. They said, "Just watch the second hand on that clock and you'll see: every minute that goes by, another car comes off the production line, fully assembled" – and it did. We made sure to watch that clock hand. That was very strange, but interesting.

We gave more performances in Detroit, but not in that same place, because I don't think Irma would have agreed to it. That was a one-off. After that, we danced in a real theatre. I gather there were a lot of young people in the audience, because we had most success with the second half of the programme, the revolutionary songs.

Why were these revolutionary songs, with our movements and the red flag – in fact the flag wasn't red; it was brown, but Irma put a red spotlight on it, so it looked red – why were these songs so interesting to them and so attractive? After all, none of the audience understood Russian. But this part of the programme was something Isadora had put on and it was something different: it was like modern art to them. Not that we liked it so much: we didn't. We liked the real thing: we liked to dance Schubert, Chopin and Tchaikovsky. The revolutionary dances didn't do anything for us, but Irma wanted them in the programme, so we did them.

And we had a great success, especially with the little dance right at the end of the programme, 'One, Two, Three, Pioneers We!' This was not the dance that Isadora created for that song, but the one Irma had taken from me a while before, when she asked me to show her a Russian dance. She didn't give the leading part to me, because I wasn't spicy enough. She gave it to the very youngest, Little Tamara, and she made me show her the steps and the movements.

The whole dance was so well done, that they even wrote about it in the papers. We youngest girls sang and danced it, with Tamara in the centre. She did it extremely well: she was full of pep and rather saucy, tossing her head.

After our last concert in Detroit, they threw lots of bouquets, and red roses for every girl, because we all had a bunch. Then, when we came out of the stage door, there were all these young men waiting; we were whipped away by these young chaps and they carried us on their shoulders through the streets to the hotel. That I do remember! It was extraordinary to have such a success, it really stirred us. We had never experienced anything like it – and we hadn't expected it.

We didn't stay long in Detroit, just a week. The next day, when we went to board the train back to New York, we were all still carrying our red roses. I still have a photograph of us, with Tamara in the centre, standing there with our bouquets. We had tremendous success there, really tremendous.

Back in New York

On our return to New York, we stayed at the Hotel A La Marque again. By that time Ninth Avenue was nearly finished: the roadway was done, there were no baulks of timber lying in the middle of the road and, outside our hotel, they had laid a beautiful pavement. I have a photograph taken outside the hotel; I am told it doesn't exist any more.

Shops were beginning to open and, in the time we stayed there, it became a very nice avenue. But we liked getting out and about in New York. We used quite often to go shopping on the very best parts of Fifth Avenue, at 46th Street.

By that time we were growing up and we were allowed to have some money. After all, we had to buy stamps and envelopes to write letters, so Irma used to give our nurse a certain amount of money; each girl could ask for some of her own earnings, and the nurse would write down where the money went. Wherever we went, especially in a big store, they knew who we were, because we went in a group, and they paid a lot of attention to us.

Sometimes in the evenings we were invited to people's houses. On one occasion, our hosts were having a small, very exclusive concert. We girls were interested, and Marsha made sure she was sitting next to me, because I liked her there. We were listening to a couple singing a duet and I whispered to Marsha, "Look at her feet, the way she's holding them – and those shoes she's wearing!'' Marsha burst out laughing, and of course that affected me too, so we were kindly asked to leave the room, which we did.

Once we were out of earshot, we laughed our heads off. Eventually we subsided, because we noticed they were making preparations for tea. They were laying out these bonbons and some lovely chocolates, so we helped ourselves to a couple of those each, and went back again and promised to behave. What the occasion was and who invited us, I have no idea, but we did enjoy it.

Worlds apart

We danced in Boston, which was a rather English, well-spoken city. Our concerts there went wonderfully well, and we were a big success. They were very intelligent people there and they could appreciate what we did. I still have photographs of us coming out of rehearsal.

We had a wonderful time in America. We took them by storm: what we did was something entirely different, quite different from ballet or anything they had seen. If they were amazed at us, we were astonished at America: it was a kind of wonderland.

Nonetheless, when we started touring to different parts, it was during the Depression. They were terrible times, with so many people out of work. We found out later how it was; at the time we never understood the system, the way it worked. We knew that in Russia we were always in want, but we thought America was the land of plenty.

We could not understand what we saw. I remember going to my aunt later, and asking her: these people come from a working-class background, but they have so many things – they even have cars – and yet they say they are in want. We couldn't make sense of it; we couldn't understand how on earth they could talk about being in want, when in Russia we were so short of even the most basic foods.

Aunt Tanya

One day in the Hotel A La Marque, some of the girls came up to my room and said, "Lilya, there is somebody downstairs for you: they want to meet you." So I went down, and there was a young man standing with an older man, who both introduced themselves. Apparently they were far cousins on my mother's side and they had seen the name Dikovskaya in our concert programme. My mother gave me her name so, wherever I went, I was known by her surname, not by my real name from my father.

Anyway, they asked if I would like to go and meet my mother's cousin. That was the young chap's mother and the older man's wife. I found out that her name was Tanya, so I called her Auntie Tanya. They lived in Brooklyn, and had lived in New York for a number of years.

She knew my uncle Isaac, my mother's brother from Paris. I think the young man had been born there in Paris, like my other cousin. My uncle Isaac married in Paris, and his wife was half-sister to Auntie Tanya. They had a little boy, Alexander, also born in Paris. That little boy and this young chap were related even more closely than first cousins usually are.

So they took me to their place and they had a little grocery shop downstairs, which, as well as food, seemed to sell almost everything else. They often mentioned that on the street where they lived was Al Jolson. I never took much notice of that; I never cared for him or the way he sang. But they were proud that he was from Brooklyn.

My auntie, I liked her: she was very lively, and she could be very funny. That suited my temperament very well. She had prepared a nice meal for me, and she had arranged for some friends to come round later. They lived above the shop and everything was nice. She had good taste, there was nice, solid furniture, and I noticed a very big bowl of fruit. That was our first meeting.

Her son asked me to go out for a walk with him. To be honest, I didn't particularly like him or dislike him, but I wanted to be obliging, so I said, "Okay." I found it very hard to communicate with him: he was rather shy, and I wasn't. I was reserved, but never shy. So we walked for a bit and we came back, and I said, "I think it is time to take me back to the hotel." We said goodbye, but that wasn't the last time I saw my auntie Tanya. I liked her and I was happy go and see her again.

Next stop, Canada

I see from one of our programmes that on our next tour we went first to Chicago and spent two weeks there. From Chicago we went into Canada, and I have some photos that I took on the train. The train journeys, they were extraordinary. These old trains – you must have seen them in old films – they were very comfortable. In the daytime you had a table in front of you, the seats were nice and soft, and there was always a restaurant on the train, so you could order anything you fancied. It was absolutely capital. Every so often there would be a stop, and we could get out to stretch our legs.

It was rather a long journey to Canada, so we had to sleep one night on the train. Out of the seats and the table, they made two beds, bottom and top bunks. Each one had a curtain across the front, and a little ladder appeared from somewhere so you could get onto the top bunk. We slept rather comfortably, though of course we had a little fun before we went to sleep. We used to crawl on everyone's bed, because it was such fun. After all, we were still quite young. I was 15, and we four little girls always kept together.

Next morning we arrived at Montreal, and I was very taken by the city. When you come into the main street, it is a beautiful avenue and there is such wonderful scenery, with that big mountain facing you. I liked Montreal very much indeed. We stayed quite a while and gave a number of concerts there.

After one concert in Montreal, a young woman came to see us at our hotel. She had entered the Isadora Duncan School in the early days, but then her mother took her to Canada. In some of those evening entertainments that Schneider had organised, the bigger girls had worn costumes – we little ones didn't – and this girl had been dressed like a Gypsy. She was one of the oldest girls and her name was Frooma Grivenskay.

I remembered her from school as being rather attractive, with dark hair and light blue eyes. Now she looked like a grown-up person, wearing a dress with some sort of pleats in tiers. I didn't care for the way she was dressed. Anyway, she came to introduce herself, saying, "Girls, do you remember me?" and we said, "Of course we do." We were very surprised to see her; she said she had admired our concert and stayed talking for a little while.

From there we went to Toronto, where we again gave concerts. However, Toronto didn't impress me as much as Montreal. On the way back to New York, the coaches were arranged just the same as before and we slept on the train again and behaved in the same way, having a lot of fun. A different kind of funny thing also happened to me on the train.

There was a special stand where you could get a drink in a paper cup whenever you wanted. I was there having a drink when our pianist happened to pass by, and he stroked my head. I was surprised and wondered why. Evidently I was beginning to look a bit more grown up, and Irma must have said something about me. So that was rather nice. But I never took much notice of it.

Travelling on those trains was quite an experience: the facilities were so wonderful. You see them now when you look at old films. It was so fascinating how they used to make up the beds in the compartments, and the next day, the way they made the beds into seats again, as if nothing had ever happened. Everything was put back the way it had been, tables were brought in and you had breakfast there on the train. Not so long after that, we were back in New York.

New York again

I've just looked up what I did when we came back to New York from Canada. Well, my aunt Tanya never forgot me, and she sent her son again to fetch me. As I liked her, I didn't mind at all. I think we went to her place by subway; when we got there, I found she had a little party arranged for me, so I shouldn't feel bored. We went out somewhere with a youngish couple in their little Ford car. I remember that because the name Ford seemed to come up a lot when we were in America.

I liked my aunt Tanya. When we were left by ourselves, she used to take me downstairs to get some fresh air, or to sit outside the shop. If any passers-by looked at us - well, we must have been a funny sight - she would say, "You see that young man? He looked at you; he must have liked you." I thought she was so funny to make such remarks. Sometimes we used to go for a little walk with her son - which I never looked forward to, but nevertheless I did it. We would come back and have a little supper and then they would take me back.

Eventually we got used to New York. We got used to a certain degree of fame too, because whenever we went out we always went in pairs and people would say, "There are the Duncan dancers going along, the ones from Moscow." We used to hear them commenting, but we never took any notice.

We liked going out together: we girls always kept together, we found it more interesting and people got to know us. As time went by, we used to go very often to Central Park; I have many photographs taken there. We liked it, but of course it was a bit different then from the way it is now. You could walk by yourself anywhere and nobody would ever interfere with you.

Once we got to know New York a bit, we used to go exploring. Sometimes our pianist escorted us, or even that man that knew Isadora, the one whose name was Jannett, who took us to Woolworth's when we first reached New York. We went on the ferry to the little island with the Statue of Liberty, and I have some photographs taken there too.

A strange story, unfinished

We hadn't been in New York very long – just long enough to know that we didn't really like the meals at the Hotel A La Marque and to find some good eating places near by where we could buy our own breakfast – when one morning, as we were having breakfast, we had a real surprise. Who walked in? A girl from school.

I had been very friendly with Lucy and my mother knew her parents too. Without warning she walked in, wearing a very posh dress, accompanied by a friend. And we said, "Well! Lucy, where did you spring from?"

Evidently she had found out that we were in New York at that time. I don't know how people find things out, how rumours get around. But apparently she did, because the person who brought her knew where we were – and there we were, having breakfast. We were amazed to see her, and pleased too.

She said, "Yes, I thought I would come and see my father." Well, that was very interesting, because we thought her father was still in Russia. So she told us her story. Her mother had taken her to Russia, but not with her father: she went with her father's brother, who was also called Flaxman, of course. It wasn't difficult to carry off and no one in Russia ever knew. I gathered that her real father didn't live in New York. He was somewhere else, and she was travelling.

126

She stayed with us for a little while, but she could see that we were trying to talk and eat, with the result that our breakfasts were going cold. She didn't want to disturb us, so she left, saying, "Maybe we will meet again."

Doing our own thing

Oh, yes I can say that we liked our food, but we never liked the restaurant in the A La Marque, so we often went out to eat. Manya, whom I was very fond of, would say to me, "Lilya, how about finding some place nice to eat?" She and I used to like savoury food very much and, of course, the place where we got the things we liked best was a Jewish restaurant. There they used to make pickled herrings and that sort of thing; my favourite dishes were potato salad with wienerschnitzel – oh, I loved that – and pickled gherkins. We used to enjoy ourselves there, Manya and I.

I don't know about the rest of the girls: perhaps they didn't mind. They somehow never complained about food, so we never troubled them, but Manya and I, we would go out by ourselves to eat. I would say it was rather seldom that we all went out together to eat.

Funnily enough, once we got a little bit more freedom, we liked going out in pairs. Very often we used to go to Fifth Avenue, which was rather chic. We enjoyed window-shopping, but we also used to make a note of various shops for the future, for the time when we would have more money. Meanwhile, as the joke says, we thought it was time we bought a watch.

We spoke to our nurse about it, and she saw no objection. She got consent from Irma and we all went to one shop and treated ourselves to the watch we liked best. I made a splendid choice: I bought a Bulova wristwatch, adorned with real sapphires, with a case made of white gold. I don't remember what I paid for it, though I know it wasn't cheap, but it was beautiful. People used to take notice of it. All the girls bought a nice little watch.

Sometimes I had an impulse to go out and I would go to our nurse and say, "May I have some money, please, for some stamps?" There were never any arguments, and she would give me a little extra in case. I would set off to look for a shop where they sold stamps, and on the way I might pass a cinema. Well, if I noticed there was something interesting on, or with some actor I was rather fond of, I would never hesitate: instead of buying stamps, I would go to see the film.

My favourite actor was Ronald Colman; oh, I thought he was just It! First of all, he was very good-looking, and secondly he was an excellent actor. I learnt afterwards that he was English. Well, no wonder he had such a lovely voice. I used to pop in and watch a film, and I remember seeing one in which he played opposite Ida Lupino. She wasn't my favourite, but he was. I would enjoy myself, and on top of that I would buy a packet of peanuts to keep my teeth occupied.

If I was lucky enough to have some money left over, when the film was finished, I would go looking for a stamp, then back to our hotel. Curiously, I would never tell anybody what I had been doing or what a lovely film I had seen. I never even discussed who my favourite actor was. Somehow, I never heard that any of the other girls did the sort of things that I used to do, and therefore I kept it to myself.

People

Meanwhile, we were constantly travelling on tour. We used to go to various places and return to New York in between. On our return, we would always go to visit Mr and Mrs Rice. Irma was very friendly with them, especially with Mrs Rice, and they were very good to us.

Unfortunately, the diary that I started when we began to go on tour, in which I put down every town with the date we went there, I destroyed it as a result of certain circumstances. It is not yet possible for me to say why, but it does make it more difficult to detail everything that happened.

When we returned to New York, we didn't always stay at the A La Marque. I don't know why, but once Irma took an apartment for us – actually, it was two apartments put together – and it was very big.

It wasn't just friends and relations who found out where we were and came to see us. We had all sorts of strange people coming to visit us. While we were staying at these apartments, amongst our visitors was a Gypsy woman, who rather surprisingly was married to a prominent Russian nobleman; she had Gypsy features and I think he married her because he found her so attractive.

Since they were White Russians, they ran away when the revolution came and finished up in New York. She had a lovely little girl with her and she thought it would amuse the girl to meet us. We didn't mind. The little girl got herself attached to me for some reason or another, maybe because I was friendly.

She was clearly well off and very smartly dressed. She came from Moscow and she wanted to know how things were now. She spoke Russian to us, and evidently it was a great novelty for her to speak Russian then. For me it was a novelty to see a Gypsy woman so expensively dressed. She came a few times, that Gypsy woman.

We also had visits quite often from people at the Russian delegation. They were anxious to keep in touch with us, so that we shouldn't go astray. We used to go to the parties they organised for young people.

Quite often I went to see my aunt; she was apparently very fond of me, and I liked her. One day when I was visiting, she looked at me more closely than usual.

"You know what, Lili? That hair doesn't really suit you."

I didn't say so, but I thought, *You can say that again.*

"What can I do? I was born with it."

I was too young to think of doing something about it. This was not long before my sixteenth birthday, because I celebrated my birthday in April, and I don't think it had quite arrived yet. So there was nothing to be done, and I never knew how to manage it. I learned afterwards, but not then.

Now Mooshya, whom I was very fond of, she also had curly hair and had problems with it, but she was blonde and I was dark. We just had to put up with ourselves the way we were. My hair wasn't the only thing about myself that I didn't care for: I wanted to be a little bit taller too. I thought I would be happier then, but of course it didn't happen. You have to accept yourself with whatever drawbacks you have, and that's what I told my auntie Tanya.

"There is nothing I can do about it. You will have to put up with me the way I am."

"No, it's fine. It doesn't bother me, but I just thought."

And I thought to myself, *No, you didn't: you weren't thinking at all. Just take what's on offer.*

But we were still very friendly, and we used to sit outside as the weather got warmer. I really enjoyed her company, and she really would have liked me to stay with her. I could feel that. She had a kind of longing for her family.

I think she married after she came to New York, but she never told me any particulars. In the course of time, though, she told me about her personal feelings. Apparently, she was in love with my uncle Isaac, who lived in Paris. She always said he shouldn't have married my other aunt, whom I didn't particularly like or dislike. I met her when they came to Russia eventually. I don't even remember her name, but Tanya I did like: she was so full of life. I don't know why Uncle Isaac married her stepsister; apparently she came from Russia to marry him in Paris. I think someone or something came between Tanya and my uncle Isaac.

But I had never realised that Auntie Tanya had been in Paris, so there was something there under the surface, a bit of unhappiness, a bit of a mystery – but that is life, and you can't help it. He was now married and had a little boy, she was now married and had a grown-up son, and perhaps neither of them was quite satisfied; but they had to get on with life. My aunt understood my philosophy. I might be young, but I was still sensible. I was old enough to understand how life could be so complex.

Taken as red

I have the programme from a concert we gave in New York, at the School of Art Dancing – our usual programme, with all our names. We gave many other concerts in New York, for which I have no programme, but I know we were fully occupied, we still had regular rehearsals and Irma still worked on us.

She rented a studio where we used to go for singing lessons. We had to keep exercising, and that is just as true for a singer as for a dancer: if you don't train the voice, you can't sing. The second part of our programme was singing those songs that we learn from Grechaninov. They were called the Children's Album and they were very successful.

After that came the revolutionary songs, which always went well with the audience. They never understood the words, of course, but that was just as well. People liked them, especially the song 'Varshavianka'. I liked the dance we did with it, from the moment Isadora created it, when we were in Moscow. So, with constant practice, our programme was always ready to be put on.

Even if Americans never understood the words, they seemed to know about the red flag and apparently it had the same effect on

S. HUROK

PRESENTS

Isadora Duncan Dancers

Under the Direction of

IRMA DUNCAN

LOCAL MANAGEMENT

Ralph MacKernan's School
of Dancing Arts

S. HUROK
PRESENTS

ISADORA DUNCAN DANCERS
Under the Direction of
IRMA DUNCAN
and assisted by
MAURICE SHAYNE, Pianist

PROGRAMME

1 SLOW MARCH ....Schubert
IRMA DUNCAN AND ENSEMBLE

2 WALTZES ....;........Schubert
a. Under the Scarf—Irma Duncan and Ensemble
b. Game with Ball—Irma Duncan
c. Three Graces—Irma Duncan, Tamara and Alexandra
d. Ecossaise—Irma Duncan and Ensemble

3 WALTZES ....Schubert-Liszt

4 PRELUDE, E Minor..................................Chopin
MAYA

5 MAZURKA, op. 33, No. 3............................Chopin
MAYA, LOLA, LILY AND TAMARA

6. VALSE, op. 70, No. 3.............................Chopin
LOLA, MAYA AND TAMARA

7 VALSE BRILLIANTE ....Chopin
ALEXANDRA, TAMARA, MARIE AND MANYA

8 MAZURKA, op. 7, No. 1.............................Chopin
ENSEMBLE

9 MAZURKA, op. 2, No. 2.............................Chopin
ENSEMBLE

10 POLONAISE, A Minor...............................Chopin
IRMA DUNCAN AND ENSEMBLE

Intermission

11 IMPRESSIONS OF REVOLUTIONARY RUSSIA
a. Warshavianka (Revolutionary Song of 1905)
b. Funeral Song for Revolutionary Prisoners in Siberia
c. Trilogy
1. Labor 2. Famine (121-22) 3. Labor Triumphant
d. The Blacksmith
e. Dubinushka (Workman's Song)
f. Russian Girl Scout's Song
IRMA DUNCAN AND ENSEMBLE

some of them as it does on a bull. So, although we wore red tunics, we had orange lights arranged to shine on us, not to show off the red colour. America didn't like red.

We really took America by storm. People couldn't get over how beautiful the girls were and the fact that everybody was so young. I think Isadora's dance works particularly well for young people. Having said that, only a very mature actress could carry off certain parts that she created, like Schubert's *Trauermarsch* or the Chopin. Perhaps only Isadora could do that.

The dancing itself was all so light and so easy, so beautiful, that you had to be young, or you couldn't really do it. Even the press commented that, while it was all so wonderful, the only pity was that Irma danced with the girls. They should have danced by themselves. On many occasions, in fact, Irma was very perturbed to find she could not do a dance the way we did. All the same, the solos she did do, she did well; and the girls really were remarkable, I must say.

But what I was trying to emphasise was the reception America gave us. In Russia – where we had spent all our younger years learning how to dance, and where we had danced a great deal in very many theatres – we had never had anything as enthusiastic as what we met in America, especially in New York. It struck me that the Russians saw us as nothing special, just another kind of dancing.

That really opened my eyes a bit, that we could be so admired in America but not in the country we came from. Even in China, where we must have seemed quite foreign, I found out later that many Chinese took movements of ours and used them in their own exercises; they liked the lovely easy movements. Much later, when I came to England, I saw the way Chinese people expressed them-selves, when they wanted to relax. After all, we were in China for seven months and it seems likely that some people did take note of what we did; but the reaction we got in America, I couldn't get over it.

The other girls took everything as it came, but I didn't. I had always to think about things. I used to feel the need to understand things and compare them. I am just like that, maybe because I am so inquisitive and I love reading about people and finding out what makes people tick.

America didn't make any difference to our behaviour or ideas, so the Russian delegation needn't have worried. We were just the same; success didn't go to our heads. We were very modest in that respect, which I think was the right way to be. I think it was our schooling with Isadora that made us understand that anything artificial in behaviour was very wrong. We loved simplicity and directness in everything, not just movements, but a simple way of feeling and understanding. I understood that very well.

'Big' Tamara

One day we were at some function and I was looking round, when I noticed another of the six original girls of Isadora's: her name was Erica, and I knew that she had broken away from dancing. She was sitting there, a rather attractive person. She was sitting with a man, who I would say was a little past middle-aged. He was quite distinguished-looking, very pleasant. And he was looking at Tamara (Big Tamara, as opposed to Little Tamara).

Now Tamara was a very lovely girl, but she was very withdrawn. She never used to come forward to people; I can't explain exactly. Was it modesty? I don't know. She was not very happy with herself. I know that, because I was close to Tamara then; we shared a room and she often told me what was bothering her.

I understood that feeling all too well, for I too was not very happy, wanting those couple of inches on my height. Tamara was dissatisfied with her legs and neck. She used to say to me, "Lilya, I am always looking at you, when you are bending down or dancing, because you have such a lovely neck." Well, I had never thought of that.

Now and then we used to find out a little more about girls and their backgrounds. Tamara came from a very well-to-do family, before the revolution at least. Her father was Lobanovsky, a very well-known surgeon in Moscow, and he was married to a woman of Polish descent. Her name was Irena; I remember her very well.

Tamara definitely had a most lovely face. She was blonde, with beautiful, large eyes, which were not exactly blue: they were pale blue. She was somehow with me, and we were walking around, looking at the guests. I had already noticed the man with Erica taking notice of Tamara, and then I noticed a Native American – as we say now. In those days we said 'Red Indian'. At least, his skin was red and he didn't look European. He also was taken by Tamara. He stopped her, I stopped, and he asked an odd thing: "Can I have your hand?" She gave him her hand, I don't know if it was the right or the left, and he studied it. "I am going to tell you about your life. You are going to have a short life. You are going to die young." I was horrified. Tamara just laughed at it, and that was that.

Nevertheless, it must have stuck in her mind. On top of that, her father had lost his senses after the revolution and was put away; and that played on Tamara's mind as well. When we got back to the hotel, it came out.

"Lilya, I know I am going mad."

"Look, darling, don't frighten me. I can't stand such ideas. Don't be silly, I know you are joking, but I just don't like such jokes."

She used to follow me, telling me these things that were in her mind.

In the end I had to put a stop to it. "Look, Tamara, I don't want to hear it; otherwise, I won't share a room with you any more."

So she stopped. She had a knack of predicting things, which could be frightening. Just before we got off the boat in New York, she was the one to say, "They won't let you in." She wasn't thinking about it – she was just teasing – but so it came out.

Philadelphia

We had been vigorously doing exercises every day with Irma, preparing ourselves for our next tour. Our first stop was Philadelphia, and that was in April 1929. I liked Philadelphia: it was very pleasant there. I noticed it was very similar to New York in the grid plan of the streets. Our hotel there was opposite a big office building, where many young people worked.

We used to share rooms, and I was sharing with Manya – Maria Toropchenova, but we called her Manya for short – and Vera Golovina. Vera was rather big and stodgy, both to look at and in herself, whereas Manya and I were very lively.

If anything, Manya was a bit too lively and I said, "Now, don't start flirting." She was such a flirt; she would flirt in front of shop windows, then catch somebody's eyes. While I was with her, she managed to do that to a young chap, and I had to pull her away. I used to say to her, "My dear, there is a limit to what you can do. Please don't embarrass me and Vera."

Meanwhile, Vera lived in a different world. She never

communicated with us, which was a little trying, so we thought we would play a prank and teach her a lesson. We decided, Manya and I, that we would quietly go out and leave her in the room, locking the door behind us. Well, we did that, and we meant to leave her just for a little while, but we forgot all about it and we went to see the other girls.

The next thing there was an SOS message. They said somebody had phoned from a certain number – the number of our room – to say they were stranded in the room. And we thought *What on earth have we done?*

We went to get her out and she was annoyed. "What on earth made you do such a thing?"

"Well, we did it just for fun."

But really we did it because she was always so quiet, and never took much notice of what was going on, and we wanted to wake her up a bit. That was in Philadelphia, but wherever we stayed we had to liven ourselves up with something; otherwise, it would become very dull.

We didn't always share with the same girls. If we got a bit tired of one girl, we would change and share with another. There were two or three of us to a room, all depending on the amount of room in the hotel that was available for us.

Pittsburgh

We had quite a number of people working for us at every concert venue, setting up the stage and the lights, and for Irma everything had to be just so. The man in charge of all these people was called Bill, and the girls often used to say to me, "Lilya, there is something so nice about him, don't you think? We like him." I would just say, "Oh. Do you?" I never took any notice of course.

One evening in Pittsburgh, after we had changed back into our street clothes, he was standing there talking to somebody as we were coming out of the theatre. As we were passing, going back to our hotel, he said to his companion, "There is my favourite," and pointed at me. Well, I was more than surprised; I couldn't get over it. I thought, *Why me, little me?* I brushed it off and took no more notice. A few days later, Lolya came up to me.

"You know, Lilya, I have just noticed that Bill is downstairs in the foyer."

"Well?"

"Lilya, would you be so kind – he's talking to someone – as to introduce me to him?"

"Look, you know him as well as I do. Why do you want me to do it?"

"Ah, but you speak English, so you can make him interested."

"Okay."

We went down to the foyer, and there was Bill standing with a man. He saw us coming, stopped us and pointed to this man, saying, "This is my brother." Just when I was going to say something about Lolya, who was with me, he turned round to his brother and said, "She is my favourite." I looked at Lolya, but she made me a sign not to worry and we walked away.

I went back upstairs and I was in the bedroom, combing my hair, trying to get it straight as usual, when the door opened and Bill walked in. He told me to come over to him, which I did because I knew the man. I felt sure he was not going to do anything unpleasant. But then he put his arms round me and said, "I would like to kiss you." I said, "Oh, no" and pushed him away.

I thought *A man of his age?* He was nearly 30. To me he was an old man. I was just 16: my birthday had just passed, because it was late springtime. So I refused him and I was really a little bit angry. He should not have done that to me, me of all the girls. Some of them were rather forward, and talked about men, but I never did. It just never occurred to me. I think it was too soon for me to think about them.

Men come in all shapes and sizes, of course. I am not sure where it was, but at one place we were told there was a little man who was determined to meet us, and he was waiting backstage. He was indeed little in stature. He was friendly towards us girls, but in a nice way.

He started by telling us that he had been following us on our tour, wherever we went. We were surprised. He said the first time he had seen us dance, he couldn't get over it. he couldn't work out what was so wonderful about us, so he thought he had to keep looking. After a while he realised there was a pattern to our dancing: no matter how lovely we looked, it wasn't accidental.

We found out he was a taxi driver, so it wasn't too difficult for him to follow where we went, as long as it wasn't too far from New York. His name was Joseph. We thought he was very funny, but we appreciated his determination not to miss a concert just because he wanted to find out what was so appealing about us.

Little did Marisha know, but ...

On our return, we were in the Hotel A La Marque, and by this time Ninth Avenue was completely finished. Time was marching on. I haven't mentioned anything about Marisha Borisova. She was now a married woman, so we never took much notice of her, but Irma did. It was coming towards May and she decided to try to persuade Marisha not to go back to Russia at the end of her six months' contract.

When we went to see Teresa and we met Augustin, with his son who was so very good-looking, Irma was rather cunning. Well, we knew that in a general way, of course, but she arranged for this young man, Augustin's son, to come and visit us at the hotel. He was trying to make himself very agreeable to Marisha.

I would say Marisha was not handsome, but there was something about her, about her figure and the way she carried herself. She was tall and not exactly dominating, but she liked to be noticed. And Irma had in mind that Marisha would like being noticed by this young man and would change her mind about going back to her so-called husband. In Russia, getting married was nothing special. It carried less weight even than signing your name.

Marisha was kind to him. I found that out, because ... well, it was like this. She had money, we knew that, and she used to buy herself various nice things. Mind, we didn't deny ourselves, but we would never go buying pineapples, while Marisha had a big heap of pineapples in her bedroom. So Lyola and I decided she wouldn't miss one and we would help ourselves. We very gently opened the door, and we just as quietly tiptoed out again, because Marisha was very busily engaged with this young chap. I don't remember his name, but he was blond, tall and attractive – very good-looking. She seemed to be deep in amours with him, so we quietly disappeared.

Irma was working on the fact that Marisha was rather liberal in making herself agreeable to men. Her looks were rather attractive I would say: she was dark and she had thick lips, a straight nose and very grey, piercing eyes. When she entered the school, she looked like what she was, a working-class girl, but our cultivating her did a great deal to enhance her.

We knew what was going on, especially we little ones, and we used to make fun of many things. Still, eventually we did get that pineapple. I remember we waited until the young chap left and then helped ourselves to it. We were rather naughty.

You had to be very careful with Irma, because she was constantly working on various little schemes; and, if she was planning something, she would do her best to make sure it came off. She wasn't very successful with Marisha, but nevertheless she tried. Marisha never objected to this young chap; in fact she liked him, and she knew that he was Isadora's nephew.

Now, we were talking about the weather getting warmer. At the beginning of June, New York starts to become very hot and humid, and Irma had in mind not to stay beyond that. She decided we should go to Europe for the summer, to Paris. We began to prepare for the journey and we found out that Mrs Rice was coming with us, bringing little Barbara. She thought it would be rather nice for her little child to be with us. When the time came, Marisha said goodbye – oh no, she wouldn't stay – so what Irma had in mind hadn't succeeded. Of course we found out more afterwards, but in any event I never thought things would be straightforward in this affair.

We were naughty girls. Marisha used to get letters from Schneider. When we were staying in that very comfortable flat, whenever she was out, a few of us started looking through her things, looking for one of the letters to read. I know we shouldn't have done such a thing, but we did. We just wanted to know what they wrote to one another.

He was rather a master of expressing himself, Schneider, which I remember from school. And he started his letter by admiring her looks, her very thick lips, which he couldn't wait until he could touch them again – and then of course we heard her coming, so we put it away; we never read to the end. We thought that was a pity, but nevertheless we found out afterwards what they were scheming. At the time, though, we were laughing so much at the way Schneider described Marisha. We thought, *If only she knew!* But we kept it under our hat, as the saying goes.

7

France, Schubert, June–September 1929

We had been dancing – practising or performing, or both – every day for six months, when Irma decided we needed a break. It was now summer, the weather was getting hot, sticky and generally unpleasant, and she felt we should get away from New York, far away: so she took us to France. At last we were going to stay in Paris; we were even going to perform there, as Isadora had planned.

Before we sailed, we went shopping and Irma must have come with us, because she used some of the money we had earned to buy outfits for us. She ordered skirts, tops, special shoes and various other little things, all the same, for us to look nice on the boat. Irma still wanted us to look as if we were in uniform. We didn't mind.

When we came to board our ship, the press were there and so was our little friend Joseph, when I mentioned earlier. He came to say goodbye, that taxi driver, and he wasn't a rich man, but we admired him for his devotion. He had come to see us so often and kept in touch with us, wherever we were performing. I think he must have been single to be able to follow us like that. Even so, he came to say goodbye and he brought us a very big basket of fruit and some lovely flowers. That was extraordinary, but then he was a remarkable man.

On the liner *Carinthia*

On the boat, we again had lovely cabins, and everything was very clean. The food was *comme çi, comme ça*, but we didn't get food poisoning. As the ship got under way, we had a good look round. Everything seemed very nice, and as usual I quickly found the library, where I could find a good book, sit and read.

140

The library faced the deck. I was sitting there quietly, very much absorbed in what I was reading, and in walked Lolya.

"Lilya."

"Yes?"

"You know there is a boy – well, not a boy, a young man – walking up and down the deck outside?"

"No, I hadn't noticed."

"Well, I've seen him before. I noticed him somewhere."

"I told you, I never noticed him."

"Lilya, do please introduce me to him."

"Fine."

So I put the book away. As we came out of the library, just as I was stepping out of the door, he came up to us. I was about to ask him if he would like to walk with Lolya, when he said to me, "I've been waiting for you. Would you care to take a stroll with me?" I looked at Lolya. This was the second time this had happened: the first time was with Bill the electrician, and now here it was happening again. I felt terrible, but Lolya said, "Don't worry, Lilya. Do as you please." And she walked away.

He and I walked along the deck. He was rather shy, and I was talkative. I often am when I don't know the person; otherwise I tend to be rather quiet. But not that time. As we were walking along the deck, I saw Irma coming towards us, and she smiled at me. I thought, *Well, she seems to be pleased*.

After that first walk, we met every day and spent a very pleasant time. His name was Frederick and he was waiting for me each day, after breakfast. As soon as I was ready to go out on deck, he used to join me and I found out he had a brother. They had been sent by their family to meet some relation in New York. They had travelled in America and now they were coming back.

They were Londoners and I vaguely thought, *I have friends in London*. I was thinking of Auntie Annie and her three young men. Had they known I was returning from America, I felt certain they would have made a point of coming to see me when we docked at Cherbourg.

We were five days on the boat and he took many photos of me and the girls. I still have them. At one point I remember Frederick saying, "You are going to Paris, aren't you?" and we said, "Yes." Then he asked, "Do you think you could let me know your address there?" The street where we stayed was off the Champs Elysées, that I do know, near the Bois de Boulogne – Honorat, I think the street was called. But I don't remember giving him our address; at that stage I don't think we knew exactly where we were going, so Frederick must have made enquiries.

At the hotel I was sharing a room with Liza, which we had sometimes done in America too. She and I got on very well, though at school we didn't, but somehow in America she was very friendly with me. At the hotel they used to bring us first thing each day a cup of hot chocolate.

A few days after our arrival, Liza and I were sipping our hot chocolate one morning when a very large, flat package was pushed underneath the door. So I went to have a look at it and I opened it. It was from Frederick; all the photos came out, with a little letter saying he was glad to send me these photos, and would I be kind enough to reply? After that, Frederick used to write to me, and send me pictures now and then, and I would write back.

In Paris

Paris was so charming, so gorgeous to us. Well, of course, where we stayed was the best part of Paris, but in any case France seemed so beautiful after America.

I remember that we couldn't get over the freedom of the French people and their feelings, compared to what we knew in Russia. For instance, as we were walking in the Bois de Boulogne, we saw a couple coming towards each other; they met, they kissed one another and they went away, arm in arm. We stood watching: it was such a novelty to us. We had never seen such behaviour, such wonderful friendship, and we were very taken by it.

We had four concerts in Paris, and they were very successful. For some reason, the Parisians didn't want Tchaikovsky's 6th Symphony in the programme, so we didn't dance that. We replaced it with some Chopin, and our programme was a really good one. The audiences must have seen Isadora dance and I expect they were ready to make comparisons, but they loved our dances: they were delighted – and, I think, astonished – at what Isadora had created while she was in Russia. Our concerts got marvellous reviews.

Marguerite Bouquet

When we reached Paris, I remembered that my mother had friends living there. She knew a family: the mother's name was Marie Bouquet, and she had two daughters, who had visited us in London. The younger daughter – though she was still older than me – was Marguerite, whom I loved very much.

My mother corresponded with Marie, so they knew that I was in America with the young dancers from Isadora Duncan's School in Moscow, and they knew we were coming to Paris for a holiday. Before we had been in Paris more than a day or two, Marguerite found out where we were staying and she came to see me.

We went for a walk by the Bois de Boulogne and all the time we were kissing one another: we were so happy to see one another. I was telling her how lovely Paris was, we walked on through the Champs Elysées and then she said she would take me to meet her mother. I had turned 16 in April, and now it was June. I felt like a real, grown-up visitor.

Marguerite's sister was a year older. Fanny wasn't handsome; she was pleasant, but not anything special to look at. Marguerite was the beauty. She was so lovely with a fine head of blonde hair, her beautiful grey eyes, with black eyelashes – oh, she was beautiful. She entered ballet school and in fact she became famous later on.

While we were on our way to see her mother, she explained to me that in Paris it was not like in England, where most people lived in houses. It seemed people lived in apartments here, and she thought I might find the apartments a little strange, but nonetheless theirs was in the centre of Paris.

I didn't notice how far we walked, because we had such a lot to say to each other. We were still chatting when we reached her place and she took me up to their apartment. The thing I found very strange indeed about their flat was that the floors were made of red tiles. When I commented on them, she said, "Well, of course, Lili: naturally there is no carpet here" – but I was used to carpets. It was a nice flat and very spacious; it just seemed odd to say that 'naturally' there was no carpet. Her mother was pleased to see me and asked about my mother. There wasn't a lot I could tell her, because I was at school all the time. But I said what I could.

Marguerite went to our first concert and of course the next day she came to see me. As usual we went out to walk and talk. I soon realised that Marguerite understood Isadora's ideas and what we were doing.

"Lili, you have no idea how taken I was by your dancing. That's dancing! Not the sort of thing I do, ballet: yours is real dancing. You were all so wonderful, you took me by surprise."

That is how we were, but of course I thanked her. She had more to say, though.

"You know what? I have some ideas."

"Yes?"

"Why don't you stay here with me?"

"Oh, Marguerite, I could not do that. First of all I have a contract, and secondly I don't know how we would arrange things."

"Don't go, Lili, and we will dance together. We will create something of real interest."

"No, Marguerite, that is impossible, even though I am so fond of you and I love the idea. Maybe it would work out, but I am not accomplished enough. In any case I can't think that way. I can't just walk out on what I am doing now. No, at this stage I have to stay with the group."

I had a practical mind even though I was so young, barely 16. At least we were fully occupied, we had a contract and everything was done for us. I knew I was good at what I was doing, and I understood movements very well indeed, but I was not capable of creating my own style and choreography, and I don't think Marguerite was quite up to it either. Otherwise she would have had a better position.

Nevertheless I understood. She had found that it is not so easy to do something in a country where you have no idea how things are run. With all her beauty, Marguerite wasn't so well off, she was still learning and getting known as a dancer, and she was seven years older than me. There was a big gap between us. So we left it at that, but she still used to come often and see me; she liked chatting with me and taking me out.

I mentioned that we got very good reviews in the press, but one thing struck me as very strange. All the papers used to talk about us, but none of them ever mentioned Irma. Of course she never had Isadora's talent in acting and dancing; nor could she follow her own mind in creating a dance. Irma could only follow what she knew.

Yet Irma was very good at what she did: she could portray ideas and feelings, and as a dancer she was a good follower of Isadora. The fact was, it was very difficult even to follow someone like Isadora. As for doing what Isadora did, nobody could, just as not a person in the world could compose as Mozart did. Such abilities are a gift that only a few people have. I understood that, but I still felt that Irma was entitled to recognition for what she did, because few people could have done it.

When we were preparing a dance, Irma always asked my opinion. I have to laugh, really. Why me? I was almost the youngest girl there, apart from Little Tamara, because Mooshya, Lolya and I, we were practically the same age. There can have been no more than a few months between us. Yet Irma always asked me.

Pontchartrain

As I mentioned, Mrs Rice and her daughter Barbara came with us. We girls, we were very observant and we found out there was a bit of flirtation going on between our pianist and Mrs Rice. The two of them went to Trouville, on the coast, and stayed there. Before they left Paris, though, Mrs Rice as usual said, "Lili, take care of Barbara for me." Only this time, if you please, I was to take care of Barbara for the whole summer.

Before I could say anything, Irma very decisively agreed. "Oh yes, Lili is just the person to look after little Barbara, and the responsibility will do her good." I thought to myself, *Irma is very quick to decide what is good for me*. I didn't mind taking care of Barbara, because she was a lovely little girl, but she was very young. And why me? Why didn't Mrs Rice ask somebody else? Why didn't Irma say, 'No, Lili has done her share of looking after Barbara. Someone else should take a turn'? No, Irma always thought I was better capable of any task that came to her mind.

Irma now asked me to help find us a place to stay in the countryside. She said, "Lili, you are very practical. Go to this village with Elzbieta Grigorevnya. Go with the nurse and see if you can find a place where you can all stay for the summer." The nurse, Mooshya's mother, was always was with us, but in America she especially looked after Irma's health and helped her backstage. I never cared for her, though. Never. Not after what I went through at school with her. Nevertheless, I was civil. I understood at a very early age that people are the way they are, and you just have to live with that.

145

So, Irma sent us to have a look at a certain place outside Paris and asked me to see what I thought. I wasn't very enamoured with it and told Irma so. She decided herself to have a look around and she found a lovely village, a very well-known place called Pontchartrain, and she fixed us up in a house there. That was the village where the Ayatollah stayed, when he was released by the French.

We used to go for walks, all of us, every day. We liked the village and not far away we found a cherry tree with those pink and yellow cherries, not red ones. I don't know if you know that type. We used to sit down underneath and ate those beautiful cherries. They were so delicious, we would eat them almost until we burst.

It was a nice *pension* where we stayed, very nice indeed, and we again shared rooms. This time I shared with Manya, whom I was very fond of, because she was so lively. She was a bit older than me, though, and once we had a bit of a tiff. I said something against Schneider and she defended him. I said, "Manya, how can you defend such a man? He is so wicked." She said, "He is not that wicked really, Lilya; don't worry."

I found out that Manya was sweet on him. Many of the girls were. I remember Schneider buying wonderful things for the eldest six girls. He dressed them so elegantly, especially two of them, Tamara Lobanovskaya and Marisha Borisova. He had that love affair with Marisha, but at the same time he liked Tamara just as well. That's the way he was, and it is why I never liked him.

I appreciated Schneider's ability as an administrator and as director of our school, because he was a wonderful organiser. In turn, I discovered that he respected me – he often said so, even when I was very young – but I was never sweet on him. I thought he treated Irma rather badly, and what happened between them was not very nice.

As we walked, we girls talked about various things. My Manya would always talk about men, at which I had to laugh. She would talk about actors, and there was one actor in particular that she liked, Adolphe Menjou. She said she wished she could meet somebody like that, and I thought it so funny. But youngsters can't help being young, and we enjoyed ourselves.

White Russians again

We were at Pontchartrain for nearly three months and we had such a wonderful time: the countryside was superb and it was a real rest. The little *pension* had a good reputation and was quite at home with Russian guests, because many of the Whites used to come there, those middle-class people who fled Russia after the revolution. These people couldn't get over it when we arrived, because we girls spoke Russian all the time. Apparently they were asking each other: Who are these girls?

One day all the other girls went out, so Tamara Lobanovskaya – Big Tamara – and I were left by ourselves. The *pension* had a lovely café with tables outside, and they served beautiful coffee. We were talking, Tamara and I; after that episode with the American Indian, and after sharing a room in New York, we had become quite close, and we were enjoying our chat.

There were a few of these White Russians sitting nearby. They were very elegant, with smart outfits and parasols shading them from the sun. Their clothes looked rather chic, so they were not short of cash. After a few minutes, they struck up a conversation with us – well, with Tamara at first, as she was older.

"Do you mind? We couldn't help noticing that you speak Russian."

"Yes, we are Russian."

"Have you come from Russia?"

"Yes."

"Oh, can that really be so?"

Now I joined in.

"Why, what is so different about us?"

"But you look so civilised, and so lovely."

"Well, you needn't think all Russians walk about with guns in their pockets, because they don't. Especially not now – things have changed a great deal."

They were very interested when we told them that Lenin had introduced the New Economic Plan. That allowed private enterprise and it came in about the time we left Russia. As a result, of course, lots of new businesses sprang up, and that was why you could now buy almost anything. Then it was our turn.

"You too speak Russian, so who are you?"

"We left Russia at the revolution. But never mind us. What are *you* doing here?"

"We are dancers; we are Isadora Duncan's pupils and we are resting here."

"So you just came not long ago from Russia?"

"Yes."

"How on earth did you manage it? And how is it you look so European? You don't look like Russian socialists."

"Well, our upbringing was entirely different. In our school, we were brought up surrounded by music and art, and we had very little to do with other Russians."

They still could not get over it. After that, they used to come there quite often just for a chat, to talk, so we found quite a pleasant little place. We also had young men coming to talk to us and we used to dance with them. That was a novelty too. We were growing up and we were having a wonderful time.

Frenchmen cause a stir

After this conversation, there happened to be two young men there, one of them extremely good-looking, and they both came up to us. Pierre, that handsome young Frenchman, got hold of me, and the other one, I don't recall his name, went up to Tamara. We went dancing, and I thought, *I like this Pierre*. I looked up at him, and he looked at me, and that sealed our friendship. From that time onwards, these two chaps came nearly every day to the *pension* to invite us out, or just to be together with us. We had a great time.

Meanwhile, my Mr Frederick from London continued to write to me. Now he wrote that he was planning to come to Pontchartrain to see me. I explained my difficulty to the other girls. I said, "Oh dear, this won't do." They said, "Don't be silly, Lilya. After all, Frederick is such a nice young man." I said, "Yes, I know, but I prefer Pierre." That was how it was. I knew there would be a bit of a calamity, but I thought, *Well, we will wait and see.*

Meanwhile, the weather was lovely in Pontchartrain, so Maria and I decided to go for a walk. We decided we would pick some wild flowers wherever we saw them, especially those marvellous blue flowers that grow with the corn – cornflowers. We came across a very big field, and went a little way into the corn to pick these beautiful blue cornflowers. We never noticed that at the far end there was the farmer.

Suddenly we heard somebody shouting at us in French. It wasn't the sort of language we had learnt in those French lessons we had before we went to China, but we had learnt a lot of new words while staying in Pontchartrain. The gist of it, though less politely expressed, was, "What on earth do you think are you doing there? If you don't get off my land now, I will shoot you." My goodness, didn't we get a shock! Manya and I raced off like frightened rabbits. Afterwards we laughed such a lot about it, but not at the time.

Boys (in various sizes) will be boys

Nevertheless, the following day we went out again, and this time I took little Barbara with me. We had a bad habit of always keeping our eyes open for food, particularly for fruit trees. We used to sit down under any cherry tree we found, because those cherries were so wonderful. We used to gorge ourselves; nobody stopped us, and we ate and ate until we couldn't move.

This day we went quite a long way and found a pear tree, which we harvested on the spot. On our way back, a couple of young boys noticed us. I suppose they thought, *These young girls, who are they? What shall we do to them?* We saw they were holding a snake, one of those grass snakes, and they were making it twist around.

The girls who were in front thought they might be planning to throw it at them. Well, boys do things like that sometimes. So they panicked and started running. It only needs one to run and the rest will follow. We all stampeded and these little boys were killing themselves laughing. They couldn't get over it. We found out afterwards they were playing with a rope.

But it looked like a snake, so we ran, and little Barbara couldn't keep up with us. She kept saying, "Lili, don't run so fast. I have got a stitch." I said, "Look, Barbara, you will just have to bear with the stitch. We don't want that snake to get us. We all have to put up with a little bit of discomfort sometimes." I was trying to explain to her, but by now we had passed the danger zone. We slowed to a walk and then we found out it wasn't a snake, and we laughed at ourselves: how stupid we were! Little Barbara was half dead, but it was a funny thing: that little girl said she had a stitch, but now it had disappeared.

Anyway, all was well and we got back as usual. We knew Pierre would come round later with his friend. They arrived before tea, and invited us all round to their aunt's, where they were staying. We had a smashing time, dancing – I remember that. And we had tea there, with lovely little home-made buns.

They were so charming, those two young chaps, especially my Pierre. He was blond, he was so good-looking, so handsome, that I forgot all about Frederick. I must say, it was very wrong of me. But then at that time I still hadn't really understood that I could have such a big effect on a boy. I liked Frederick, but I never gave my heart to him, or to anyone at that age. The other girls did, but somehow I didn't. That came to me much later in life.

After that, we went back to our place. We were very glad of the big spread their aunt had laid on for us, because we always had problems with food. The food at the *pension* was delicious, but there was never enough. The husband and wife who ran it started complaining that they could not keep up with us. At dinner, they used to bring a very long plate loaded with beans, those lovely French runner beans, but in two ticks the beans were all gone and they would have to replace them with another lot.

Irma visits

When we heard that Irma was coming to see us, we were very pleased. She had been tucked away in Trouville with the pianist and Mrs Rice, who had left Barbara with us. Irma arrived and found us all in very good health, but she had to make some new arrangements with the owners about the food.

She had to pay a little extra for them to feed us properly, because even the meat was never enough. Otherwise we were very contented with our *pension*, but we were always running about or walking somewhere, so we had very good appetites and the food was delicious.

While she was there, Irma went out with us, and it seemed she was always next to me, either talking or just walking side by side. I really don't know why. I was fond of Irma in my own way, and she was fond of me really, to be honest. I know she respected me, because she often used to say, "Lili, you have more sense in your little finger than all the other girls put together." I never dwelt on that, but I knew from experience that if she had anything to discuss, she would discuss it with me, not with anybody else, not even with Elzbieta Grigorevnya.

This day, Irma was walking next to me, and I was wearing a necklace in the form of a little snake, which I had bought for myself. I didn't like it on my neck, so I twisted it round my wrist. As we were walking, Irma took my wrist and said, "Lili, you have very good taste." Well, I was very pleased she liked my bracelet. Like all of us, I suppose, I remember anything particularly pleasant – or unpleasant.

Irma left us all in good shape, saying, "Girls, you are doing very well" – because we were there for three months, and that was quite a stretch – and she went back to Trouville. She took Barbara this time – her mother wanted to see how she was. And since she didn't think Barbara would have much fun by herself, she took Little Tamara to keep her company.

Tamara was away for three days. When she came back, we were eager to find out how it went. "Oh, girls! You have no idea!" She started describing Mrs Rice putting her swimming costume on, and we were in fits of laughter. Then Tamara told us about Moise Borisovich Shane, our pianist, because he and Mrs Rice were very sweet on each other.

Tamara may have been young still, but she was also very observant. She came back on her own, without Barbara. Perhaps Mrs Rice wanted to see more of her daughter or perhaps Barbara had had enough of being with us, especially as her little legs couldn't keep up with ours.

Life gets a little complicated

Meanwhile, we were having a nice time with these two young chaps. I really liked my boyfriend, Pierre, but as the day came closer when my Frederick was due to arrive, I began to get alarmed. I said to the other girls, "What am I to do?" They said, "You are going to meet him bravely. He is a very nice young man, and if you are thinking of trying any tricks, we will see that you don't get away with it."

The day came and the girls kept a lookout for him. They saw him coming from the railway station and they rushed to tell me, "Lilya, prepare yourself. He is on his way." I thought, *No, this cannot be. I must do something.* So I ran upstairs to one of the bedrooms, not mine, and there was our big travelling trunk. Well, our clothes were not in the trunk: we had taken them out, apart from our dancing gear, and there wasn't much of that. There were just tunics, so I hid myself inside where we hung our clothes and managed to close it from the inside.

They were looking for me, when he came. He asked, "Where is Lili?" The girls were incensed; they knew I had hidden myself somewhere, but where? They couldn't find me. Then it dawned on Valya, who knew me well, where I must be. She said, "I bet she got in the trunk." They came upstairs, opened it and started to pull me out.

That was very naughty of me, but they got me out and I faced the consequences. I came down and said, "I am sorry, Frederick, but I was a little bit detained." He said, "It doesn't matter. How are you?" I said, "I am fine, we are all fine. You know all the girls, don't you? I expect they have entertained you." He said, "Yes, yes." He knew Lolya well, and he knew Marsha and Little Tamara. We were always together, as you can see in many of the photographs he took of us.

He ordered a dinner for us, a special one, and I found out he was very well-to-do indeed, but that in itself didn't attract me one little bit. We had a lovely meal – it was not dinner, actually; it was lunch, as the English call it, so it wasn't meant to be the main meal of the day.

Then it was time for him to walk to the railway station, which was some distance away, and I went to see him off. I told him I would go only halfway; he agreed. I said it was too far for me to walk; he agreed. So we walked and we talked of this and that.

He got the message all right and we stopped corresponding. He was only 21 or 22, no more, a young chap and rather nice. I felt a little guilty, but you can't help events. After all, Pierre was here on my doorstep and Frederick was across the Channel, in London.

Back to Paris, back to New York

Well, we had been nearly three months in Pontchartrain and time was marching on. We had been so busy, we hardly noticed the time passing. Just before we left, a fair came to the village and we went to

152

that too. We had had a very good holiday, but now we had to pack our things and return to Paris.

I don't think we stayed in Paris very long, but I must just mention one thing, which I didn't know at the time. Many years later, after my return to England, I found out that my father was alive and was then living in Paris. I could have got in touch with him. You may think that he could have got in touch with me, except that my mother changed my name and my birthday. She never wanted him to find out where we were. So I had her surname, Dikovskaya, though my father's name was Lotterbach; and I celebrated my birthday in April, when really it was in March.

When I discovered all this, I also learnt that he was married, with a big family. Since he had never divorced my mother, it might have caused a lot of trouble if I had suddenly turned up. I didn't want him to think I was going to intrude on his life, so I never made any attempt to get in touch with him. Perhaps I should have done, but that is another story.

We didn't stay long in Paris, so beautiful as I remember it. We travelled to Cherbourg, boarded the boat and sailed back to New York. On the boat there was a whole group of boy scouts travelling, and of course a couple of boys made friends with me. They made the first move; I was never the first to approach anybody. That is not in my character, even to this day.

So they approached me and we all got quite friendly with them. The two boys were Frederick – another Frederick, a tall chap – and his friend Bill. I liked both of them, but I preferred Fred. In the photo, Fred is on the right – he was *sympatiya*, I liked him and he had a soft spot for me – and his best friend Bill is on the left. We had a lot of fun together.

Shura Aksimova, that beautiful dancer, told me later on that they came up to her and asked if she could foretell the future. She said, "What do you want to know?" Freddie said, "We would like to know about Lili. What is her future?" So she made up all sorts of stories about my future. When she told me afterwards, I was laughing my head off. So that was quite a pleasant crossing and we were back in New York.

Schubert's 9th

Of course by that time the first six months of our contract had elapsed, but in the contract Irma signed with Hurok we had agreed to perform for another six months. So we had to continue dancing and travelling. I don't remember all the towns we visited, but I know exactly what we and Irma were rehearsing.

It was the 9th Symphony of Schubert and, even though we had been working on it before we left Russia, she worked us very vigorously. She hired the same rehearsal hall again, it was a very spacious place, and we had our own pianist, but there was just one problem: Irma had forgotten the choreography of the last movement.

We didn't dance the first movement, but we four younger girls danced the scherzo. The music changed in character from the scherzo to the trio, which the bigger girls danced. It was very lovely, I liked that part, and the movements to it were so beautiful.

Then the scherzo came back again, but after that Irma couldn't remember the movements. She had to ask Anna Duncan to come and help her out. Anna did come – she was very good in that – and showed her how the last movement was danced. I watched her very carefully. To be honest I didn't like her movements. Perhaps that's how she was taught to dance the Schubert in Isadora's first school, but by the time Isadora came to Moscow she had gained new insights and developed new techniques. That's why Isadora always used to say we danced better than her first pupils: we had nicer movements. The first six girls had great success, but not as wonderful as we did.

Well that was the episode with Anna, we came to the end of rehearsals and our performance was ready for Carnegie Hall. Irma told us to dress and look our best, and then she added, "That was our last rehearsal so, when you are ready to go, you go home and rest." We didn't say yes and we didn't say no; we just listened, as we always did. We never agreed or disagreed with Irma; we just listened.

Flying feet

We all left together and we never thought to eat anything – no, no. But on our way back, we passed a cinema that was showing a film called *Flying Feet*, and who was in the film? Ramón Novarro. Well, of

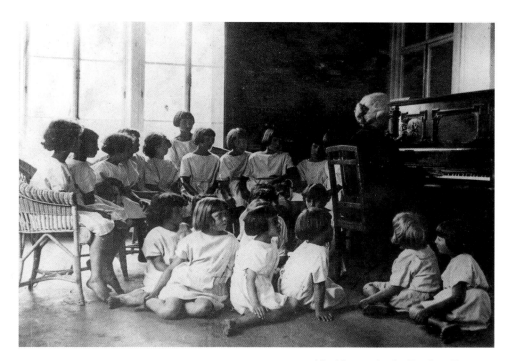

10. Above: At the Isadora Duncan School in Prechistenka street, pupils listened to live music every day. The rooms of the Ushakov mansion seemed huge, but beautiful, to a child of 8. When this picture was taken in the school's first year, Lily was absent – probably ill with malaria.

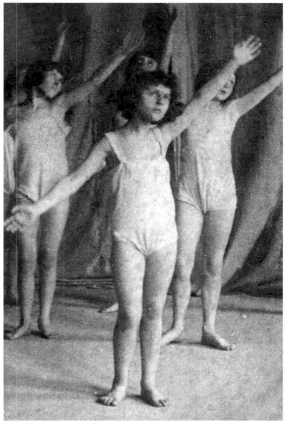

11. Left: Lily concentrating, but looking relaxed, aged 8, shortly after joining Isadora's school; the girl behind, to the right, is Galya Antonova. Lily found that Isadora's dance movements came naturally, even though – or perhaps because? – she had never had dancing lessons.

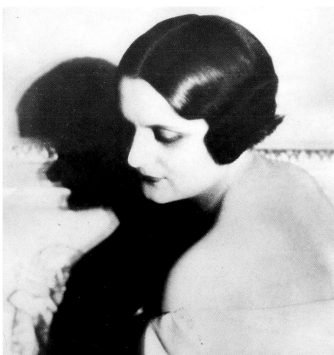

12. This picture of Irma Duncan was taken in the entrance vestibule at Prechistenka 20. Irma was a good dancer, though not outstanding; but she was a gifted teacher, whereas Isadora would simply show you what she wanted and then expect you to understand and follow her. Many girls couldn't do that, so usually it was Irma who actually taught them.

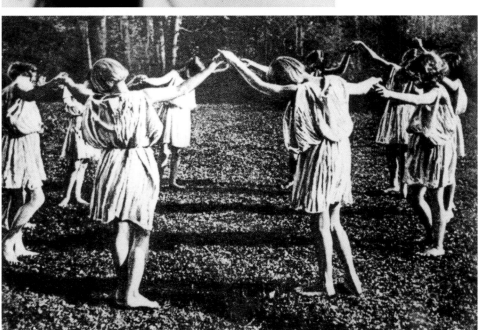

13. After malaria in her first year at Isadora's school, Lily fell ill with pneumonia in her second year. Even so, she felt the pupils lived a healthy life, with plenty of exercise and fresh air whenever the school's director could arrange it. They always danced barefoot; this picture was taken in the garden of Krasneya (The 'Red' Mansion), which belonged to a nasty woman called Soltichvicha.

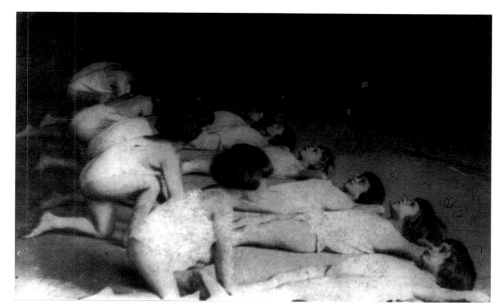

14. Isadora's ideas about clothes for any kind of movement were a good fifty years ahead of their time. On the other hand, they weren't ideal if the school central heating boiler broke down, as it often did. In this gymnastics lesson, the nearest pair are (left) Lyola Terentieva and (right) Lucy Flaxman; behind Lyola is Lily.

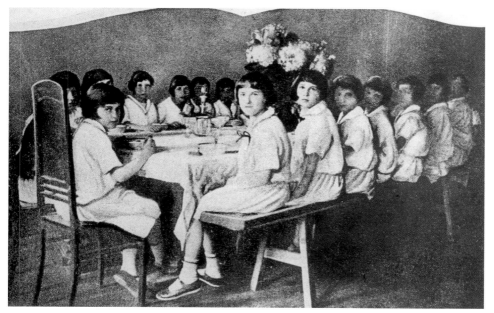

15. Just like her dancing, everything about Isadora's school – from uniforms to meals – was simple, yet done in style. Eight-year-olds were not too young to appreciate a spotless linen tablecloth or flowers on the dining table. If you sat on the end of this bench, you had to beware! The girl on the chair is Lucy Flaxman. At the back, leaning forward, is Manya Toropchenova.

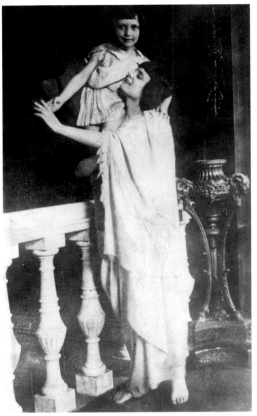

16. Irma holding Lida Lozovaya on the balustrade of the landing overlooking the entrance hall. Lida, the youngest pupil, looks quite calm considering what a long drop there is behind her.

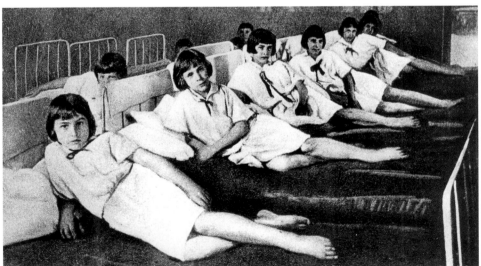

17. This was where Lily first slept at Isadora's school. Compared to the school in Lincoln, the dormitories at Prechistenka 20 were spartan; but, compared to what other Muscovites had, these living quarters were literally palatial. The nearest girl in the picture was better at reciting than dancing, and did not stay long. Behind her are Manya Toropchenova, Lucy Flaxman and Marousha Borisova.

course, he was one of our heart-throbs, so we decided quietly to go and see the film.

We went in, bought tickets, found seats and watched the film – and, at the end, we stood up to leave and what do you think we saw? Irma was sitting there at the back! She smiled and didn't say a word, but we were on flying feet. We just flew out of the door and went back to the hotel to rest, before we had this fantastic concert.

Carnegie Hall was constructed only for orchestral concerts really. It wasn't suitable for stage shows, though people did sometimes use it for such things, especially dancing. I don't know about Isadora, but we were told that Teresa Duncan had danced there, with success.

Everything was arranged, though we didn't have an orchestra, which I would have preferred. There were two pianists playing the symphony and, well, I think that was the best experience I have ever had on the stage. The dance itself, the scherzo, which we younger girls danced, is my favourite bit in any event from the whole symphony. It is so vivid. It is so fast, so full of joy. I loved anything that was fast.

It was so successful because we danced wonderfully. I must say that, because we were at our best. The big girls, too, were lovely, but we were exceptional in being so young and so alike; and we used to fly about, in the most extraordinary way. We didn't need a film to show us flying feet.

The film people begged Irma to let them shoot some film of us doing this symphony. She refused, because Isadora had always said, "No one must ever film my dance." That was silly – and a really bad mistake – because as a result people completely lost sight of what Isadora had created; and that symphony was one of her most wonderful creations.

We had four concerts at Carnegie Hall, and every one was a huge success. Out of that whole wonderful episode of my life, that time in America, there were two evenings that stand out: that concert at Carnegie Hall – the 'first night' of our new season – and our very first concert in America, at the Manhattan Opera House.

At the Opera House we had an orchestra. They didn't play everything, because there were some things that only a pianist could do, like Chopin or Schubert; but for the rest of our programme we had the orchestra playing. We so looked forward to that very first concert – and so did the audience, because they didn't know what to expect.

Every other concert we danced well, but that night at Carnegie Hall we were really at our best. And that is why I feel so disappointed that Irma followed Isadora in not allowing the cameramen to film. Isadora wasn't always right in everything she said, but what she created was unique. After her, nobody created such wonderful dancing and movement. So she was very wrong to deny it to those who came after.

At the end of the symphony, we all danced together. That wasn't my favourite bit, but the fact that we all finished together, the whole group, that was impressive really. It is a pity they never took that film of us at Carnegie Hall: I would love to see us dancing when we were young, very much so. But there is nothing of us anywhere.

I also wonder now what our American audiences saw, what they were so enamoured of. Whatever it was, we were very surprised and it rather pleased us to find that our dancing was not only appreciated by those who understood what we were doing, but was also admired by the wider public.

Press Comments

"There is recaptured here more of the spell of Isadora herself than in any previous appearance of her disciples, not even excepting the six "Isadorables."

New York Times.

"These lissome light-footed, exquisite creatures were seemingly as dainty as fluttering butterflies."

New York American

"It is hard to realize this effect of joy and spontaneity as the result of careful training."

N. Y. Eve. Telegram

"An untrammeled lightness and fleetness and bodily exultation which is often imitated but rarely reproduced."

N. Y. Herald-Tribune.

"An entertainment sufficiently diverting to make one wish to see these young people again."

New York World

"Singing as they danced, these alert youngsters embodied the eternal spirit of youth afire."

Chicago Herald Examiner

"There is an abundance of grace, charm and enticement in what the girls do."

Chicago Tribune.

"In the dancing of the girls there is an heart-rending loveliness."

Chicago Daily News

"For the first time I felt that exhilaration of whole-hearted approval and enjoyment that comes from spontaneous appreciation."

Herman Devries,
Chicago Eve. Press.

"Vital flesh at one with rhythmic spirit, disciplined abandon, fluent gesture, light, quick harmony of motion—these the Isadora Duncan Dancers gave."

Boston Transcript.

"Throughout the performance the large audience showed every sign of pleasure."

Boston Herald.

"Their art was of the innermost plasticity and freedom."

Boston American.

"Isadora Duncan Dancers get ovation at appearance here."

Phila. Public Ledger.

"Isadora Duncan lives again in these dancers."

Phila. Record.

"Their rhythms and movements brought rounds of applause."

Phila. Eve. Bulletin.

"Curtain calls were frequent."

Phila. Enquirer.

"The audience was moved to tremendous applause."

Detroit News

"You will come away with the experience of an unusual night in the theatre."

Detroit Eve. Times.

"Brought forth shouts of 'bravo' and insistent applause".

Detroit Free Press.

"The girls are all extremely young and each is beautiful."

Hartford Daily Courier.

"The Isadora Duncan Dancers etched out an evening of beauty."

Pittsburgh Press.

"Music's beauty and imagery interpreted by Isadora Duncan Dancers."

Pittsburgh Sun-Telegraph

"Combine personal beauty with their grace and dramatic effectiveness.

Newark Ledger.

"It was an unique entertainment every minute of which the audience enjoyed keenly."

New Haven Times Union.

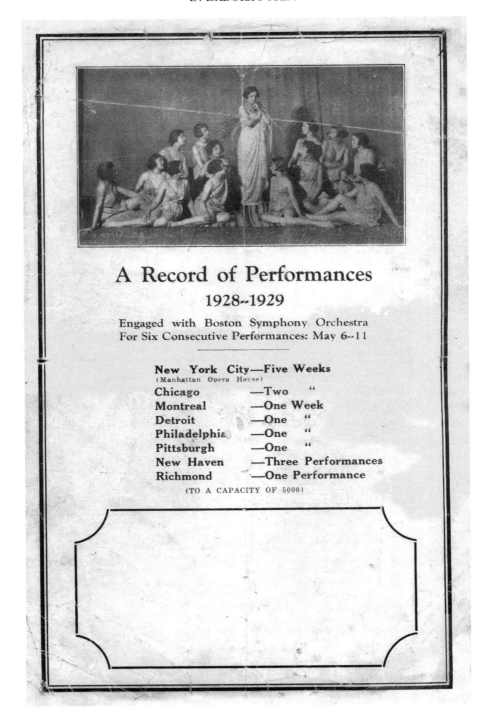

A Record of Performances

1928--1929

Engaged with Boston Symphony Orchestra
For Six Consecutive Performances: May 6--11

New York City—Five Weeks
(Manhattan Opera House)

Chicago   —Two   "

Montreal   —One Week

Detroit   —One   "

Philadelphia   —One   "

Pittsburgh   —One   "

New Haven   —Three Performances

Richmond   —One Performance

(TO A CAPACITY OF 5000)

8

The Most Important Thing, 1929-30

Until the time came when we had to leave America, we were very friendly with the Russian consulate. They never had an embassy in New York, just a consulate. They used to get in touch with us and invite us round, quite often for tea. It seemed quite natural at the time.

Among these people was a young woman in her late twenties. Now, I don't know quite how it came about, but she became very friendly, especially with Big Tamara and Shura, the two big girls. She had beautiful clothes and I remember she passed on a dress to Shura and one to Tamara, because they were the same height, and her clothes fitted them.

But the rest of us were always a bit suspicious. How is it that she speaks fluent Russian? And what does she do for money? If we met Russians abroad, they were usually exiles or else people starting a new life. They scraped by; they had to make do and mend.

This young woman seemed to live a life of leisure. As well as expensive clothes, she had a beautiful apartment, which she invited us round to visit, but who she was, we had no idea. She clearly knew the people at the Russian consulate because, whenever they invited us to tea, she was always there too. I wondered about her even more when odd things happened later on.

Fame and fortune

We were the talk of every town we visited. Wherever we went, people with big houses invited us as a group to their homes. At one place a very well-to-do couple invited us round one afternoon and

159

made a beautiful spread for us. Irma made fun of them, which I thought was very wrong, and she whispered to us all to follow her.

"Just watch me, girls, and do the same. You watch: they'll all do what I'm doing."

There were quite a lot of people there as well as the owners, who looked quite young – I don't think they had any children. Irma went down on her knees and everybody followed her. We followed suit; well, we had to, but I thought at the time it wasn't very nice of Irma to behave like that. Still, she was right: they all did what she did.

After that we had tea and then we danced – ballroom dances – and in fact they had a ballroom. I noticed that the husband danced remarkably well and Irma noticed me noticing it. She was always rather observant of what other people were about, and on this occasion she was standing not far from me. I don't think the other girls had noticed him, but I was admiring his dancing. When that dance finished, she went up to him and very gracefully asked him to dance with me, I thought, *That's nice of Irma*. He and I danced, and he danced beautifully. I wasn't so bad myself.

For a year we performed all across North America, to attentive audiences and packed theatres. When we were on tour, those were the most important things to us: the audience, the theatre and of course our performance – our work, if you like. It was fun to see new places, of course, and have people making a fuss of you. But grown-ups do like to make a fuss of children on stage, don't they? That was nothing unusual – in fact, for us it was normal.

By now we had got used to fame. Whenever we went out, we always went together, in pairs, and the people would say, "There are the Duncan dancers from Moscow, going for a walk." We didn't think of ourselves as rich and famous – but we were, all the same. We were young and we were used to people arranging everything for us, so I suppose we were unaware of a lot of things. Probably we were on tour in October 1929, but the Wall Street Crash didn't make a big impression on us, even when we got back to New York.

Irma handled all the money. We were given pocket money, but that was all: we didn't really need anything more. Everything was paid for – meals, hotels, apartments, train and boat tickets, taxis, clothes, shoes – even if everything wasn't always just the way we might have chosen. But we were not grown-ups and we did as we were told.

After each tour, we used to come back to New York, but we didn't always stay at the Hotel A La Marque, as we had at the beginning. We stayed in various apartments that Irma used to find for us. Sometimes they were nice, sometimes they were not so nice. But we never ever complained, we girls. Now, when I look back, I think we were wonderful. We never demanded anything: we just accepted whatever Irma decided – except for the very last thing she decided, because she got that so wrong.

We are the last to be told

Whatever really happened, I still don't know, but that episode was extraordinary. Perhaps Irma thought we would just do whatever she said. Even so, whenever I look back, I can't really get over what Irma did. What persuaded her to do such a thing? But perhaps I know the answer to that. We had been brought up in Russia to be egalitarian, to live simply and to work hard, whereas Irma – though she too loved music and dancing – always looked to see what was in it for her.

So what *was* in it for her? A lot of money. She was already getting $250 a week. We girls were being paid $60 a week, though we never saw it; but then, as I said, we didn't need to. We didn't know then – I found this out later – but our contracts with Sol Hurok were coming to an end. Naturally other impresarios scented an opportunity, and one of them offered to double our pay – and Irma's. She was to be our director, but the contract allowed for us girls to perform without her. It was us they really wanted.

We knew nothing of this until we heard somehow – maybe through our nurse or one of the stage managers – that the newspapers were saying Irma wanted to sign a contract with someone else. In fact, she had already agreed terms for a new tour, but she never said anything to us about it.

Even worse, by the time the story reached us, we discovered that Irma was no longer talking to Sol Hurok, our agent, and was in trouble with the Soviet authorities. Before that, we had only had to worry about unwanted approaches from young men; now we were the centre of unwelcome attention from newspapers, lawyers and government. This was what we read in the *New York American*:

SOVIET BUREAU ORDERS DUNCAN DANCERS HOME

The Isadora Duncan Dancers, a group of ten young Russian girls on a professional tour of America for the last year, have been summarily ordered to start back to Moscow this week by Soviet representatives in Washington, it was revealed yesterday.

The order, it is understood, was the result of a break between the unofficial Soviet representatives in America and Miss Irma Duncan. She is the adopted daughter of the late Isadora, who has been training and managing the youngsters for several years.

Baggage seized

Miss Duncan told the New York American last night, that local representatives of the Soviet have sought to embarrass her by seizing the company's baggage and passports, and had used threats to frighten her young charges into agreeing to return home.

Miss Duncan declared that if the girls were forced to return to Moscow they would in all probability become public charges, as none of them had funds.

Clash with agent

Back of the altercation, it was learned, was a misunderstanding that Miss Duncan had with her American booking agent, S. Hurok of No. 1560, Broadway. Miss Duncan said she had refused to play further dates under his management because of a money dispute.

Hurok countered by declaring that Miss Duncan had an objectionable 'red flag' dance on her programme. Papers were served on the young woman last Friday in a breach of contract action filed by Hurok. He demands damages of $64,500.

It was interesting that Irma said none of us had any funds. I'm sure none of us gave much thought to that, but did it really cost $60 a week to keep us? Or was that just one of her bargaining chips? And why did she say the Soviet representatives were trying to frighten us? They can't have been trying very hard, because they didn't say anything to us. We girls knew only what we had heard, but certainly

162

something odd was going on. Was it anything to do with that young woman with the beautiful apartment, the one who spoke Russian so fluently?

A meeting is arranged

We had been away on tour – to Florida, among other places: I have some photographs showing the palm trees – and we had just got back from a couple of weeks in Montreal, I think, when Irma decided to gather us together.

We were sharing a flat, a very spacious flat with two bathrooms. Well, as long as we could have a bath, the rest of its facilities didn't matter. When we wanted to eat, we knew our way about – all the best delicatessens, and the restaurants where you could get a really good main meal – so we had the important things sorted out.

Irma had been staying with some people in a lovely apartment overlooking Central Park, a place she stayed quite often, and she told our nurse to bring us round there from our apartment. Apparently, she had something very important to tell us.

We didn't know what to expect. We never did know, because Irma always kept a little distance from us and never spoke about her intentions beforehand. So we had no idea what she was planning to do.

Irma gets it all wrong

When we entered the room, there were chairs waiting for us and on one of them sat a man. Somehow he looked like a lawyer. Irma started by saying she had decided (*now that it's in the newspapers*, I thought) to tell us what had been happening.

"I have arranged a new contract for you, with a new impresario, and it's all ready for you to sign – there is only one difficulty. I have been told that the Russian Government insists you must all return home."

Why? She didn't say. We went very quiet. She went on.

"The point is, the government say that if you don't go back you will never see your parents again."

Well, that frightened us. It was certainly the wrong thing to say if she wanted us to sign the new contract.

But we were surprised too. Why did we have to go back? Why now? She didn't go into details. Irma made so many blunders with us, and they were mostly because she never explained what was going on. Really and truly, what she got, she deserved. I know it isn't nice of me to say that, but how could she keep us in such ignorance? I didn't understand it. It was true we were young and far from home, and we depended on her, but we were not babies.

Anyway, she started to explain - at least, she evidently thought she was explaining. We were still wondering why the government had demanded our return, but we didn't ask Irma why; if they said we had to go back, there had to be some reason. It seemed to be nothing to do with Irma, so we didn't ask any questions, but as she went on she could see we were bewildered. She was telling us what a wonderful life we could have in America, that it was the land of plenty, that she would take care of everything and that we would all be rich. But that still didn't explain things to us.

To her the answers were obvious, but to us none of this made sense. In any case, we girls wanted the answers to different questions: When would we go home? What about our families? What had gone wrong? Irma never mentioned our mothers and fathers, nor Mother Russia, nor even Mr Hurok, who had brought us to America and looked after us really well. Didn't he want to be our agent any more? Why not? Our tour had gone so well. We were more baffled than ever.

Now Irma made her worst and final blunder. She saw that we still hadn't got the message. By way of explanation, she pulled a green dollar bill out of her purse and said, "Don't forget!" And these were her exact words - I remember them so well - as she waved that dollar bill in front of us. "Don't forget: this is the most important thing!" I was surprised, because we had been brought up never to think of wealth. We all thought art was the most important thing, and money came some way behind. Nobody can be without money, because you can't live without money: we understood that. She didn't have to emphasise it.

And that was the most stupid gesture she ever made. Of all the girls, I especially was very surprised at her saying such a thing, and of course I was translating for the others, who never spoke English that well, whereas I had spoken it from infancy. So I translated her words and then looked at everybody. She could see we were not with her -

even when I had translated her words, most of us didn't see where this was leading – and she was exasperated that we couldn't see the point.

"You fools! Don't you understand, you stupid girls?"

Well, I was really annoyed. It didn't take me long to translate that.

What happened next changed all our lives for ever. Perhaps if I had been just a little older and had seen a bit more of the ways of the world, I might have waited to hear more, but I wasn't going to stay to be called a fool, by Irma or anyone. When I had translated her words for the other girls, I looked at everybody and I added a few words of my own.

"Now, there's something not right about this whole business. The thing is, if we do sign, we won't ever see our parents again, and now Irma is telling us we are stupid."

I stood up and walked out; and the others all spontaneously stood up and followed me.

To call us fools! For what reason? Because we didn't agree that the dollar bill was almighty? Because we didn't understand things we had never been told? She never explained what had happened with Sol Hurok; she never told us what the government had actually said; all she told us was that the Soviet authorities said we must return.

That was where she went wrong. We could do nothing about the government order; if that was what we had to do, what was there to discuss? Yet she was holding out a dollar bill to persuade us to stay. It didn't make sense.

We all felt there must be more that we hadn't been told and Irma was not being open with us. Nor did we feel she was really on our side, if she could call us 'fools'. To make matters worse, as we were going out, she said:

"And if you are thinking of staying in America, but you don't want to come with me, it will make no difference. If you decide not to go back to Russia, you will never see your parents again."

Now, how were we supposed to take that? It was a real insult. She could only think of one motive for us walking out: money. She evidently thought that, now we knew we could get a new contract, we would cut her out, forget about the school and make a better deal of our own. As if we would.

What now?

It was like a bombshell. We all went back to the flat and the other girls, they were all really bewildered. I remember that Shura, Tamara, Valya and, I think, Liza as well decided to stay, but I had already decided to go back, because I couldn't leave my mother by herself. How could I? It was impossible for me to think of doing that. I was her only child and she had sacrificed so much in life for me, which I well understood. And I was always very soft-hearted.

So I thought, *No: I can't leave my mother on her own*. I knew she had family in Russia still and they would look after her, but nevertheless who could tell what might happen later, when she was getting on in age? That was the first reason. The second reason I couldn't explain then, but later on I understood.

The other girls asked me what I was going to do. I said I couldn't leave my mother for ever, I just couldn't - even though I was very, very happy in America. We all were happy there, I must confess, and, as I said, some of the girls were thinking of staying.

When they went out, Mooshya's mother, Elzbieta Grigorevnya, who was our nurse, asked me - one of the youngest girls, though I had been the leader of our group in this crisis - for my advice.

"What would you suggest I should do?"

"Look, you can't ask a girl of 16 to advise you. I think you're old enough to know your own mind. In any case, what can I say? I can only remind you that in Moscow you have a lovely husband and three beautiful sons, and that is your home."

And I left it at that.

We had bought ourselves a Pet-o-phone, a new kind of portable gramophone, and someone bought a recording of a Russian song called *Ochy tchornye* - 'Black eyes', a Gypsy song, very well known. We all liked it and every girl bought themselves a copy. Now we were lying on our beds listening to it. When the big girls came back, they started to listen too and we played it again. We all began to feel very homesick. We didn't play it for that reason; it just came to hand and we were using it to try out our new gramophone.

But, from listening to that record, some of the older girls - Tamara, I remember, and Shura - decided No, they could not give up Russia, they couldn't, and they decided we should all go back. Funnily enough it was four of the youngest girls who were seriously thinking of staying.

Meanwhile my aunt in New York found out that we were thinking of going back to Russia, and she despatched her son to ask me to come round and see them, so I did.

"You know, Lili, I hear you girls are discussing going back?"

"Well, circumstances are forcing us to, Aunt."

"Think twice before you go, because they have a five-year plan over there now."

I had no idea what that meant and I don't think my aunt had either, but everyone in America had heard about Russia's new plan and who was in charge now. It didn't sound very sinister to me, though it might have done if anybody had told me in plain language what lay behind it.

I said to her I would think about it, and that's all I said. I knew she was very fond of me, and she wanted me to stay there, but even so I was a little bit suspicious. After all, I really knew nothing about her or her family. She had seen my name in the paper and approached me. I had never been told there was anybody related to my mother in New York. I didn't much care for her husband or her son, but I liked her all the same.

A wonderful appearance

After that, it turned out that we had ever so many friends, though where some of them came from, I've no idea. Maybe they were from the Russian consulate, keeping an eye on us. It was almost Christmas, New Year was coming soon and we realised we would be returning to Russia in winter.

We were taken to a fur shop and every girl was allowed to choose a fur coat. Of course, we couldn't have the really expensive furs, but they looked good all the same. They were coney, I think – rabbit fur, dyed – but the collars were fox fur. I chose a grey coat; it looked a bit like squirrel. We bought fluffy berets too. We looked capital, and we felt warm, all geared up for winter. God knows where the money came from.

We were looking forward to the big farewell party that Sol Hurok was giving for us. Earlier the same day, though, Irma invited us all round to her place. I don't know who she stayed with, but she lived very smartly in someone's house, and she really put on a show on

167

this occasion. Knowing Irma, I guessed there would be a purpose behind it.

When we arrived and she came to greet us, I had never seen her look so wonderful. She was wearing a *moiré* silk dress, beautifully cut, and long, beautiful earrings to match – granite, I think. She looked wonderful, with her black hair and really white skin. I was very taken with her appearance, because I always notice what looks well.

There was music and she started dancing with us. Soon she got hold of me and started talking, and I think that was her real purpose in inviting us. But it wasn't the only purpose, because before long she commented on the way we were dressed.

"You cannot go to Sol Hurok's party dressed like that! I will give you some clothes to wear. You can't go to such a big event as that – the whole opera house is going to be there, and a very well-known opera company from Germany: what would they think? You just can't appear looking like that."

She began pulling out trunks full of clothes, finding dresses and fitting us all up.

I know what she put on me: an ivory dress, with beautiful pendants of mother-of-pearl. I remember thinking, *Yes, I do look well in this; it suits me*. She put clothes on all the other girls too. Well, we had never had such clothes to wear! Maria particularly I recall, because she was one of my best friends. She had beautiful, long blonde hair, and for her Irma made up a kind of a tunic.

Irma knew from previous events that I liked ballroom dancing. She invited me to dance with her and as we were dancing she talked.

"Lili, I want to speak to you very seriously."

"Yes?"

"Stay with me. Let the other girls go, and you stay with me."

"Yes?"

"You're a fine teacher, Lili, and we will teach together."

Well, the idea would have suited me, but I could see one or two little drawbacks.

"Who? Who are we going to teach?"

The way we were brought up, the doctrine was always that everyone should have the same opportunities, whether they could pay or not. I knew that wouldn't be Irma's way. So I asked her again.

"Who are we going to teach?"

She stopped dancing.

"Well . . ."

I knew she couldn't answer. We could only find pupils through advertising, and who would we get? It had to be people who could pay: you can't live on nothing, and Irma liked to live well. So the first thing we'd be looking for would not be talent, but money. And who would we get? Children with doting parents. I knew Irma: she'd take anybody as a pupil, if she could make money from it.

We left it at that. She understood that, at the least, I was sceptical of her motives. And how could I trust her after the way she had behaved? I didn't mention this conversation to anyone else, not even to the other girls. She never asked any of them to teach with her; she only asked me because she thought my approach was similar to hers: she felt that I understood her way of teaching. I did, but I also understood Irma herself, all too well.

I could never trust her after seeing the way she behaved, the way she invited us to that meeting, never giving us any idea what was coming. Why wasn't she straight with us long before that? Why didn't she tell us there might be problems? Had she wanted to, she could have asked the consulate to get in touch with the Russian Government and ask whether it was true that we all had to break our contracts and go back. She could have tried to negotiate or persuade them, but she didn't, so there must have been some intrigue going on, which she kept from us.

I used to think about things and I always put two and two together. Some people you could trust, and certain people you just couldn't trust; and amongst those was Irma. Neither of us ever spoke about it again.

By now, it was time for Sol Hurok's party. We all dressed up against the cold and set off to the opera house, intending to have a very good time, which we certainly did.

A wonderful evening

Hurok organised a marvellous evening. The food was so plentiful, it was like a delicatessen and you could just help yourself to anything you fancied. Thanks to Irma, we girls looked lovely too, but we were not the only people invited for what was really a New Year party. The other guests included the entire cast of a touring German opera company, who were booked to perform at the opera house.

When we arrived, an orchestra was playing and the whole opera company was standing there, waiting to greet us. The orchestra struck up a dance tune and we girls were whipped up by young men – I had a partner immediately – and we all went straight onto the dance floor.

I really remember that gathering, it was so enjoyable. There was something nice about it, spontaneously nice. None of us knew one another, but it didn't take long for us to mingle and feel at home with people. The music never stopped and we didn't stop dancing.

We never drank alcohol at all normally, but this was a very special occasion and in any case it was New Year, so we all had a glass of champagne to perk us up. Marsha – Manya Toropchenova her name was, but I called her Marsha – was a little bit intoxicated and she suddenly darted out onto the dance floor. Irma had fixed her a kind of Grecian outfit, fastened on one shoulder, to show off her lovely skin.

As she ran out so suddenly, what was pinned up on the other shoulder fell off and exposed her breast. I have to say it didn't really matter, since she had so little to show. But we couldn't get over it; and she was so embarrassed, she flew straight back again.

"You be careful next time, Marsha. Don't run around madly like that."

"Lilya, I just had this impulse to rush out."

I don't know what she was doing; it wasn't even a Russian dance. Whatever it was, she just flew out.

At the end of that wonderful evening, we all said goodbye to one another. We thanked Sol Hurok very warmly for all he had done. Yet he never mentioned anything about the fact that we hadn't renewed the contract with him and he said not a word about us going back. That was very odd, when I think back. The whole thing made no sense. Irma kept us in the dark from beginning to end, but why did Sol Hurok never say a word to us, even when we were about to leave? Had there been some sort of arrangement between Hurok and Irma?

Last days in New York

At the end of the evening, we went back to our place. The next day we returned all our dresses to Irma. She wanted us to keep them, while we were saying No, no, we couldn't possibly keep anything. Most of us didn't want to keep them, even if the dresses did look beautiful on us. After that experience, I couldn't trust Irma - to me she wasn't straight, she didn't treat us as she should have done.

Nothing like that would have happened with Isadora, never in a million years: she would have told us everything. But then she wasn't devious like Irma - it's also true that Irma was very practical, whereas Isadora was just the reverse - but you had to face up to reality. We all felt that, after what had happened, we would never know where we were with Irma; we were better off returning to Russia.

In the time we had left, we went shopping. We were given money to spend, though it was never clear where the money came from. I know Irma had a lot of our money, so that is probably what it was. I was certain she wouldn't give us money from her own purse, because that would be too obvious. She said we had made up our minds to go, despite her efforts to persuade us to stay.

Well, I wouldn't really say what she did was very persuasive: it wasn't. She never explained anything - how all this had come about and why, what would happen or what choice we had - she didn't even suggest that we think it over. All she did was pull out that dollar bill. That was vulgar; it wasn't the way to talk to such lovely girls. We had been brought up to be straight, we could think for ourselves and we liked to know what was really going on.

Another bit of 'persuasion' that Irma tried, this time on Shura, was the same thing she had tried with Augustin's son and Marisha: she arranged for this handsome young man to meet Shura. Well, they were both quite grown-up, old enough to marry, so Irma invited him to come and get acquainted with Shura. But when Irma introduced them to each other, Shura wasn't remotely interested. She wouldn't even contemplate chatting him up; she looked on him as an irrelevance. How can you just walk up to someone, a person you have never met, with the idea of asking them to marry you - not knowing the person, not knowing anything about them? Shura just said, "No, no!" and she left. Irma couldn't get over that.

That happened while we were still deciding whether to go or not. Well, I had decided straightaway that I wasn't staying for various reasons, my mother being Reason Number One. I was still very obedient and I would listen to my mother, so if my mother had been in the picture, and if she had written to me and said 'Stay there!' I

171

would have done; but she didn't. As far as she knew, we were coming back to Russia, though she didn't know exactly when.

When word got around that we were returning to Russia, there were some rich people in New York who decided to buy us clothes and presents. They took us to the big stores and told us to choose what we liked, fur coats and all. And I still don't know who they were, even to this day.

We went shopping on Fifth Avenue. Among other things, I was looking for a certain type of shoe that I knew I wouldn't be able to get in Russia. We knew that in Russia everything would be in short supply, but little did we guess just how short of everything we would be.

The *Ile de France*

When the day came that we were to sail, a few of the friends we had made in New York came to see us off. We said goodbye to them, and they seemed to be genuinely sorry that we were leaving. Perhaps we were too, but we still had each other; we had stayed together, the whole group. Irma stayed in America, so our nurse Elzbieta Grigor-evnya took charge and showed herself really capable of managing things. This was the first time in all the years I had known her that she really did help us.

Irma had booked and paid for our passage on a ship called the *Ile de France*. All we knew before we boarded was that we were sailing to Cherbourg, as we had before. We expected it to be much the same as our previous transatlantic passages, which we had so much enjoyed. We were in for a surprise, and it was not the last. The boat was unbelievable – nothing like the *Caronia* or *Carinthia* of the Cunard Line.

The cabins had two bunks, one on top of the other. That wasn't so bad, having just two sharing, but the cabins were awful – tiny and dark, because they had no windows. They must have been below the waterline. Evidently Irma had bought the cheapest berths there were. What was worse, we hardly went out on deck, because we had such a rotten crossing. It was January, of course, but for five days our boat was constantly pitching and tossing. I was sharing with Liza, I think, and nearly the whole time we were being thrown from one end of the cabin to the other.

172

There were a couple of better days when we got out a bit, but meanwhile we found there were many Russians on board, going back home. We became friendly and they kept us company, especially one engineer who was rather *sympatiya*. We liked him and he used to come to our cabin every day to chat. I think he liked my company. Otherwise, the time went slowly, day after day. That boat was most unpleasant and we were glad to get to Cherbourg.

Paris: all change

We made our way to Paris and there we got another surprise. That was as far as Irma had booked us and she hadn't given Elzbieta Grigorevnya any money for our fares beyond Paris. This was the end of our journey, unless we wanted to walk to Moscow. When I look back, it sounds so funny and so awful too.

We arrived on a Sunday. We found ourselves a hotel and we had a little money between us, so we knew we could pay for a few nights at least. Now we had to find out how we were going to get back to Moscow. Here our nurse was very resourceful. She could have just sent a telegram to Irma, asking what to do. Instead, she said first she'd go to the Russian embassy and off she marched, taking one of the older girls with her.

Meanwhile, I liked Paris so I went off to look at the shops; we still had some money left from America. Paris was marvellous, just as it had been in the times of Balzac or Flaubert. When Flaubert was asked how he liked the Eiffel Tower, he said he liked it when he was inside it.

The following day Tamara Lobanovskaya asked me if I would like to come with her, because her mother had some friends in Paris, and I could come with her to meet them. I said Yes, I'd like that, so off we went and found where they lived. The two women turned out to be Whites, which perhaps I should have guessed. I've mentioned before that Tamara wasn't like some of the other girls; she came from a very well-to-do background. In Russian they were called *bevshel*, which means 'they were' – short for 'they were once well-to-do'.

These two ladies were rather nice and very friendly. In Russia they had never had to work, but in order to live they had had to learn a trade, so they used to make fine underclothes. I remember they were showing us these nice things they'd made. We chatted about this and

173

that, and they were very interested in us, but one of them said a strange thing to Tamara about me.

"The way that girl talks, she must have a very lovely voice."

Tamara laughed and said "She has: she sings beautifully."

So that was the very odd compliment I got, just through talking. We stayed a little while longer and then we left. Tamara was pleased that, when we got back to Moscow - if we ever did - she would be able to tell her mother about her friends in Paris.

Tashkent for bread

This was on the Monday. I have an idea the embassy could not - or would not - help us, so our nurse decided the best thing was to go and speak to a railway official at the Gare de Lyon, since that was one of the biggest termini in Paris, and find out about trains to Riga. Before she went, we all got together and decided that, if we could get to Riga, we would be able to stay there a few days, because the people at the ballet would look after us. We had got on very well with them when we stopped there with Irma, on our way to America.

If they could help us arrange some concerts there, that ought to raise enough to pay our fares to Moscow. We no longer had Irma with us, but we had had great success in America, and in Riga they liked us anyway. So Elzbieta Grigorevnya negotiated with the railway official.

"If you can manage to give us free tickets to Riga, we will pay for the journey when we get there. Whatever the cost of it, we will send you the money."

He agreed - by this time he had found out who we were - and after three or four days in Paris, we packed, marched off to the railway station and boarded the train for Riga.

After a couple of days' travel, we arrived in Riga and found a hotel. As soon as we had settled in, our nurse was busy organising things. When we were little, she always slept beside us, the youngest ones, and she used to tell us about the famine there was immediately after the revolution. There was no food to be had, but she was very resourceful - well, she was a nurse and she came from a very good background - and she used to go to Tashkent. Apparently there was a saying that Tashkent was the place for bread, so she used to travel there and bring back some bread or flour, whatever she could get. In those areas, Kazakhstan and Tajikistan, they grew wheat, so she knew about buying such things.

Riga for friends

So, as soon as we got there, we got in touch with the ballet and explained our situation. Could they arrange for us to give three concerts there? They gladly arranged everything and to our surprise – considering the short notice and limited publicity – each of the three nights was a great success.

We did 'Missimo', because the bigger girls knew all the choreo-graphy; they knew because Irma had shown them. Lately Irma had done very little dancing, so she had coached them and they were very confident. After the three concerts, we sent the money off to the railway official at the Gare de Lyon, to pay for our journey, and then bought our tickets to Moscow.

But how incredible that Irma should have done that. She was the one who arranged our passages, so she must have known what she was doing. Was it her revenge on us and Hurok? Or was it an idea thought up by the two of them? To pay our fares just to Paris, knowing that we had no money to buy tickets from there onwards, not even to Riga, never mind to Moscow?

We would have to stay in Paris, but how would we manage? Irma knew what money we had and what would happen when we got to Paris, with no tickets booked. I think now she must have calculated that we would see how foolish we had been, how we couldn't do anything without Irma and the thing to do now was send her a telegram, asking her to forgive us and book our passages back to New York. If that's what she thought, we gave her a big surprise.

And yet it was no bigger than the surprise she gave us when we reached Paris. None of us was told a thing – not even our nurse – and that is so odd. I always think, when things like that happen, it's so funny and so awful at the same time. Still, we managed. We liked Riga very much, but within a week it was time to board the train again, for the last part of our journey through the winter, back to Moscow. Home – wasn't that the most important thing? But now nothing seemed the same after America.

9

In Russia, in Love, 1930-3

Schneider's Five-Year Plan

When we got back to Moscow, we all went straight to our own homes. There was no thought of going back to school; in fact, I don't think the school existed any more, though Schneider still lived there. Later he moved into what had been our dining room and divided it into living and sleeping areas. He took all Isadora's furniture, including that very beautiful screen, made of mussel glass, with brass sphinxes (I think that's what they were) at the ends.

After a few days, we got in touch with the authorities and now we got another shock. They were as surprised as we were: "Why on earth did you come back? We never thought for a minute that you would; we've already formed a new group of Isadora Duncan Dancers."

This new group was led by Marisha. That, too, was a surprise to us, especially as she was hardly any older than the rest of us, but now a lot of things began to fit together. When we were reading Schneider's letter to Marisha, back in New York, we just thought how funny they were. Now, in retrospect, we saw that the scheming had begun even before we left Russia.

Schneider had gone down on his knees, asking Irma to let him go with us to America, but she wouldn't. Had he gone, he would have smelt a rat long before Irma got far with her schemes and we would have stayed in America. He must have guessed that Irma would be tempted to stay in America and she would try to get us to stay too. Schneider was not the man to stand by while someone took away his position, his income and his home. He must have had a plan.

Luckily, he had Marisha - or perhaps it wasn't luck at all? - and he

176

made sure her contract freed her to return to Russia after six months. As a result, she got paid for her dancing in America; no one else did, because Irma claimed we had broken our contracts. We were young and inexperienced; what could we do or say?

Irma

For all that Irma was so clever, it seemed Schneider had been cleverer. She never deceived him at all, though perhaps she thought she had. Why did Irma make such a mess of things? She lost everything, except money – but then she did say that was the only thing that mattered. Apparently it didn't matter that she deceived us. She deceived Hurok too, letting him think we were going to sign a new contract with him, while negotiating behind his back with other people. That was why he caused her all that trouble, with the court case and the publicity about it.

Yet the new contract she signed, though it would have paid her twice as much as before, did not pay her to dance. She was to be our coach and manager, but she was specifically excluded from appearing on stage as a dancer, and I think she resented that. She was jealous of us girls, our youth and our abilities as dancers. From then on, I think, there was a bitterness to whatever she did.

Later she wrote a book about her experiences. It is very interesting, but reading it you might easily get the impression that Irma toured on her own in the 1920s and we girls were somewhere else. In China she talks about where she went, what she did and the people she met, with no mention of the girls of the Isadora Duncan School, who were the reason she was there at all. It is the same when she writes about Paris, where she says "misfortune struck me" – but that was later, in New York. You could call it 'misfortune', but sometimes people make their own luck.

Once she saw that we were not going to join her, Irma gathered together dancers to form a new group in America, and they went on to become very famous there, but they were not the best. Margot was not so bad, but she was never going to be really good. When she visited Russia and came to see me, she asked my advice, saying, "I want to perfect my dancing." The kindest thing I could think of to say was, "We haven't enough time to do that." She didn't stay.

Anna and Teresa Duncan joined Irma's group, but they were

dreadful dancers. And Anna too made a mess of her life, even more than Irma. She was so beautiful and lived to a good age, yet she died in a nunnery. The only decent one was Teresa. She had soft, dark auburn hair; she was a better dancer than Anna, and Augustin, Isadora's eldest brother, adored her.

None of this should have been any surprise to Irma, because she and Isadora had picked out the very best dancers as children and trained us over a number of years. The only surprise, perhaps, was that we had different ideas about the most important thing.

Crimea and Astrakhan, 1930

We were all dreadfully disappointed to find that we were not expected and apparently not wanted. But then we were approached by Basmanov, who had been our manager at one time. He wanted to arrange a tour for us to the Crimea, and we agreed. We went as a group and he paid us very well. Then he offered us a tour down the Volga to Astrakhan.

Meanwhile, our pianist, the one who said he would never leave his parents, well of course he never returned. But that didn't matter because we got a very good pianist to replace him. Apart from that, he was so nice and all the girls became very friendly with him. We did not even call him by his surname: his first name was Vladimir, but we gave him a pet name and called him Vovachka, because he was so charming. Now we started to work with him and he was very happy to be with us.

He was with us when we started that tour down the Volga. It was a most beautiful trip and it came in very useful; later I will tell you why. We were glad to be dancing again. We knew we were at our best, not just because we had trained so hard or because we were now seasoned performers, but also we were young and lovely, and now we were getting plenty of fresh air and the most marvellous food. Those Volga boats were famous for their food.

On the way downriver we stopped a few times, though I don't recall anything about our concerts. What I do remember is that the trip was just as charming as the ones we had made a few years earlier, with the school. We went right down to Astrakhan, where we gave several concerts.

Astrakhan is the home of caviar. Just below the city, the Volga

178

ends in the Caspian Sea, where they catch the sturgeon from which caviar comes. So we found out where the factory was and managed to buy a kilo of caviar. That was marvellous because there was such a shortage of food in Russia. That caviar was very useful when we brought it home.

Following this very successful tour, the government approached us: they wanted to make one group out of the two. Schneider was to be manager, which was fine, and Marisha was to be in charge of the rest of us. We flatly refused that. Tamara was the leader of our group; we were used to her and she was much more intelligent than Marisha, and *sympatiya* too.

So Marisha left the group and stopped dancing, but she found that she missed us all. She and Schneider had a big flat, on a street parallel with Prechistenka where the school was, and we used to visit them quite often.

This was when Elena entered the group; she didn't go to America, not being good enough then. Next we had some concerts in St Petersburg and met Lunacharsky again, with his secretary; they were about to go abroad. He asked us the same question as the government: "Why did you come back? You must have been mad!"

Mooshya's party

Mooshya was feeling very down, so she decided to have a party. What made this easier was that she had three brothers, and two of them were very handsome. The first brother, Aleg, was a sportsman, tall and beautiful looking; the middle one, whose name was Slava, was a lawyer or something like that; and she also had a very young brother, called Meega.

We all arrived, all the girls with their boyfriends, and we all sat down and started talking. The young men naturally wanted us girls to join them, and I sat down along with two other girls. It was much like any other party. Young people are much the same all the world over, aren't they?

But they were all smoking, and I was surprised. I had never even thought of smoking. Somebody offered me a cigarette and I said, "No, thank you. I don't smoke." And they all shouted, "Spoilsport!"

People talk about youngsters today and what a bad influence they can be on one another; but it was no different in our youth, and how

179

many years ago is that? I am talking about the early thirties, 1931, getting on for 1932, just shortly after we came back from America. And of course they forced me; it seems extraordinary, but if you found yourself outnumbered like that, you would think: *Well, I can't stand out against the majority.*

So I tried a cigarette. I didn't particularly like it, and I didn't dislike it. So they left me alone after that and we began dancing. Mooshya lived in a very big flat, because her father had some high position. Her mother had been our nurse. Originally they lived on the third floor, but some important official who lived on the ground floor liked their flat better and he decided they should switch flats. That was how they treated people in Russia, at least until the system changed.

When they moved downstairs, they had to put iron bars on all the windows because it was so dangerous to live on the ground floor, but they made the flat nice. It was a rather prestigious block and the flats were spacious and well equipped, so really they couldn't do anything but accept the change. There were plenty of rooms – I think they had three bedrooms, a lounge, a dining room, a kitchen and their own bathroom – and they had lovely furniture. They always lived well.

Anyway, we had a smashing time at this party – quite literally. There was something about my Marsha: things always seemed to happen to her.

"Lilya, you know what? My watch slipped off my wrist and somebody trod on it before I could pick it up, because we were all dancing. And they smashed it."

"Marsha, really! Aren't you careless! So, can it be repaired?"

"I don't think so."

"Marsha, why can't you be more careful?"

"Well, things happen; you can't help it."

That was a sad episode, because watches then were a bit of a luxury. I felt sorry for her, and I said so, but she didn't dwell on it. She used to laugh things off.

Otherwise, we had all rather enjoyed ourselves. I certainly had, except for that smoking. Grigori – whom I shall say more about in a moment – used to smoke, and after that he would always offer me a cigarette. I did take to it a little, but I never smoked more than four in one day. I didn't care for it much and I wasn't addicted to it, but I had a little puff here and there.

One too many

After New York and Paris, Moscow was bound to seem a bit dull. It wasn't just that life was difficult in Russia; it was more that in America we had been admired, talked about, fussed over and constantly invited to events, to people's houses and to splendid parties. We weren't so special in Moscow, though we still had plenty of invitations.

Shortly after we arrived back from America, I got to know a young man called Grigori, and he often invited me to go somewhere with him. Well, it was amusing after all, and as an escort he wasn't bad to look at, but, to be honest, at times he got on my nerves. He was an economist, and there were plenty of those in Russia, so he had quite a big circle of friends.

His best friends lived outside Moscow: they invited him round and told him to bring that girl from America who had just arrived – which he did. They had a nice spread with plenty of booze, as they called it. That was something I wasn't used to.

His friends were not dull, and certainly they were not ignorant, but they just didn't appeal to me, because they never talked about the arts, which were what I liked and what I did. They didn't seem to be very interested in that or even in what I had been doing. All they were concerned about was to get me drunk. Of course, I didn't realise that; but afterwards, when I did see it, I couldn't get over it.

Well, they kept on pouring more wine, which I knew nothing about really, only that it helped the food down. After all, they had provided a nice supper, plenty of lovely home-made dishes, but each time I had a sip of wine they used to top up my glass, so I didn't realise how much I was having, until I really felt awful. I couldn't stand it any longer and I said so to Grigori.

"I feel sick."

"Don't worry. I'll take you outside. You'll soon feel better."

So he took me out and I relieved myself of all that wine and that feeling of nausea, which was ghastly.

That did teach me a lesson, once and for all, not just to be careful how much wine I drank, but also never to trust people. How could they do such a thing? The audacity of it, to do that to a young person – I wasn't even 17 at the time, still 16. So young, so innocent. But you get over it.

A blue-eyed boy

The party continued all night, so I just had to wait until it was over for Grigori to take me home. The following morning, I was all dressed to go home and thinking, *I never want to see people like that again, however wonderful their parties are*. As I was standing waiting for Grigori, a nice young chap came up to me and introduced himself as Ivan Ivanich. I noticed he had beautiful blue eyes.

There were so many young people at the party, I hadn't noticed him, but funnily enough he had noticed me. Now he showed great interest in me: Why had I come here from America? What was I doing now? I told him I was a dancer. When I mentioned the name Isadora Duncan, he knew about her. I discovered Ivan Ivanich was rather intelligent and we walked about while I was waiting. He asked me for my telephone number and I thought, why not? He seemed rather nice, and his face – a real Russian face – was what I would call *sympatiya*. He had a nice smile and those lovely eyes, and blond hair. He did attract me.

Grigori got me home safely, and of course my mother was very anxious to know how I had got on. I didn't say much. I had got into the habit of saying very little about myself, because she had a tendency to take charge. She never looked on me as grown up. She pushed Grigori at me because *she* liked him; she never asked if *I* liked him. I resented that. He was very persistent, but I had started thinking about this Ivan Ivanich.

At this time, our dance group was not very happy. Mooshya, our nurse's daughter, dropped out, because she had so many problems, but we had plenty of girls, so we could always manage well enough. Nonetheless, we had to rehearse much more frequently now with our new company.

One day we had a rehearsal and my Marsha, of whom I was so fond, was on her way there by train. She was telling a friend that she had to hurry because of this rehearsal, and she mentioned to her friend that we were dancing something of Isadora Duncan's. When we met, she mentioned this to me because of a little episode that followed.

There was a nice young man sitting not far from them. As soon as Marsha mentioned Isadora Duncan, this young man began listening to what she was saying. She noticed his blue eyes too.

"Marsha, I met a young man like that the day before yesterday. I

182

was at a party and there was a young chap that I liked. He had blue eyes."

"I'm sure it was the same young man."

"What makes you say that?"

"Because he was suddenly so very interested in what I was saying to my friend."

Shortly after this I had a phone call from Ivan Ivanich.

"Do you remember me?"

"Yes, I do."

"I was travelling on a train and I am certain I met one of the dancers in your group."

"What makes you think that?"

"I heard her say, to the friend she was travelling with, that she must hurry or she would miss the rehearsal – and I'm sure she mentioned Isadora Duncan. I just put two and two together. I thought your friend would tell you about me."

"You're quite right. She told me she had seen somebody who looked like you, taking notice of what she was saying."

The next time I saw Marsha, I told her she had been right all along: it was Ivan Ivanich that she saw. From then on, Ivan Ivanich quite often phoned me and asked me to come out. That was nice. I liked a little walk in the evening.

Grigori has his uses

It was wintertime, there weren't so many things you could do and it was interesting to have some new company; Ivan was rather intelligent too. That's not to say Grigori wasn't: I just didn't like the sort of person Grigori was. He was too demanding – in fact, he was obsessed with me. I don't know why. Perhaps he fell for me the first time he saw me, as a girl of 15, before we went to America.

I have no idea why he took such a great fancy to me. He was always wanting me to go somewhere with him; even if it was a street demonstration, he would ask me to join him. One day we walked nearly down to the Kremlin and I was very thirsty. One of our girls, Lulya, lived not far from there. She had a big family, so I felt sure there would be someone at home.

"Let's pop in at my friend's house; she will be pleased to see me."

So we popped. It wasn't a very big building where they lived, though it had a big yard, and that's where her entrance was. I knocked at the door and she came out.

"Lulya, I'm so thirsty! We were just passing; I wonder if we could have a drink?"

"Who's that with you?"

"That's my boyfriend."

"Really? He's very handsome."

She told all her sisters, and they ran out one by one to have a look at him. I couldn't get over it. I thought: *How funny - they like him and I don't.*

For all that, he filled in the time for me. When you are young you want to do things and a girl needed someone with her, to take her to places. We used to go to concerts, but culturally I think that was about his limit and he only did it for me. He had no interest in music, but he soon got interested if anybody looked at me. Our conversation would get quite animated at such times.

"I am just going to speak to that man and ask him what he thinks he's doing, looking at you all the time."

"Look, Grigori, if you don't behave, I'll walk out. Calm yourself and sit down again. I mean, everybody can look where they want and you have no right to feel bad about it."

We often went to see a show and met friends there, so I didn't have such a dull time. But I never felt complete.

Tamara

Although Big Tamara was still in charge, we already knew she was ill. She had started to feel weak and they diagnosed tuberculosis. Her mother had had TB before the revolution and recovered - but things were different then.

Her mother had managed to get a place in a sanatorium where the patients slept in the pine woods. They rested there day and night - they never lived indoors at all - and all that fresh air did help to cure them. They had various remedies as well. They used to pick the very thick stem of a cactus and boil it with chocolate to make a kind of stew that they drank. We told Tamara to make that to help her.

But now things were not so easy in Russia, and Tamara lived in such dreadful surroundings. You couldn't believe that, with such an opportunity to stay in America, this beautiful girl in the prime of life would come back to live with her mother. Does the place where you were born and bred always draw you back? Perhaps she missed her mother too, but they lived in a basement and it was awful.

Because of that I very seldom went to see her. I used to arrange to meet her somewhere or else she would pop in to see me. If she met a friend, a girl or a boyfriend, and she was passing, she would always come up and introduce me.

We all had a very good relationship with Tamara, but I was particularly fond of her and I saw how brave she was. I often thought of that American Indian, telling her she was going to die young. It never quite left my mind. I don't think any of the other girls knew about that episode and Tamara would never mention it. She would never make any fuss, but also she wouldn't want to admit she was even a little superstitious. Nevertheless, I understood the idea was in her mind, deep down, because she couldn't seem to fight her illness.

It didn't help that she was in love, though you might think it would. The trouble was, she fell in love with a man whom you really couldn't trust. She brought him round to see me and afterwards asked me what I thought of him. I said, "Look, Tamara, you are happy and that is all that matters. Just don't ask me about it." She was quite happy with him, but I never liked him. I don't like people who aren't sincere.

More fish in the sea

Before we'd gone to America, Ivan Ivanich had come to see us dancing. Afterwards he came backstage especially to see me and praised me: "You dance so softly." Well, I was very light and very supple from an early age, and I never lost that lightness. I used to jump the highest of any of the girls; I know that, because Irma had noticed it.

She had once come into the studio when we were doing some exercise that involved jumping on the spot and then doing a frog leap. She watched us for a minute and then said, "Lili, see how high you can jump on the spot." So I did, and I went up really high in the air, so high that Irma couldn't get over it. She always said, when I did something particularly well, "Girls, just try and do the same as Lili." But often, of course, they couldn't. That ability was part of my make-up; the others were light, but they could never jump that high. So,

185

when Ivan Ivanich said to me how softly I danced, I was not surprised. He and I used to meet periodically. I was fond of him and we used to walk out in the evenings sometimes.

One day my mother told me she had had a phone call to say that Auntie Annie's eldest son, Barney, had come to Moscow to work, along with his wife, and he wanted us to come and see him. "That's lovely" I said, and we went round.

I always liked Barney's wife, Tanya – she had a certain charm that appealed to me – but they were both pleased to see me. Barney said, "By the way, did you know that Moss, the middle one of us brothers, is coming to Moscow too?" Apparently they had been invited by the Russian Government because they spoke English and Barney was working in a research field that the Russians were interested in. At that time the Depression was bad in England; in fact all over Europe work was scarce. It was very difficult to find a job, so Barney quickly took up that offer.

But why did Moss come? They invited him too, but he already had a good job in England. He worked in a bank and earned quite a good salary. Nevertheless, they were a close-knit family, and Moss was very fond of Barney. There was something more than that, though, because one day after rehearsal, when I came home, my mother was waiting for me with a question.

"Guess who has been here?"

"No, I don't know; I can't guess."

"Moss came; he waited for you."

"Oh? That's odd."

I knew him, of course, but we were never close, not the way I was with Freddy, the youngest brother. I was surprised that he dropped in like that. In fact, I was rather intrigued when my mother told me about Moss having called to see me. "Um," I said, "that was interesting." But I never gave it any thought. It never occurred to me to go round and see him.

By now I was getting terribly tired of Grigori. His behaviour towards me was so persistent. He wouldn't let me breathe, let alone have any freedom. It was as if I was his property and now he had got hold of me, he wasn't going to let me go. Well, I was fed up with being his trophy.

Barney phoned and invited me to go round there one evening. We fixed a date and he added, "Bring your boyfriend with you – don't come by yourself." I told Grigori, who knew the family a little. He remembered Freddy, but he had never met Moss, Barney or Tanya. I know it's a funny thing to say, but I never really liked Grigori, but I will say this for him: he was certainly rather striking in appearance. So Tanya sat up and took notice of him.

Moss had a streak of humour that I liked very much. He had only recently arrived from London and he had brought all sorts of funny gadgets with him. He had a piece of sugar with flies on it and, whenever Tanya put sugar on the table, he would add that piece to the sugar bowl. Tanya would try to brush it away and the fly wouldn't move. Then he put out a box of matches: when you went to pick it up, the box would shoot away from you. These things were novelties then and they really made us laugh.

Naturally, he had to play a joke on Grigori. Under the cushion of the armchair he put one of those rubber cushions that made a raspberry sound when you sat down. Grigori sat down and it made that very rude sound, but it wasn't a novelty to him and he didn't blink an eye. That's what Moss was like sometimes.

That first evening, I noticed Moss looked at me a great deal and I couldn't understand why. After that, though, he used to come and see me quite often, and I really grew to like him. He was full of fun, but he was also intelligent and knew such a lot; no wonder they called him 'the walking encyclopaedia'.

I had been going out with Grigori for over a year, because when I came back from America in January 1930 I was still 16. I had celebrated my 17th birthday that April and now I was turned 18. I thought to myself, *I must part with this man. No matter what happens, I don't care. But it is going to be very difficult without some help. This is my opportunity, because I will have a man to help me.* I also had to tell my mother.

"Mother, I have had enough of Grigori. Now I am 18, I know my own mind and this is what I am going to do. And don't you interfere with me."

"All right, Lilya, I promise."

"Speak to Moss while I am out at rehearsals – he will come, I know he will. And tell him I want him to escort me whenever I go to a concert."

When I got back from the rehearsal, my mother said she had spoken to him and, when she had explained what was wanted, Moss had said he would be round like a bullet when I said the word. So that was agreed.

187

The following day Moss came round, so I got hold of Grigori. He came round to our flat and I told him the news that I had decided we should part.

"Remember, Grigori, there are plenty more fish in the sea. With your looks and position and everything, you can meet lots of nice girls. Just forget about me, for good. I've always said I didn't want to marry you. If I wanted to, I would – but I don't. So I insist we part. Look, be a man: stand up and face facts."

I had to add that last bit because he couldn't seem to get over it. I was talking to him in the kitchen, because there was nobody else there, and he went down on the kitchen floor on his knees. But I was firm. I thought, *I've made up my mind this time to break up with him*.

He had made my life quite unpleasant: I couldn't stand the way he was so obsessed with me. It seemed I couldn't go anywhere without him. And when we did go out, even if I did meet people, nobody got a chance to speak to me or be friends with me, never. He was there all the time like a hawk. But this time he was dumbstruck. I was firm, I walked out, I went to my room and I closed the door. That was how it finished. Or so I thought.

The first sign

Every time we had a concert, Moss used to come with me, and even when we didn't he used to come and see me. After a while it was every day. I used to wait for him, and we would eat together whatever food my mother had prepared. She and I never sat down to our meal without him, and he so appreciated it.

To be honest, we fell in love. It was the first time it had happened to me. I think in everybody's life, there is never anything quite like the first time you fall in love. We found we had to be always to-gether, whatever we were doing, even if it was just to eat.

When he finished work, he would come home – Moss was living with his elder brother and his wife – and then he used to disappear. Barney and Tanya wouldn't ask him where he was going; they would never do that, but they talked to one another and wondered where he went. Tanya used to prepare a meal and Moss would say he had been invited out. And so he had, in a way. At any rate, he always came to us to eat. It wasn't just that my mother cooked very well, because Tanya wasn't a bad cook either.

If I was performing, Moss would escort me to the concert and wait for me afterwards. One night, when we had finished, the other girls must have finished changing before me. Our dressing room had a big round table in the middle, and round the walls each of us had a dressing table, a mirror and a chair, so we could put on a little make-up.

All the others had packed their things and gone downstairs, and I was just packing up, when one of the girls came running in to warn me.

"Lilya, you have a problem! I think you've got trouble."

"Now what?"

"Grigori is here, downstairs, unshaven, and he looks ferocious."

"What?!"

"You had better hurry."

And she disappeared. Before I could finish packing, Grigori walked in. He got straight to the point.

"Now I am going to kill you."

I was very frightened, because he looked so awful, so pale, and I thought, *I bet he will too – he will choke me or something. What am I going to do with a big chap like him?*

He came round the table and I dodged the other way. He ran round the table after me, but I was quicker. I was so quick on my feet, being a dancer, and that really helped me. I even found time on the way round to pick up my little bag with my tunic and I darted to the door, flew down the stairs and ran right into Moss's arms.

"What now?"

I told him what had happened.

"Don't worry. Leave it to me."

Grigori had followed me down, and now Moss went up and spoke to him.

"Look, there is no point in behaving like this. A man like you, a handsome man, can always get himself a girlfriend. There are plenty of nice girls, but this one doesn't like you. She never did. She told you that, so it's hardly news to you. She never wanted to marry you; she said so. What's the point, lingering like this? Trying to hang on and just upsetting yourself? Why don't you just go away and forget about her?"

Moss managed to calm him down, which I could never have done.

189

I didn't know how to deal with it myself; I really needed his help. It was such a relief when he saved me that night, and then persuaded Grigori never to come back, that I can't put it into words.

After that, we were out walking nearly every day, and Moss came round every evening. We knew what time he would come, and we would be ready to have dinner at that time, usually about half-past six. Then we would sit down to our meal. We both understood how the other felt, without saying a word. I think that's the first sign you are falling in love, when you both want to be together all the time.

A proposal

One evening after dinner, we went for a walk. Moss said something that got me interested, and made me rather intrigued.

"You know what, Lilya?"

"Yes?"

"I am going to start a new page in my life."

"Oh?"

"I am going to tell you something. I must confess that I so love you so deeply, and so truly, that I want you to be my wife. What would you say to that?"

"Oh yes! That is what I would love best of all!"

We were so happy. When we got home, my mother had just finished washing up. We told her we had decided to get married and she was pleased. I don't think she was overjoyed, knowing her, but still she was pleased.

Moss and I thought to ourselves, *Now we have to tell Barney about this, and Tanya. What will they say?* All that time, they never knew that Moss was coming to our flat for dinner every day. But they were both very happy for us.

So, in the spring of 1933, we married.

A bad move for Uncle Isaac

Luckily enough, not long before this, my uncle – my mother's elder brother, the one that she followed, who fled from Odessa and settled in Paris – my uncle Isaac moved to Berlin. He had married in Paris, but returned to Russia after the revolution, just as my mother had, along with his wife and their little boy.

Their boy was nearly grown up now, but from birth he had had some little deformity in his shoulder and neck. It meant he couldn't turn his head very far to the left. That was all. I remember that, when I saw him, he was a nice boy and very pleasant to look at. I liked my uncle very much and I often used to go round to their place. My cousin was fond of me too, so we all got on well.

Uncle Isaac was a member of the party, and they offered him a job in Berlin, running a bank, which he took. He was a very capable man, so running a bank was not a problem to him, and he thought that he might be able to get treatment for his son in Berlin. His son didn't look Jewish, being tall and blond.

This move was lucky for us, because they were selling their furniture. I bought many things from them, even before Moss came along: a beautiful double bed made of mahogany, since the one we had was so awful, a table and dining chairs, and a kind of sideboard where we kept glasses and cutlery. My room now looked a lot nicer and it was really comfortable.

Life upside down

After our wedding, we had a party, and from Moss I had a basket of the most beautiful flowers. We had a lovely spread, with salmon, caviar and all sorts of delicacies because, funnily enough, you could buy such things in Moscow then, even though some Russians could hardly get enough to eat. But, if you were a foreigner invited to come to Russia – there were quite a few from England, very few from France – you could buy groceries at a special shop on the square.

That shop was E. Ilyasevsky's. It was a beautiful place and very prestigious. They sold all kinds of food, but only for hard currency, not for roubles. Moss had brought quite a bit of hard currency with him from London and, by the terms of his contract, he was paid half in sterling and half in roubles. So he could buy freely in Ilyasevsky's, and that made life so much easier. You could get the best of everything there.

Later on, one of our favourite occupations was to go to the shop and indulge in certain little pastries that we liked. They also had lovely little flaky pastries with meat inside, rather like the one I had on the street as a cold, hungry little girl on my first day in Moscow, when my mother and I went for a walk to get away from that awful hospital. Now Moss and I had some real comforts.

When he came to live in our flat, he brought some furniture out of store. He had a leather two-seat settee, called a put-you-up, which you could make into a bed at night. That was very useful when we had visitors. He brought an extra wardrobe too. I already had that mahogany bed, and he liked that.

Well, we had a lovely party and so began our married life. Moss and I got on really well; we were just so comfortable with each other. Now everything seemed entirely different. I felt as if my life had been turned completely upside down, yet in a lovely way. I had never before felt as happy as I did then.

My new life changed everything. Wherever I was, whoever was with me, whatever I was doing, the thought kept running through my head: *Now I have somebody with me, and I love him so much.* Even when I was travelling to rehearsals, he never left my mind; and when I was going home to him, I felt so happy. I had never experienced anything like it before.

Of course, the other girls noticed. One by one, they took me aside and asked, "What has happened to you?" And I said simply, "I am so happy." That was all I said. I didn't want to exaggerate my feelings. I just wanted to hug them to myself.

The neighbours

We had a neighbour downstairs called Mahmet, who worked in the Kremlin. At first he lived on his own and then one day he told me that his wife was coming to join him. Soon after she arrived, I met her – this was before I got married – and we became very friendly.

She was a lovely little woman. She was older than me, but that didn't make any difference. We never stopped talking, because she liked talking as much as I did. We were both very pleased to meet somebody in our block who was willing to stop and chat, because everybody else seemed to live their own lives and keep themselves to themselves. By contrast, she was very open.

She used to pop in to see me, and I used to pop down to see her. Sometimes she would even phone me, to ask if I would like to come down for a little while, and I'd tell Moss, "I won't be long." But of course we used to get carried away and talk for ages.

She told me all about her life. She came from Baku, and Mahmet came from Tiflis, and their backgrounds were very different. How they met was remarkable. She came from a large family, all girls and not just good-looking, but extraordinarily beautiful. Their parents were very rich; they owned two oil rigs and about ten big blocks of flats. Mahmet was a Communist, and after the revolution he was sent to requisition their property, to take everything away, in fact.

Nevertheless, he became friendly with one of the daughters. Her name was Sonya, and he told her that he was going to Moscow, to work in the Kremlin, and if she wanted to come, she would be welcome. He would be very pleased to see her. She said to me that, because of what had happened in her personal life, she had no option but to come to Moscow and get in touch with Mahmet.

They decided to get married. She always told me she didn't really have a choice; it was a question of circumstances. She wasn't unhappy, because he was a kind man. He was a big man too: tall, I would say, but very light on his feet, because all Georgians are. I mention Sonya not only because she was so lovely, but because Mahmet was so kind to me always. If ever I was in need, he would always offer to help. He was highly placed in the Kremlin.

This was such a happy time. Moss and I had a wonderful circle of friends, particularly in the world of literature and the arts generally. It was stimulating to know people like that, and we went out regularly too. It was our system of living: once a week we went to see a film and once a week we went to see an opera, or sometimes a ballet if it was something of interest.

I remember especially the Stanislavsky theatre; they had extraordinarily beautiful dancers and they used to put on some wonderful shows. They produced a new ballet about the Bakhchisaray Fountain, the Fountain of Tears that I saw when I went to Samarkand, the one in Pushkin's poem. It was in that theatre that they put on *Sinbad the Sailor*. The ballet was magnificent. The stage set made the sea and the boat quite real. One thing I must say about Russia: perhaps they starved, but they had the most wonderful theatres.

Barney and Tanya

So time went by, and Moss and I enjoyed life very much. Our closest friends were Moss's elder brother, Barney, and his wife. I liked Tanya, and she liked me; in fact, she was very fond of me. Moss, she looked on very much as if he were an elder brother, except that she was in charge.

We met up twice a week. That was absolutely a must. Once a week they used to come to us for dinner, and once a week we went to them. They had a lovely flat. It didn't belong to them; no one in Moscow owned their own home, with a few exceptions. One of those was our flat. It was called a co-operative flat; my mother paid for it gradually out of her earnings, and therefore it belonged to us.

But Barney and Tanya were given a flat when the government invited Barney to work in Moscow. There were lots of flats like that, for officials and their families. It was a very nice flat in the centre of Moscow, in a very nice part of the city near Pushkin Square, where his monument stands.

Tanya was delighted with Moss's choice, and in fact for our honeymoon she and Barney suggested we should take a house in the country and they would share it with us. It was coming round to that time of the year when anyone who could manage it moved to the country for the summer. They so wanted that, and we agreed.

We found a very nice place in the country, with two lovely bedrooms, a very good kitchen, a pleasant sitting room, a big veranda and a pretty garden. Very often her mother used to come down to visit, and so did my mother. Tanya's mother had got married for a second time, to a very pleasant man. We all liked him. In fact, we all got on very well. I still have photos from that lovely summer.

10

Life Opens Out, 1933-8

A walk in the birch forest

Meanwhile, Moss went off to work each day, and so did Barney.
Tanya and I stayed at home, or rather at the house in the country that
we were renting. She used to cook, and very well, but I found
cooking difficult. Luckily, I was allowed a honeymoon in the kitchen
as well. It lasted about three months altogether.

In the summer, nearly everybody left Moscow. It was a habit; not
only did Moscow get too hot, but the countryside around it was so
lovely in the warm weather. And it wasn't difficult to reach, so you
could still go to town for work. It was convenient and pleasant, and
we were all very happy, until one day in July, only a few weeks after
our marriage.

Moss came home with some news. "You know what, Lili? They
want me to go to London. We are buying some machinery, and they
want me to help arrange it." He was an obvious choice, because he
spoke both Russian and English, and this contract was something to
do with his department. Naturally, I was pleased for him.

Everything was booked and paid for, but they gave him some
money for expenses, about £25. It was in £5 notes, I think, big black-
and-white notes, nearly the size of handkerchiefs, and he kept them
in his wallet. He always carried this with him, even if we just went
for a walk. It was the height of summer and you don't wear thick
clothes then, do you? I was in a summer dress and he wore a summer
shirt, so he would stuff the wallet in his trouser pocket.

It was not long until he had to go and our time together was
precious, so nearly every day the two of us would take a walk in the
forest, not far from the house. He was very good at whistling – he

used to imitate the birds – and I was charmed, really. Then we would run about and he used to chase me.

One evening we got back and found he had a hole in his pocket: his wallet had gone. What were we to do? He was setting off shortly and he couldn't go without the money and his documents, but how do you find a thing like a wallet in a forest? Even if the forest is very open, as this one was. It wasn't dense and overgrown: it was a beautiful forest, all birch trees, pleasant and easy to walk through.

Now it happened that not far from us was a place where a party of schoolchildren were spending their holiday in the country. This gave my clever Moss an idea. He went to see the head teacher and told her what had happened. He asked her whether they went into the forest very often and, if so, would they keep a look-out for his wallet? She promised they would look, and there were thirty or forty children there, so, if they all looked hard, there was a chance.

A few days passed and then we heard they had found it. This was an absolute miracle, but it was all the result of Moss's bright idea. We went out to get them the largest box of chocolates we could find, to thank them. So they were pleased and we were pleased – or, in my case, pleased and not pleased at the same time.

First parting

I realised that I wanted to go too. I said to Moss, "Take me with you." "Oh, it is too late to arrange that." I begged him. "Please take me with you." I thought that, if I went with him, I would never come back. I never told him that, but he must have sensed it and he put me off. He said, "It's too late; you can't arrange things like that overnight."

I saw him off at the station. I think it was called the Alexander Station, the one where people arrived from the West. There were many such foreigners, coming to Moscow for various reasons. The biggest number came from England, and Moss was in charge of looking after them, so he often went down to the Alexander Station to meet them and introduce them to one person or another.

At the station there were many foreigners. It was autumn now and these people all had expensive-looking topcoats. They all looked so smart to us, entirely different from the Russians. They always attracted me and reminded me of America.

196

Moss could see I was a little bit sad and he said, "Don't worry. I am only going for a month." I couldn't do anything about it, because he hadn't asked his department if I could go, and by the time I begged him, it was too late, I suppose. But I don't think he wanted me to go with him, because he sensed what I would do.

Three deaths

Never mind, he went. I was left with my mother, Tanya and Barney, though not for long. We soon moved back to our own places in the city. Our dance group had some bookings and I started touring with the girls. I kept busy and the time went quickly.

Besides my Sonya, I had another neighbour downstairs in the block where we lived. Her name was Olga, Olga Lynch. I liked her; she was friendly. She used to distribute tickets for various shows and, knowing I was on my own, she once or twice asked me if I would like to go with her to see an operetta or whatever was on. We used to go out together when I was at home.

Among our nearest neighbours – very near, because they even shared the same toilet – there was a couple with four children. I wouldn't say they were old, but they weren't young either. They had one grown-up son and another a bit younger, then a little girl, a lovely little girl, and a very young boy who was a cripple.

At first, the two older boys – they were rather good-looking boys – were away in the country, staying with some relations, but they came back early and they came back very, very ill. They had caught a terrible disease, a stomach illness. It was dysentery, but in a very bad form.

We found out that the relations grew their own vegetables; apparently they had picked a cucumber and never washed it before eating it. A fly or something must have landed on this cucumber and the boys fell ill. They both came home with this awful disease. Then their sister got it from them. I was terrified, and Moss was away.

I was always in touch with Barney and Tanya. When I told Tanya how frightened I was, she said, "Well, Lilya, come and stay with us. We have plenty of room. You can sleep on the put-you-up. Come for a few days." She didn't mind at all; in fact, she liked my company. They had two bedrooms, but their lounge had this bed-settee.

I told my mother and she thought it was a good idea, because

197

dysentery was such a dangerous disease. Perhaps she thought she was immune to it. Anyway, I stayed with Barney and Tanya. Tanya was fond of me, of course, and Moss was very attached to his elder brother, much more than to his younger brother. I don't know why. They had this mutual friendship.

When a week had passed, I went back home and learnt what had happened to our neighbour. Two of the children had died; the eldest boy and the girl, who was so lovely. It was very sad. I really felt so sorry, terribly sorry. And of course there was great grief in that home. The mother had a sister who lived somewhere far away, not far from the Caucasus Mountains, though she was Russian. This sister, when she heard the news, travelled to Moscow to console her sister; and, when she went back, she took one of the other boys with her, a very nice boy, and she said she would adopt him.

For the mother it was a relief, because she had other problems. Her husband was a drinker. He used to get so drunk, so often, that I saw it would end badly, and indeed shortly after that she lost her husband as well. He was run over on the street, because he was too drunk to get out of the way, and she was left by herself with one boy.

The rolling stone returns

Time went by and one day I came home to find a letter from Moss saying he was just setting off back to Moscow. Of course, before he left, he was given a very big list of things to bring back. On that list was tea, Indian tea, because you couldn't get it in Russia – they drank only China tea – and there was a special cheese I liked, cheese that came in little round boxes and wrapped in pointed pieces in silver paper. And of course I put clothes on the list, because my good clothes from America were getting worn now, and you couldn't buy anything like them in Russia.

My mother and I went to meet him. When he got off the train, we could hardly see him for all the parcels and things he was carrying; and then we hardly recognised him, because he was all dressed up. Winter was approaching and he had on a fabulous new coat with an Astrakhan collar. I looked and said, "You look so smart!" He laughed.

We had such happiness being together again, and then there were all the presents to look at. To celebrate, we went and took a photo with me in my new outfit. He brought material for me to have a coat made, and some beautiful knitwear, a skirt and a top, which I thought very attractive.

He brought the cheese, too, that I loved. My mother wasn't interested in that type of food and Moss wouldn't eat any of it either; he would say, "I had plenty when I was in London. You never have anything like that here, so that is for you." I would try to insist, because I knew Moss liked it. "Try one piece, just to please me." But he would say, "No, that is for you." No matter how I fought, we used to end up laughing. He brought a huge tin of tea as well, because he liked English cups of tea. The Russians couldn't get Indian tea, but in any case they never drank tea with milk.

It was autumn now and the concert season had begun. The Isadora Duncan Dance Group were booked to appear here and there, so I had to go away for concerts. Wherever I travelled, I always had Moss's photo with me. Whenever I was staying in a hotel, he was always there on a table by my bedside. The other girls used to laugh at me, but I only said, "Well, there will come a time when you do the same."

All the same, it didn't please Moss that I had to go away, especially so soon after his return from London, and he was reluctant to let me go; we had so seldom been parted. I had to work a bit to persuade him. It wasn't just that he missed me; he missed my housekeeping too, because I have to admit that my mother was not as particular as I was.

I kept everything at home just so, and he liked the way I looked after him and did things. He was delighted with the way I did his shirts. He told me that his elder brother had said to him, "The way she does your shirts is incredible. Where did she learn it?" Well, I was very adaptable and I liked things to be as perfect as I could make them.

Home improvements

When I got home from that tour, I found there were alterations going on. Moss had got permission to make our main room 10 feet larger. The communal hallway was very much bigger than it needed to be and the other flats had made use of it to enlarge their main rooms. Theirs were much larger than ours, so we had permission to move our wall the same distance as the one next to us. Moss was very good at arranging things.

The builders hadn't quite finished, but the wall was built and the door hung, so we could close the door and sleep there. The floor wasn't ready either, but they were doing that as well, and I was very pleased about it. I thought it was fantastic. The work was coming to an end, so I must have been away a little more than two weeks.

The room now looked a lot bigger, and I rearranged it. I decided I didn't care for our dining table. So I went to a big department store at the start of Petrovska, a very well-known shop, to find a replacement. On the top floor they sold lovely furniture, and I found a beautiful round table, quite a fair size, made of walnut with a beautiful pedestal. The table had a flap that you could take out, to make it smaller. When you had people coming, you could insert the flap to make it larger, so I bought it.

Our room looked lovely, and many friends and acquaintances came to see it when it was finished. Even Mahmet from downstairs said, "Well, you've put on a really lovely show." Whenever I came back from a trip, I used to make everything shine and look beautiful, and I would buy flowers to put in the centre of the table. When Moss came home, he used to say, "I knew, once Lili was back, everything would be just lovely."

We had a very good social life, and not just dinner parties. We used to go regularly to shows and, if there was a premiere, no matter what it was, we would be there. Besides that, we read and talked about books, except that Moss liked English writers. He never took any interest in foreign literature.

My uncle – Uncle Peter, the youngest – was well read and very intelligent, I have to say – as well as being fond of me – and he lent me books. He was a great book-lover and a connoisseur of certain writers. Through him I read very widely. He used to bring books to me, rare books that – in Russia, then – you couldn't just go and buy.

He knew I was very fond of French writers, as he was. I liked Guy de Maupassant especially, having read a few at school and acquired a taste for them. Uncle Peter used to borrow them, one volume at a time, from one of his wife's relations. Before he gave a volume back, he would bring it to me, and in this way he and I read our way through the whole of Maupassant. He also got me many stories by Balzac, which I relished for their humour – or is it comedy? – but that is beside the point.

A *dacha* with Susanna

That summer, the summer of 1934, Barney and Tanya wanted to do as they had done the previous year and share a house with us in the country, but this time we said no. Moss and I wanted to have a place of our own. We rented a very big *dacha*, a country house. The family who lived there moved out – they had another house they could live in – and they let the whole *dacha* to us.

We had lots of space, so we gave one room to my aunt and my mother's younger brother, and a room to my mother. She came with us to look after the food because I never had time. In any event, I knew nothing then about cooking. We all got on very well, we enjoyed life, we went for walks and we met various people. There was a pool nearby, on a small river, and we went swimming there. It was really very pleasant.

By that time Moss had introduced me to his friends, and I got on well with them, even though I was a lot younger. One of them, Susanna, was the same age as Moss, but she hadn't married, though she did flirt a bit. She and Moss were 29, whereas I was 19, but she became very friendly with me. She was blonde, fashionably dressed and very keen on clothes, especially Western styles.

Whenever we started talking about shoes or coats, or fashion generally – and it didn't take long for Susanna to get the conversation back to clothes – she would ask, "Where do you shop?" And I would say, "I find it very difficult. I don't really know where to go. I can't find my way about." So she introduced me to a very good dress-maker and told me, "All you have to do is find the material, and then get in touch with her."

When we rented this *dacha*, she said to Moss – not to me, but to Moss – "You know, I would love to come with you." He asked me if I would mind, and I said, "No." She had a man friend, though he didn't join us in the end, but nevertheless we gave her a room. We didn't ask her to pay anything; we didn't need to. We were rather well off, I would say.

Something cooking

So Susanna came to stay. Then one day, I don't know how it happened, I came home and went straight into the garden. When I came into the house, I saw Susanna sitting on Moss's lap. Well, I thought that was odd, but beyond that I took no notice.

The next thing was a day or two later. My mother always cooked for us – she always had, before Moss moved in and after – but this day she had to go to Moscow, so Moss asked me: "Who is cooking the dinner? You know, *you* should be doing it." At that point, Susanna offered to do it and that was that. It was time for him to set off for the office and my mother was catching the same train. As they were walking to the station, Moss re-opened the subject.

"You know, I am surprised Lili doesn't cook. She does everything else so well, and yet she can't cook."

"Look, dear, you married a dancer. You knew she wasn't used to doing the cooking."

"Even so, a wife should be able to cook."

"Well, you should have thought of that before. It's no good telling her that now."

He didn't say anything more. Of course he knew what she said was true.

My mother didn't stay long in Moscow. She always made sure I was looked after, and we had a very large place there, but also she had put two and two together. When my mother got back, she told me about this incident; and when Moss got back I started looking round and seeing things I hadn't noticed before – and I didn't like the things I saw and heard. Susanna never missed a chance to show up my weaknesses and belittle my good points. She was trying to get my Moss.

Of course, she was never going to get anywhere, because he was never in love with her. Apart from anything else, he knew her too well. But, for her to tell him all my minuses and none of my pluses, I didn't like that. I don't like schemers. It was very wrong of her when she was our guest.

I felt it was also very wrong of Moss to complain to my mother that I couldn't cook. I wasn't made to be a cook. But to him I said only how I felt about Susanna.

"I don't want Susanna to stay with us any longer."

"Fine, I agree with you. I agree with you completely."

He didn't like her behaviour either. So we went together to tell her.

"Susanna, we are sorry, but you will have to leave."

That night we listened to records. We had some marvellous

records, a really good collection, and Moss had brought a gramophone – well, what we called a gramophone then, but actually it was just the turntable, a Pet-o-phone – and I had a wonderful Brunsvig amplifier. So we had a concert all of our own. Very early the following morning, Susanna left us. It was only the next night that we discovered she had taken ten of our best records with her. I thought, "What a cheek!"

It didn't spoil my holiday, because I wouldn't let it. We went on enjoying ourselves, just as if nothing had happened – I have the photographs to prove it – but we were rid of a source of friction, one that had started to vex even Moss. He could see I wasn't making a fuss about nothing when I said I didn't want her to stay.

On top of that, to take our best records, that was shameful. But that is how some people are. So you have to be really careful who you become friends with. Never mind, it didn't matter: I had plenty of friends besides her.

Music – and a discordant note

I will say, though, that the dressmaker Susanna put me in touch with was excellent. She made me two beautiful frocks, one black and one red, of chiffon – I was fond of chiffon. Whenever we went out, I always liked to dress nicely and wear good clothes. I suppose that comes of having a mother who was a seamstress in *haute couture*, but it has never left me, right down to the present. I remember wearing that red dress, though not at the *dacha*, of course; I had dressed up to go to a concert.

When we came back from that holiday, I saw there was to be a performance of *The Magic Flute*, the opera by Mozart. I had never heard of it, but the name 'Magic Flute' appealed to me, so I bought two tickets. When I told Moss, he said, "Oh, that is marvellous." We went to see it, but we were disappointed to find it was not a proper production. It wasn't a theatrical show at all: it was a concert performance, or rather an undressed opera.

Apart from that, I was too young to appreciate the music, I must confess. I never knew any Mozart at that time, because Russian orchestras never played Mozart. Moss and I used to go to concerts. We heard a lot of Tchaikovsky, and I liked his music very much, especially his piano concertos. I still do. In our dance repertoire, we had Beethoven, Schubert, Chopin, Liszt and others, but no Mozart. Only later did Isadora put on that dance based on the Turkish march, which is a movement from one of Mozart's piano sonatas. With that exception, I never heard his music in Russia.

Now, though, Mozart is my favourite composer, partly because I am much more mature now and partly because, when I settled in England, I was sort of introduced to him. They play a lot of Mozart in England. Once I understood what he was about, I couldn't get over the beauty of the music. After that I never stopped playing him.

That evening that we went to see *The Magic Flute*, I was wearing my lovely red chiffon dress, with a pretty little hat. I liked to wear a hat because it covered up my hair, which I never did like. Well, I couldn't very well shave it off, could I? So I had to put up with it.

Vanya Weinstein

When we got back, we were both astonished to find a stranger sitting in our room. He stood up and came forward to greet Moss, and my husband was so delighted. He introduced us, saying, "This is my wife." We had not been married long. It turned out that this chap who had just dropped in to see us was a very old friend of his from London, who had suddenly decided to come to Moscow, to start a new life. He looked at me, I remember, and said he was very pleased to meet me. That was all he said, but I noticed he couldn't take his eyes off me - or perhaps it was my red chiffon dress.

Of course they talked between them. Eventually I found out that he was a jeweller, and the reason he had come to Russia was that he had suffered a great misfortune. Insurance wasn't so readily available then as it is today, and he wasn't insured for all his goods. He had to take a big collection of jewellery somewhere, and it seems somebody was watching him - and had been watching him for some time. It had all been planned. He was robbed, lost most of his stock and found himself in grave financial difficulty. He had almost nothing, so he couldn't start afresh in London.

He came originally from some village in Russia, with his brother. So he had Russian blood in him. His name was Weinstein, but we never called him by his full name. His first name was Arnold, but we thought that was too flowery. Instead, we called him Vanya, a name he liked very much.

Moss asked him what his idea was: what was he hoping to do in Russia? He said, well, he could do some mosaic work and perhaps something more interesting. He soon got some work, engraving, I think. He was very talented and had lots of skills.

He came by himself, leaving his family in London. His wife had come from the same village as Vanya, years ago, and they had three sons, all born in London; the eldest boy was nearly grown up. Weinstein wasn't very young and he wasn't very old. You would say he was middle-aged, but he had a very good face. His features were prominent and somehow very direct. I liked him, and he and I became friends.

He came to see us regularly. Moss and I were very often out, but he was quite happy to be with my mother and help her with the household chores; they became very friendly. She often used to buy some special cream and he used it to make butter for us. He was a very adaptable person, I would say, but we had to tell him how things were.

"You are going to find it very difficult. For one thing, you can't find anywhere to live: it is awful."

"I will manage. I'll rent something for the time being."

Such things never worried him. This is something the Russians have, a determination deep down, that means they never worry greatly about where they are going to eat or sleep. They expect to manage somehow.

Vanya often used to come round and he would listen to music with us. One day he told us that he had managed to find a big room to rent, big enough for him to share, and he had decided to bring over his wife and one of their sons – the youngest son, whose name was Gerard. The other boys wouldn't come.

Shortly afterwards his wife came to Moscow to live with him and we met her, but I didn't like her. And I wasn't the only one. Vanya Weinstein was so pleasant, and she was so – well, it's hard to find a single word for it, but when she talked to you, she never looked straight into your eyes; she used to look all around. That's one thing I don't like, somebody who doesn't talk to you directly, but keeps looking somewhere else. That was the thing I didn't like about her.

Vanya was a sensitive man and he saw at once how we felt. He found it very difficult, of course, but he still came to see us – only less often and on his own. I think Moss encouraged him to visit. After-wards, years afterwards, Vanya told me that Moss was very kind to him. Well, Vanya was an old friend, and he was such a nice man. I know Moss helped him a great deal financially, but then we had quite a lot of money, so it really didn't hurt us.

Throwing away the key

As part of his job, Moss came into contact with many senior people in the Kremlin and elsewhere, and his abilities were known and respected. In 1935, he was flattered to be offered a new, highly paid job in the government's Translation Bureau.

The nature of the post made it very sensitive and whoever took it on had to be completely reliable politically. There was one simple way of achieving this. Purely as a formality, Moss was told, he would need to take Russian citizenship before he was appointed. His elder brother Barney had done the same, for the same reason, not long before, so to Moss it evidently seemed nothing of special significance.

He came home to tell me that he had accepted the job offer and then, by the way, mentioned that they had asked him to take Russian citizenship and he had done so. I was horrified. As British subjects, he and Barney were safe from Stalin and the KGB; as Soviet citizens, they had no more protection than any peasant. The first, dreadful result of their folly came only three years later.

"My wife doesn't need to dance"

Each year, I would be away travelling for part of the concert season, and each year Moss got a little more restless. He didn't like me constantly going away, especially without him, and he hated it when I was away for two weeks at a time. Once in a while, when he could manage it, he would come with me.

Every so often Schneider, who had been our director at the Isadora Duncan School, would arrange some one-off performances at places that didn't usually aspire to anything out of the ordinary. He did it so that we could earn more, because these little events paid a lot of money. However, the venues were sometimes rather shabby.

Moss came with me to one of these performances – it wasn't really a proper concert – and when he saw the makeshift kind of place it was, he was disgusted.

"How can anyone expect lovely girls like you to dance in such a place?"

After the concert, if you can call it that, was over, he told me what he thought; then he went up to Schneider and told him the same.

"That's it. My wife isn't coming to places like this to dance. She doesn't need to."

From then on I stayed at home. About this time, Auntie Annie came from London to join her boys in Moscow. She was delighted to see me. Whenever she came to see us, she would teach me some new thing about looking after a home. I took notice of whatever people told me. I never said 'I know' – I have always been willing to learn.

Moss was now very happy, but I was a little bit – how can I say? – not bored, because I loved Moss too much, but I had a lot of time on my hands. He had to work; he couldn't always be with me. One day I was out walking in Moscow – there were some very attractive parts of the city, where I liked to walk – and I bumped into Schneider. We chatted for a few minutes and then he looked at me.

"Lilya, you have become a housewife."

"Well?"

"Well, you are not meant to be a housewife."

"It's all right; it doesn't matter."

We left it at that, and I came back home, but he was so cunning in planting that idea and then just leaving it to grow. He probably already had things planned.

A few days afterwards, I had a bit of real luck. At least it felt to me like luck. There was a phone call and Moss answered. He began asking questions – I was really puzzled what it was all about – and then he told the caller to hold on: he would bring me to the phone, so they could ask me. It was one of the girls and she had asked Moss to let me come back, because they really needed me. While I was talking, he nodded his head, so I said yes; but, after I had put the phone down, I wanted to reassure him.

"Look, I'll write to you. Really, I can't refuse. The other girls have specially asked me to join them."

"I know – and you should go. After all, you have danced all your life. It was not fair of me to uproot you like that. You can go, providing they are decent concerts. No more of those dreadful, seedy places. I know you made a lot of money at those events, but you are not short of it. Perhaps the other girls needed it, but you don't.''

Nearly the North Pole

So I began dancing regularly again. This concert they needed me for was at the North Pole, they said, which wasn't quite true, thank goodness, because there's no land there, is there? Still, it was interesting, because the place was inside the Arctic Circle.

Off we went – just six girls, with our pianist, because that was as many as they wanted – to Polyarniy, which is a port a few miles north of Murmansk. It was so strange when we got there, because at that time of the year it was always daytime. The air was very, very still, there was deep snow lying and it was so quiet.

The Russians are extraordinary where art is concerned. They had built a lovely theatre in this remote city and the facilities were first-class. Our concerts in Polyarniy were very successful. The programmes were a mixture: there was a violinist and a cellist, there was a singer and I think there were other people; and Vovachka, our pianist, played for our dances.

We did enjoy that visit. I still have a big photograph of us there. We stayed there about two weeks, but we never saw the night sky: it was always daylight. But we did see the aurora borealis, the northern lights, and they were moving about from side to side. That was a wonderful sight.

A child

I must confess that events set me off. Our neighbour had a little girl who was now two years old and very sweet. She was jumping about the whole time, wanting to show her mother things, calling, ''Mummy, mummy.'' Well, suddenly it dawned on me – I had been married about three years then – and I found myself thinking, *This has gone on long enough. I also want a little child to call me Mummy.*

Now this seemed the important thing. It started really playing on my mind. I tackled Moss about it.

''Moss, don't you think we ought to think of having a child?''

208

"No, not really. I don't particularly want any children."

"But you cannot live through life without any children."

"No dear, we don't need children. We are happy as we are."

But I could not let it rest: the idea had gripped me. I wanted a little child to hop about and call me Mummy. So how could I get Moss to want a child too?

When we used to walk out together, I used to stop in front a big store from the olden days; it was called Murmalise, I think, and belonged to the French. Its window displays were full of beautiful things – the best in Moscow, I would say, – and it was just at the end of our street. I used to stop and make him look at the children's wear. I would say "Look at those beautiful little things: aren't they pretty? And those little knitted boots – I think they are gorgeous." I tried that for quite a while and gradually it worked.

In the evenings, when Moss was free to walk, we liked to go for a walk because we lived in such a pleasant street, one of the best streets in Moscow – Petrovska. There is a delightful short story by Chekhov, 'The woman with the dog', that mentions our street, because the hero lives in Petrovska. That was most interesting. We used to meet all sorts of people there.

One day we met a couple – I knew the husband from our concerts, because he was an administrator – and he was so pleased to see me. He had a lovely little wife, they had never met Moss, and we introduced one another. He said, "What a coincidence to see you here," and I said, "Not really, because we live just up the road." We got chatting and it turned out she was expecting a baby. After a few minutes, we parted, but it got Moss to think about having a child.

That was strange: now I had got him really interested.

"Well, of course, I wouldn't want a boy."

"It's no good saying that; you have to take whatever comes."

But if it was a girl he would absolutely delighted, and deep down I wanted a little girl, because my neighbour's little girl was hopping about every day in front of my eyes. She was so sweet, and I was very friendly with the mother. They were quite ordinary Russian people, not of any particular intellect or anything, just nice, open people. The mother was a lovely, friendly woman; her name was Tanya.

A month passed and Moss started to ask me, "Well, anything happening?" and I said, "No, not yet, but it will come." Another month passed and he was really anxious. I had to reassure him: "Now don't start worrying about it." And in another two months, a baby came along. This time, when he asked, the answer was yes. Oh, he was so pleased. Now isn't that odd, how one can persuade another person?

Moss told Barney, his elder brother, and Tanya what was on the way and they were delighted. Tanya told me a little secret of hers, how she had wanted a child, then both of them did, but nothing came of it. Well, they had waited too long; they waited ten years before they tried, and you can't. Even with Moss and me, waiting three years made a big difference: otherwise I would have become pregnant straightaway.

Now he looked forward to the baby's arrival. He used to run about, making sure I was comfortable. I said, "Don't fuss." I was still dancing and I was fine. I was just excited. Things were happening. It was early 1938.

Barney disappears

One day in early spring, we got an urgent phone call from Tanya. Within an hour or so, she and Auntie Annie came to see us, with such expressions on their faces. Their news was extraordinary. They told us that during the night the KGB had come to their flat and taken Barney away; they had no idea why, nor where he was.

How on earth could this happen? We became very alarmed – we couldn't see any reason why they should have taken him. I assumed Barney was being used as a scapegoat, like my uncle Isaac: they had picked on him because he was Jewish. I was trying to work out how it was they had spared Moss, my husband.

We found out the real reason later on, but at the time I thought it must be because the brothers had different surnames. Barney kept their father's name, Isaacs, but Moss could never forgive his father for what he had done to his mother, and he took the name of his stepfather, Muscat, the man Aunt Annie came to Russia with.

To each according to their need

Of course, Tanya was distraught, but one has to be realistic and adapt to the situation. Life goes on. We cheered up Tanya and Aunt Annie as best we could, but what were they to do now? The flat in the city was allocated to Barney; it would probably be given to someone else now, so they would have to move. That was not a major problem for Tanya, since she was still in the prime of life, but Aunt Annie was getting on – in fact she was getting old.

I liked Aunt Annie and I would have been quite comfortable having her living with us. If anything, she wasn't so helpful as my mother was, but she was pleasant and sensible, very clean and very ordinary – and Moss liked her very much. But she couldn't come to us. We had no room and, even if we had, she and my mother would have clashed sooner or later, though they were very old friends.

I was very fond of Tanya's mother and her husband; they were both of them lovely. They also would have been happy to take Tanya in. It might have been a bit of a squeeze, since they had their son living with them at the time. But even if they could have managed Tanya, there was no room for Aunt Annie – and Tanya wouldn't leave her mother-in-law on her own.

Of course Tanya could have gone with Aunt Annie to the new flat in the country that she and Barney had bought; but it was too remote to be safe or convenient. Luckily she had some very good friends – old friends from before the revolution, that her mother knew and that Tanya herself had known since she was young.

The husband was an architect and before the revolution he had designed and built for himself a beautiful house. I remember the house: it had columns downstairs and it was full of character. Parts of Moscow were very nice, including the area where our school was. Do you remember that I mentioned when we were at school and we marched off to the sports arena? Well, if you kept straight on, you came to the street where these friends lived.

At the time Barney disappeared, this friend of Tanya's – the architect – had just died. One room in their house was rented out, but his wife – she was called Varvara – was afraid that the authorities would force her to share her lovely house with someone else, someone she didn't like. Varvara herself had a bedroom and a big lounge.

So she said to Tanya when she heard of this terrible misfortune, "Tanya, you must come and stay with me. You can't go to your mother – she has no room. I have plenty of room and I don't want to share with strangers." They had a luxurious bathroom and a beautiful kitchen, which was very large. They also had a big dining room.

They arranged a bed there for Aunt Annie, and Tanya settled in with Varvara in the lounge. One good thing was that Tanya was able to bring her furniture, because the people who wanted their flat didn't need their furniture. She was allowed to take everything except the big gun that hung on the wall.

We all worried about Barney, especially because we heard no news of him, but things could have been worse. The rest of us each had a home, with decent people. I liked Varvara; she was friendly and easy to get on with. We used to go and visit her. Meanwhile, time was passing and I was growing a bit. It was early spring when they took Barney, and now summer was approaching. At seven months I gave up dancing. Moss wouldn't let me go any more, though you couldn't see much on me. I was so round, and everyone said that a round look meant it would be a girl.

From each according to their ability

The reason why Barney was taken away lay in something that had happened earlier. One day our neighbour upstairs came to see us and said there was a very beautiful flat for sale in the country. It was in a new building built for officials, but they wanted to sell one flat privately. We didn't want it – we were happy where we were; besides, we were too busy with other things – but we told Barney, and he was very interested.

The person who knew about it wanted to be paid for the information – such people always wanted commission – but Barney didn't mind. However, he didn't have quite enough cash, so Moss said he would help. He gave them quite a bit of money – which I didn't mind at all – and they bought this lovely flat in the country. That summer we were invited there and we liked it very much. But they kept on the rented flat in the city for the time being.

Now they had taken him away. Eventually we found out that one of their neighbours wanted their flat in the city. It wasn't in a prestige area, because they had to go where they were put; they never had their own place. They lived in whatever the government allocated them, whatever came vacant when an official was posted somewhere. But their flat looked special, because Tanya had very good taste and they had done a lot of work and made it very nice.

Even before they bought their country flat, Barney liked hunting, and he had a very big gun hanging on the wall. The neighbour had seen this gun and had heard him type. Well, that was nothing unusual: Moss and Barney were both translators, from Russian to English, but Barney not only worked for the government; he translated books too, foreign literature. He made quite a bit of money at that, so he gave up his job in the ministry to concentrate on this work.

The neighbour, though, who was some kind of official, said he thought Barney might be a spy. That was enough for the KGB or NKVD - whatever they called the Secret Service then - and they bundled him off. In reality, this man liked Barney's flat better than his own, so he just concocted the story. He never tried to find out why Barney had a gun or why he was using a typewriter. He just made sure poor Barney was sent to Siberia. That was a terrible misfortune to us, yet - despite their grief, wondering whether they would ever see Barney again - they all worried about me: would the anxiety affect me having my child? We went through quite a bad time then.

Preparing for a big event

I knew it would not be long before my baby would have to make its move out of me, and I thought, *What I will do now is rent a big* dacha *for the summer*. I took this very big place and I said to the others - Nadeyda, Tanya's mother, Aunt Annie and Tanya - you are all going to move there for the summer, and my mother will stay with me until the baby comes.

Strangely enough, they all settled in together at our *dacha*. They were quite happy. They made jam, I remember. Tanya used to make blackcurrant jam, because the fruit was coming ripe. It was very nice, the place I had chosen, and we even had some friends staying not far from there. They also had come for the summer.

The time came when I had to look after myself a bit more because my little child was due, but the weather was so hot that I couldn't go out during the day. Moss was so worried. But we used to walk out late in the evening, just to get some fresh air. So I managed somehow - well, you do when you are young.

Then during the night there was a bit of an emergency, when the waters broke and I put out an SOS. Moss arranged to take me straightaway to the maternity hospital. When I got there, they gave me a bedroom to myself and told me to lie there quietly until the pain came.

213

I didn't understand them. I said, "But I feel fine," because there were no contractions at that point. Nonetheless, Moss couldn't sleep for the rest of that night, because he was so worried. Every half an hour he came to the hospital to find out what was happening and they told him, "Don't worry; it is coming."

The time came when they took me into the main ward. There were many other women there, all about to have their babies, and there were doctors walking up and down, and nurses on duty. That is how it was done in Russia then. Things were organised for the common good, in theory at least, and you were expected to accept it.

Funnily enough, the doctors told us that childbirth was very painful, but we could just express our feelings and there was no need to worry about it. This was extraordinary.

Something wonderful

Before I went into hospital, Valya, one of the dancers in our group, came to see me. By that time she had had a little boy and she told me all about it, explaining what to expect and how I should behave, whatever happened. She really prepared me for how it would feel. That was really and truly such a good deed that she did, because what she told me came from experience and it helped me a great deal.

Yes, it was difficult. It was very painful, but at last my child came. And once the baby was out, everything went away, the pain went and I felt so terribly happy. At that moment Moss sent a big bunch of red roses, just when she was delivered. I couldn't forget that, because it was such a happy coincidence.

The doctor came to examine me, to see how things were, and announced to the other beds – I don't remember how many exactly, but there were eight or even ten mothers there – that I was absolutely wonderful and this was how women should have their babies. But really it was all thanks to my friend Valya. The dancers in our group, we were all like sisters to one another.

When they brought me Moss's bunch of red roses, I was more eager to find out what I had. "You have a most beautiful little girl." I thought, *Good gracious! To be given this little wonder and then to get exactly what you want as well.* They wrapped her up and brought her to me. I took a look and said, "Isn't she funny?" Well, she was. The two nurses went for me then. "How can you say that, when she is so lovely?"

After that we were taken on the ward and looked after. I got a message from Moss – "I'm told we have a little girl, which is marvellous. What sort of eyes does she have?" – but he wasn't allowed to come and see me. That was the rule, in case a visitor brought in an infection. They were very, very strict.

I am telling all this because the experience of childbirth was so different in Russia in those days. I don't know what happens there now, but I think many women will be interested to compare it with their own experience. I must have stayed in hospital about a week – doctor's orders. I was so happy. My only worry was that they might mix up my little one with someone else's. But they didn't.

Each time the nurses came in, they brought me my little girl – she had no name yet – to be fed. She was always hungry, I noticed that. I used to wake her up, her little neck would stick out and she would be looking and looking for me. She would stay awake until she had satisfied her hunger. Apart from that, she hardly opened her eyes; she used to eat and then go off to sleep again.

For me that week in hospital was all very positive. I was getting well again too, but the doctors were very disappointed in me. I don't know why. After five days, I felt really well and I told them so.

"I don't need to stay here any longer. I would rather go home. My husband is dying to see her."

The doctors consulted and they agreed. There were quite a few women ready to go at the same time as me. The doctors met us together before we were discharged, and we were given a little lecture before we went home.

"Look, all of you, I don't want to see any of you here again in the next three years. You should not have children one after the other. It doesn't do women any good."

Now we are three

Then we all went home. My husband came to meet me; his delight was extraordinary, and I felt as if I was in heaven. As usual – it's the way I am made – as soon as I got home, I overdid things. I was doing everything that needed doing with nappies and so on; my mother wanted to help, but I said I would do it all myself. Not surprisingly, I developed milk fever. I had to go to bed again, for another two days, but my mother did everything that was necessary and I fed the baby. I had plenty of milk to give.

Our happiness was extraordinary. The days passed and now I really felt stronger. We began to think about that place in the country waiting for us, and all my close people, that I was very fond of. They were all waiting to see her and they would want to know what we had called her. But Moss and I still hadn't found a name. She was two weeks old and opening her eyes now; she really needed a name of her own.

Before we went back to the *dacha*, we went to see Verdi's opera, *Il Trovatore*. In the troubadours' duet, I heard the name Leonora. At the interval I told Moss.

"There you are. Now we have the name. Leonora!"

"You're right."

"It suits her, because she has those beautiful big, dark eyes, not black but very dark, and they flash when she opens them."

So we named her Leonora and now we were ready to take her to the country.

Proud parents

Moss and I travelled down to the *dacha* and everyone wanted to come to see Leonora. Tanya came to greet me in great delight. She looked at Leonora, and Leonora opened her big eyes. Tanya spotted the resemblance straightaway and drew my attention to it.

"Lilya."

"Yes?"

"She is so lovely, but you know she looks like Barney, rather than Moss."

And funnily enough, it was true in a way. She had his eyes, which was strange. Moss too had nice eyes, but they were different. Barney had flashing eyes, like Leonora's.

Tanya looked at me and laughed mischievously.

"Lilya, are you sure it isn't Barney's baby?"

"Tanya, don't be silly."

I never forgot that, but we all settled in together beautifully.

However, some of the neighbours were taken by surprise and the rest pretended to be.

"Where did that little baby spring from, then?"

"Why? Didn't you notice Lilya was pregnant?"

"No, she was always so neat, such a trim figure, you couldn't see a thing. So tell us, where did this little one come from?"

Well, I wasn't all that neat. You should have seen the things I'd been wearing to hide my bulge.

Moss stayed with me at the *dacha* for about two or three weeks, and then he had to go to Moscow. He didn't know how long he would be away. He had been asked to act as compère at a series of concerts, because they needed someone to translate from Russian to English, for all the tourists from America. They felt Moss was the right man: they knew the quality of his work and they knew he always looked immaculate. I saw to that.

Not so hot

I was just beginning to think it was time he came back to see me, when a strange thing happened. I never normally wake up at night, but this night I did. And that was the strange thing. It always happens – why, I have no idea – but I always wake up before something untoward happens, even if there is no warning.

Every evening, I made up a kind of nightlight, in case Leonora awoke in the night or needed anything. She didn't wake that night, but I did. I woke up in the middle of the night and had to go to the bathroom. I came back and was just putting my foot on the bed, when there was a little blow and I turned round to see what it was. That nightlight contraption I had made, it had just burst into flame.

It flared up and lit the whole bedroom. I could hear little crackling noises. Still, I didn't lose my head. I pulled the pram, with my little girl, out of the way; she woke up then and smiled. I took a blanket to smother the flames. They had already gone a little way towards the door leading to the owners' rooms, but I managed to stop them. At that point I came to and suddenly I felt shattered.

That was such a silly thing. If I hadn't been awake, we would all have perished without any doubt, because a wooden house like that would have gone up like a match. I decided to wake my family up. I

217

told them what had happened and they couldn't get over how lucky we were.

Thank goodness, they didn't mind, but they all came to see what there was to see, and of course they had to check how my little girl was doing. When she saw them all, she smiled. After all she was so young, she was only about a month old. I went back to bed and slept as if nothing had happened.

The following morning, I thought, *It's time Moss came.* I was really starting to miss him. In any event, it was nearly September and the weather gets less reliable then. It loses some of that lovely heat and the evenings get much cooler. I said all this to my sister-in-law.

"Tanya, I think we should all go home."

"That's not a bad idea."

I told the others then. We didn't wait for Moss, we all packed and arranged transport and everything, and we went home the same way we had come.

Return to Moscow

When we got into Moscow, we parted. The rest of the family went their own way, and my mother and I went back to our flat. Late in the evening, Moss came home and of course he was surprised to see us.

"Oh, how nice! I thought it was time you came back."

"You're very late, Moss. Where were you?"

"Well, I couldn't help it. I was kept back."

But there was a little hesitation in his reply.

Something wasn't quite right, and I began to take a little more interest in what he did. And I found out by various means that he had been carrying on a bit of a flirtation on the side. I was very angry and I confronted him with it.

"After all I've been through, all that pain to give us a child, and you've been out enjoying yourself."

"Oh, Lili, I'm sorry. Do forgive me, dear."

When I had got over my anger and calmed down, I did understand his situation. First of all, when one is carrying a child, for the man it is not so wonderful; and then, after the baby is born, the mother and baby are the centre of attention and the husband gets even less than

218

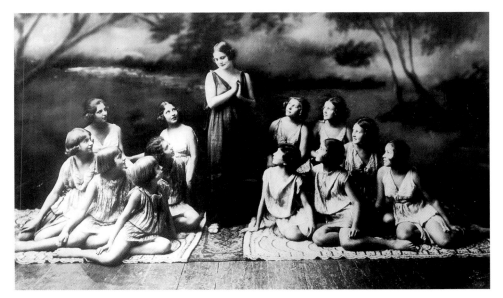

18. Rehearsing in the theatre at Harbin, Manchuria, Irma was looking straight at Lily, aged 13. From left (back left) Marousha Borisova and Liza Belova, (back right) Manya Toropchenova and Shura Aksimova; then (middle left) Lily and (middle right) Tamara Lobanovskaya; and (front left) Valya Boye, Doda Ozhegova and Tamara Semenova, (front right) Moushya Mysovskaya, Lyola Terentieva and Yulia Vashentseva.

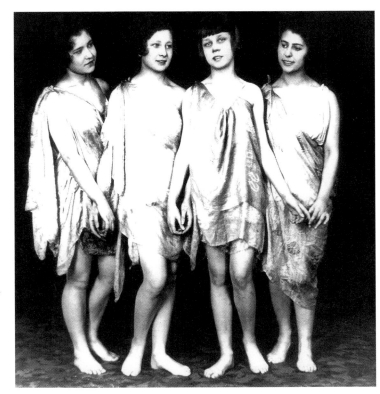

19. The Four Graces: Lyola Terentieva, Moushya Mysovskaya, Tamara Semenova and Lily Dikovsky. Tamara's costume is what they all wore to dance Schubert's 9th Symphony in America.

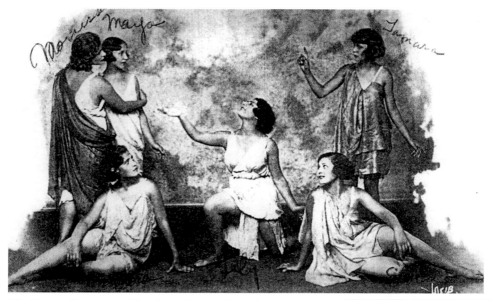

20. Above: Dancing a Chopin waltz are (from left) Manya
Toropchenova, Liza Belova and Vera Golovina (seated),
with Lily (centre), Moushya Mysovskaya (seated) and
Tamara Semenova (on the right).

21. Below: The girls of the Isadora Duncan School in front
of a gateway in Peking (Beijing). They saw some
wonderful sights, but China was more exciting than anyone
expected. At times it was too dangerous even to go out.

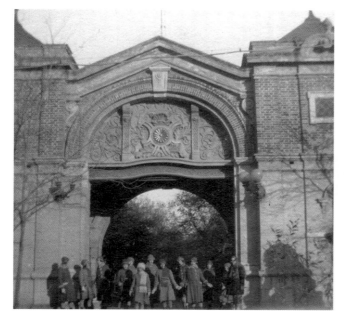

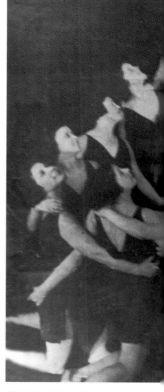

22. The New York
newspapers wanted to
give the story a new
angle, and this shot was
Irma's idea. Busby

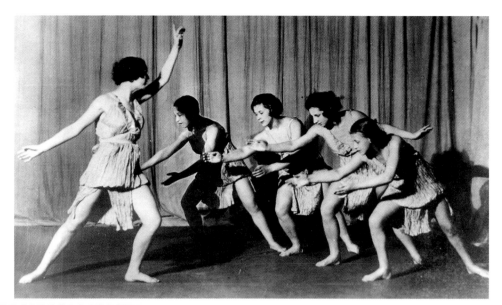

23. Above: In the studio at Prechistenka 20 preparing for their tour of the USA are Shura Aksimova, Liza Belova, Manya Toropchenova, Marousha Borisova and Tamara Lobanovskaya, rehearsing 'Ball game' to music by Glück.

24. Below: Tientsin seemed more like a Western city than a Chinese one. Here (from left) are Shura Aksimova, Tamara Lobanovskaya, Manya Toropchenova, Lyola Terentieva, Yulia Vashentseva, Valya Boye and Marousha Borisova, with (at front right) Tamara Semenova and Lily Dikovsky, who is trying to coax a smile out of Moushya Mysovskaya.

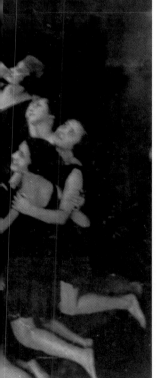

Berkeley began using the kaleidoscopic 'top shot' in films with Eddie Cantor about this time.

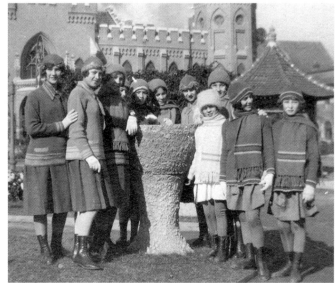

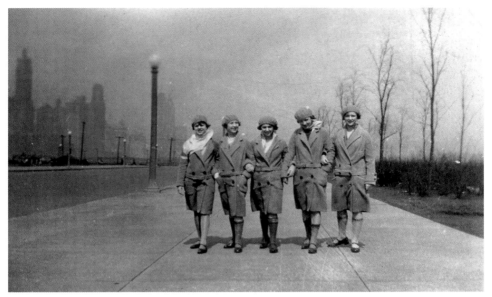

25. The Isadora Duncan Dancers are the only sign of movement on this section of Michigan Boulevard, Chicago, in 1929.

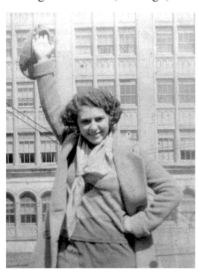

26. Lily on Ninth Avenue, being a model for the Statuette of Liberty.

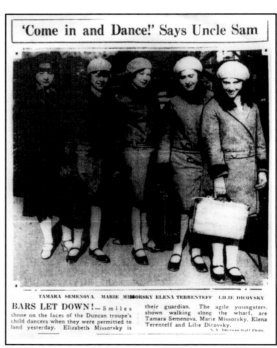

'Come in and Dance!' Says Uncle Sam

TAMARA SEMENOVA. MARIE MISSORSKY ELENA TERRENTEFF LILIE DICOVSKY

BARS LET DOWN!—Smiles shone on the faces of the Duncan troupe's child dancers when they were permitted to land yesterday. Elizabeth Missorsky is their guardian. The agile youngsters, shown walking along the wharf, are Tamara Semenova, Marie Missorsky, Elena Terenteff and Lilie Dicovsky.

N. Y. American Staff Photo.

27. Being locked up on an island for Christmas didn't seem much of a welcome to the younger girls, but Uncle Sam made up for it later. This newspaper cutting shows (from front): Lily Dikovsky, Elena Terentieva, Maria Mysovskaya, Tamara Semenova and their nurse, Maria's mother.

usual. So I was very understanding. I thought, *I can't be angry for long*.

Meanwhile, he got tickets for the theatre. He knew at once how to win me. It was a ballet with Ulanova, who was a wonderful dancer. Moss had got tickets for the opening night of this new production of *Giselle*, which we enjoyed very much. He was rather cunning, but all the same I was pleased. And I must say he was genuinely delighted that I was back.

11

The Absence of War, 1939-41

Enyukidze

While my daughter was a small baby and still needed me constantly, I couldn't really rejoin the group yet. Then, one day I had a telephone call from our director. He told me, "Lilya, we need your help. It is important. We have been asked to dance in the Kremlin and we need you with us." I at once said yes, because this could be our chance to get recognition and funding.

There was a minister of the arts, it seemed, a Georgian man called Enyukidze. Now we had been to Georgia a number of times and whenever we went to the Caucasus - especially to Tiflis - we had found that the Georgian people responded far more than other audiences. They were enchanted with our dancing, even more than the Russians, I must confess. We couldn't quite understand why that was. Perhaps it was because they danced in a similar way; they danced a lot and Georgian women were very graceful. So we felt a Georgian would appreciate what we were doing.

Enyukidze had seen the other girls somewhere in a concert and was very taken by what he saw, so he arranged for us to perform at the Kremlin for an invited audience, just arts administrators and party officials, to show them what he had in mind. Well, we danced there and he liked it even better than before. He said he was charmed and he offered to help us.

"How is it you have been so many years in Russia, and no one has done anything to help you to continue your work? You have no schools and no pupils to teach. I am going to arrange everything for you - you are going to get premises and you are going to develop your art."

It seemed that at last someone was going to support our efforts in the way they had supported Isadora.

Kozlovskiy

Not long after that, the girls got in touch and came round to see me.

"Lilya, we know you have your little baby now, but you have to help us out."

"What is it now?"

"Well, you know the famous tenor, Kozlovskiy, who sings at the Bolshoi? He wants to put us on stage, us dancing, with him singing. He remembers us dancing something from *The Blessed Spirits*, that thing by Glück, and he got in touch with our director and asked if we would oblige him by coming to a rehearsal and showing him the whole dance. Go on, Lilya, you can't let us down!"

"No, of course not, but I am feeding the baby."

"Don't worry: we'll arrange things."

And my mother said, "I'll look after her and bring her to you."

So we performed our dance, to that wonderful music of Glück, and he was enchanted.

At the end, we went to the dressing room and sat down to rest. My mother brought me my little girl to feed, and Kozlovskiy came and sat down beside me.

"What a lovely child! You know, I am married, but my wife doesn't want any children. It makes me feel very unhappy. You don't mind if I watch her?"

"No, not at all."

I mean, after all, there is nothing new under the moon – that's what I always say. So he watched me feeding the baby. He commented again how lovely she was. Mind you, Leonora really had eyes when she opened them; they were delightful.

He told us he was going to stage the opera and he wanted us to perform the Dance of the Blessed Spirits, because the ballet wouldn't do. He felt we were just perfect for the opera. In the end, though, the Bolshoi Theatre would not allow him to stage the opera. They didn't want somebody else straying onto their territory. Now this seems so strange, and of course it was petty.

If Isadora had been there, there wouldn't have been any argument, but she wasn't; so he had to give it up. It was a great pity because we so fitted in to that opera. Isadora had such marvellous ideas in her choreography, especially the part where the spirits came. The flute played that wonderful tune, we entered the stage from one side with a very slow movement, saying goodbye to Faust, and then we began dancing. It was enchanting.

Fallen angel

Whatever Isadora wanted to achieve, there was always something to prevent it, one thing or another that could not be done. Now, with this support from someone high up in the Kremlin, we felt we had a wonderful opportunity to do what we had always wanted to do, to teach, to continue that wonderful movement that Isadora began.

But we heard nothing more from Enyukidze. Eventually, we found out he had been dismissed by Stalin for corruption and executed by firing squad, even though they came from the same country, Georgia, and Stalin tended to favour Georgians; but there were always intrigues in the Kremlin, always. Apart from that, Stalin himself was rather a moraliser. He liked things done decently, he never made any fuss about his own life and he expected everyone who worked for him to be the same.

I wouldn't say that Enyukidze was an angel – far from it. Nevertheless, there are many people in the world who are no angels where morals are concerned, but they achieve good things all the same. However, Enyukidze disappeared and all our dreams were shattered.

The summer of 1939

The next summer, Tanya asked me if Moss and I would like to come and stay with her at the flat. They had this flat in Malakava, a lovely place in the country, one of the nicest places around Moscow. And I said yes. I went and so did Auntie Annie, and Tanya's mother too.

It was coming up to Leonora's first birthday, in July, and Tanya said we should have a birthday party for her. She was so delightful, my little girl. She hadn't started walking, but she could stand up very straight. I bought her a beautiful little dress and one of our friends, who was marvellous at embroidery, she embroidered a lilac on it. I bought a bunch of ribbon because she had such a lot of fair hair, ash-coloured, and I tied a little ribbon on her head. She looked lovely, and we all enjoyed ourselves.

Tanya had given Moss and me her best room. He spent a lot of time in Malakava that summer, and we all had a good time. Before the end of our stay, though, we heard that England had declared war on Hitler. We knew that, no matter what Stalin did, something would happen. War was going to come to Russia sooner or later.

A trip to Poland

When Stalin made the pact with Hitler that the Nazis were not going to invade the Soviet Union, the price was that Poland would be invaded instead, and the Germans and the Russians would divide Poland between them. The Soviet Union hadn't yet got the appetite for war, or simply wasn't prepared, and that averted for the time being the destruction and the horrors that came later. So there was a period of unnatural calm, during which the Soviet Union tried to appear friendly towards Nazi Germany. That may be why we were invited to give some concerts in Warsaw and Kraków, which we looked forward to very much.

Now Moss was very excited: he thought this would be rather an interesting trip, and not just for cultural reasons. He told me this was my opportunity to make us both very well-dressed. He gave me a little suitcase full of money, something which it had never entered my mind to ask for. I thought, *Fine, that is very generous of him*. There was quite a bit of money there – I would say there was about 10,000 roubles, which was a lot of money then.

I had read a lot about Poland, partly through Russian literature – Gogol especially wrote a lot about it – and therefore I was always interested in Poland and its history. I read a lot about Polish women and various stories set in Poland, so I was rather excited to go. Schneider didn't come with us for some reason. I think he couldn't get away and so somebody else came with us. The tour manager was somebody I didn't know, but he knew about us.

We got there safely, and I managed to get in touch with certain people who were to help me, to guide me to the places where I could buy certain things. I don't recall who they were, but they did it willingly. I also approached our administrator and said I would like to buy some goods, but I didn't know where to go because I had never been in Poland before, so he introduced me to people. There were good shops there and they were well stocked. I bought a lot of clothes.

The city showed signs of Russian influence, though of course they hadn't put their foot in it yet and wouldn't for some years. This was very shortly after the signing of the agreement, and therefore Warsaw remained much as it was before, with plenty of wonderful things. The money had changed, of course: the Polish money had already been replaced by German currency, but the shops accepted Russian money and I had quite a bit of that. So I managed to get my little girl some outfits – wonderful, knitted woollen clothes and warm leggings.

Also I ordered a beautiful suit for Moss, because I had taken his measurements. I chose the material, grey flannel. Before I left, he had stressed that I should get myself a winter coat. He wanted me to have a new fur coat, because the one I had was getting tatty. He said try to get a Persian fur coat, and I did try, but I couldn't get hold of one. Instead I had little outfits made for me – dresses, beautiful, elegant things. I bought a dozen hats too, because I always liked hats and you can't have too many, can you?

We didn't go for very long – about ten days or a fortnight, I think – but Poland made such an impression on me. Warsaw was so wonderful; it was the most beautiful city I could ever imagine. I took a great interest in the buildings and the streets. The architecture of Warsaw was most beautiful. I was very much taken by it. We had several concerts there and the audiences seemed to enjoy them very much.

We had a splendid time in Warsaw and then we went to Kraków, also a very beautiful city, but I had been so taken by Warsaw. It just reminded me of Europe – what I thought of as the real Europe, I suppose. Those performances in Poland were our last for some time. I tried again in Kraków to get a fur coat but I couldn't. I imagine they had stopped making them as soon as it was occupied. That was the usual thing: the one-party state arrived and everything else stopped. As a result, when I got home, I had some money left over, the money I was going to spend on a coat for myself.

Moss was astonished that the suit fitted him: the length of the trousers, the fit of the jacket, everything was just right. He looked so smart. It may seem extraordinary that he should have been surprised, but the fact was he had tried twice before to have a suit made to measure. He had bought some marvellous material when he was in London and had it made up for him when he got back to Moscow. Each time, when it was ready, he couldn't wear the suit, because nothing fitted. The trousers were so baggy. I don't know if he had any idea why it was, but the cutting was dreadful. So each time he had to sell the suit and this was the first time he had got himself such an elegant, beautifully cut suit.

Tamara

Not long after Leonora was born – it was when we returned from the country, so it would be September 1938 – Big Tamara came to see me.

"Lilya, I had to come to see your little girl. Everyone told me how delightful she is. Do you think I might hold her?"

"Yes, Tamara, of course."

She was very diffident in asking, because she was frightened that the baby might get this illness she had. Well, I knew an illness like tuberculosis could travel, but none of my family had ever had that illness, so I was not concerned.

"I will try and not kiss her – don't worry. I just want to hold her."

I thought Tamara was sweet really, and very thoughtful in this.

The following year, she again made a special journey to see me, just before we moved to the country for the summer. That would be May 1939. She wasn't well at all and she was getting worse. All the girls were very upset and we did everything we could to help her. We danced for her, and the money we earned went to help her.

Unfortunately, Tamara had a mother who didn't understand what was needed, and perhaps didn't understand how serious it was. Their flat was damp and the heating and ventilation were poor. Tamara used to smoke too, and that didn't help. But, worst of all, instead of trying to persuade her to give up smoking long before, her mother used to buy her cigarettes. Now that is such extraordinary behaviour.

Moss kept in touch with our director and asked him about Tamara whenever he saw him. He would come and tell me what he had found out. When we went back to the country and I was busy with my Leonora, Moss came from work one day with the news that she was a lot worse, and they now had no hope that she would recover.

Our director, Schneider, was very kind. He took her into his flat and gave her his bed, and he slept on the settee.

I remember I made a special journey to say farewell to her, because I was still in the country. It was so sad. Moss came home and told me.

"Lili, I don't like to upset you, but there is sad news. Tamara has died."

"Well, we were prepared for it. Even so, when it does come, it's very sad."

She was prepared for it, too, because I remember she said she wanted to be cremated. When she died, I felt so sorry for her. She was so young, not even 28, and so beautiful. Life never treated her properly, but there was nothing anyone could do about it. We all gathered at Schneider's place and said goodbye. She was lying there so peacefully. It is sad to think of it even now, but one cannot dwell on these things. That is life. It comes and it goes.

Juakina

We had a wide circle of friends, all involved in writing or translation in all sorts of languages. Among them Moss had one particular friend, whom he had got to know through work, and he brought him round to our flat. His surname was Gomchervich; I have forgotten his first name. I liked him, he was very nice and easy to get on with. He used to come to us quite often, because he lived near the end of a side street almost opposite us.

He told us something of his life. He had been in Spain during their civil war. The Russians were anxious to keep the flames going there and, since he spoke Spanish and Russian fluently, he had been very useful to the Soviet Government. He told us about the war and about the people he met. He had met a lovely young woman there, and married her. We wanted to know: Well, where is she? It seemed he was waiting to get permission for her to come to Moscow to join him. He particularly stressed the point that he would like his wife to meet me. He liked me and he thought she would be rather happy to meet me. And he was right.

In the summer of 1940 we rented a place in the country, near Tanya's flat. We didn't want to trespass on her space. I felt it wasn't right, now that my little girl was running about, getting into everything. Anyway, I liked to be independent, but I also liked to keep in contact with Tanya, and she felt the same. She liked our presence and even more so our little girl, who was growing. Leonora was lovely to look at and great fun to have around.

So we rented a lovely little *dacha*, quite small, with two bed-rooms, a kitchen and a little dining area. We could go back to our flat in Moscow when we wanted. My mother of course lived with us in the country. She had one bedroom and we had the other; there was also a little dining room and a nice kitchen. Tanya was nearby, so we used to go to her very often and sit in her garden. Her mother was staying with her, and they both liked Leonora. She was getting quite a little girl, running about and making mischief. She was delightful.

Before this, though, Gomchervich told us that his wife was com-ing. At last they had given her permission. Just before we moved to the country, she arrived and he brought her round. Her name was Juakina, a lovely name. We fell for one another, because she was delightful to be with and gorgeous to look at – and she liked me too. I invited them to the *dacha* we had rented. When they came, we walked, ate something and had a splendid time. No one could not like Juakina. She was a year or so older than me, dark with grey eyes – I always think that an attractive combination – and a lovely smile. She had a good figure and she was three or four inches taller than me. Oh, I did envy her there. We became very friendly and soon we met nearly every day, because she didn't live far from us in Moscow.

I mention her because I liked her so much. There were never many people that I really liked. I don't count the girls in our dance group, because we were more like sisters to each other. No, Juakina was different. She was a new acquaintance with a fresh outlook, and I was always interested in Spain, its history and its national dances.

I didn't invite Juakina at the same time as Tanya, because that would have been awkward for Juakina. She was still adapting to Moscow and Russian life. She and her husband had a splendid room – not an apartment, but a beautiful room – in a nice block of flats. He was absolutely in heaven, because he was so in love with her.

The journey to Ashkhabad, June 1941

Our group still danced whenever we were asked, and one day in early 1941 Schneider, our director, told us that they want us to dance in Ashkhabad, which is over 2,000 miles from Moscow. I had always had a premonition that if anything happened, if war were declared, I would be miles away from home.

Why I thought that, I don't know. Call it a superstition if you like, or a premonition, but in much the same way Isadora used to say that, if anything happened to her, it would be through being in a car. She always said that, even though she loved travelling in an open-topped car. It was always in the back of her mind.

Now it is a very long way to Ashkhabad, but we had the option to fly there. Whoever wanted to fly, they could, but Schneider warned us that the firm would not pay for us to fly; they would pay only for travel by train. Moss told me not to worry, but just to tell them that I was going to fly; at least then I would have five more days at home. So I told Schneider that, and he agreed. When the others set off, I remained at home, because their journey by train took nearly a week.

I must confess I am not so brave as I made myself out to be. I thought, *Flying all that way, how long shall I be up there, up in the air?* The feeling came and went, but I hardly slept the night before, I was so worried. I thought, *This is an adventure, and not the kind I ever thought I would take on.*

So we went to the airport. Moss saw me off and it was only then that I realised I had forgotten to ask him for some money for the journey, just in case, because they said I would still arrive before the other girls. Their journey on the train took a week, and I had stayed on in Moscow for only five days before flying out on the 6th of June. It was possible there would be nobody there to meet me.

When I went to board the plane, I found I was the only woman there. All the other passengers were men, not only on my flight but on the others. They all seemed to be officials who had gathered for a meeting in Moscow. I suspect they had met to talk about what they would do if war came, and now they were flying in various directions back to their posts.

My neighbour on the plane took an interest in me, as I was the only woman there.

"Where are you going? Why are you taking this flight?"

I explained that we had a concert, that I belonged to a dance group and that the rest were coming by train.

"Oh, you are brave."

"Don't worry, I hardly slept all night."

"What will you do when you get there? The rest of the group

won't be there. Have you some money, in case no one comes to meet you?"

"Well, I haven't, but nevertheless I think I will manage."

"No, no, no, that won't do. I insist on giving you some money."

"But how can I return it to you?"

"Don't worry about that."

Well, I took it; one never knows. We had two stops on the way, to stretch our legs and to refuel the aircraft, I suppose. It gave me a chance to talk to people, but I talked mainly to this neighbour of mine. He was rather nice and very friendly.

So the time went by and finally we arrived, but it gave me such a funny feeling when I stepped out of the plane. It was as if somebody had put me in hot air, because it had been so much colder in Russia itself, and this country was far to the south and east, on the border of the Soviet Union. I didn't even know what it was called. I said goodbye to my neighbour and by luck there was somebody to meet me. They took me to the hotel and of course I had a bath and I felt much fresher. I went to bed and I slept beautifully.

The following day, the other poor girls arrived, quite worn out. They were rather envious of me looking so fresh. The train journey had been very long and very hot.

"Lilya, aren't you lucky?"

"Well, if you had scrimped and saved a little bit, you could have flown too."

They were flat out. Elena Fidaroskiya just said, "I can't even talk" and then lay down on her bed. Elena had joined our group quite a while before. I haven't mentioned her until now because, though she was at school with us, Irma didn't take her to America. That was because her dancing wasn't good enough, I would say, but she had good looks and she fitted in, so we managed.

I don't remember if I shared a room with somebody, but they all fell into bed and I was so fresh that I didn't need to. I felt so sorry for them. It took another day before they came to, and the next day after that we went out to explore the place. It was still very hot, and we were all wearing sundresses, sleeveless dresses. Well, we had to eat and we found a nice restaurant; we went in and sat down, but no one took our order. Instead, the manager came over to speak to us.

"We can't allow women coming in and exposing themselves like this."

We looked at one another, thinking, *Where on earth have we*

229

come to? What a strange thing to say. If they all say that, there won't be anywhere for us to eat. I think he could see we looked baffled.

"Well, put on a little blouse or something."

So we had to do that. We were guests in their country, so we had to obey their rules. And of course we discovered that these people were not Europeans. This was Turkmenistan: they had their own customs and I think they still do. With them, time didn't count; nothing had changed in the way they behaved.

Return from Ashkhabad

We had rehearsals and soon it was the day before our first performance. The strange part was that on that day there was an announcement on the wireless. Molotov, the Foreign Minister, said that Germany had declared war on Russia. I said to myself, *There you are, Lili – just what you always thought would happen. You get all that distance from home and then it happens.* We never had time to give even one concert.

We all said we were going back home, and our manager agreed. He bought the tickets for the train, and there was no difficulty getting first-class seats, because the train started from there. So we managed to get comfortable seats, which was just as well on such a long journey.

On the way, as we came further into European Russia, we started to notice people running. God knows where they were going, but they seemed all to be from the Baltic countries, and there were thousands of them. They all wanted to get on the train but they couldn't, because this was a passenger train, on which you had to book seats. But I thought, *Good gracious, what disorder!* Overnight, it seemed, the whole of Russia had been turned upside down.

It was awful, being besieged like that. The other passengers felt the same. There were a few men travelling home to Moscow, and they couldn't get over it either. We still managed to get food because it was a train equipped with tea – you could have that at any time – and every time the train stopped you could buy food. At each stop, there were always peasants coming out with various nice things they had made. You could buy cheeses, boiled eggs, things like that – even fresh bread sometimes.

So we were not short of food, but at the stops there were these big crowds of foreign people. They seemed to be from the Baltic states, but anyway they were not Russians. We knew that from the way they spoke to one another. I was horrified at this rapid onset of disorder. I thought, *Good gracious, I wonder what is happening in Moscow*. The journey dragged on, much longer than before. It took us over two weeks to get back to Moscow.

Back in Moscow, July 1941

We finally arrived. Of course Moss couldn't get in touch with me; everything stopped and I could imagine how worried he was. My little Leonora was in the country, and I knew she was going to be all right with her auntie Tanya, because Tanya just adored her. She was just two years old, a lovely age, full of spirit, full of fun.

When I got home, I phoned Moss at work, and he didn't recognise my voice.

"I have got a message from your wife."

"Oh, really, I am so desperate. Tell me."

"Moss, darling, it is me – Lili."

"Oh, Lili, you pulled my leg there."

He never forgot his English expressions.

"Yes, I did."

"Never mind, I will come home straightaway."

"Lovely."

I was already at home, and I had a look round. There was no one else there. I think my mother was still in the country. I could see a helmet lying on the settee, with a gasmask and other bits of equipment, and I thought, *No, they cannot send him to fight – he isn't capable of fighting. And I won't let him go*. At that moment he arrived.

How happy he was to see me! Before long we were exchanging news, and then the next question was what we should do now. Moss was unsure.

"I haven't made up my mind. What are you going to do?"

"Well, first, let's go to the country and get Leonora and then I'll tell you, because I have decided what to do."

"Can't you tell me now?"

"No, not yet. And, before we go anywhere, what's all this stuff? Are you preparing to go to war?"

"Yes."

"No, you're not. You won't."

"Why not?"

"You aren't capable of picking up a gun and shooting. They must be barmy to take you – it's like sending a professor. You just couldn't do it."

He laughed then, because luckily enough the government had said, No, he is not going to war; he is staying here. We need him for translation work, especially now with the war. We need somebody who speaks English and Russian fluently. It was already decided, so that was one good thing.

We went to the country and the weather was still marvellous. When we arrived at the *dacha* and opened the door, I could see Tanya crawling under the table with my little Leonora. Tanya did everything that little child wanted. It lifted my spirits to see them playing in the midst of all these terrible events. They were very pleased to see me and Moss. Once we had all exchanged news, they asked what we were going to do. Tanya naturally wanted to know, not just because she had been enjoying looking after Leonora, but because I had many of my belongings in the room Moss and I had occupied. I felt that, now we were all together, I could say what I had decided.

"Well, I have concluded that we should evacuate. I am going to take my mother and Auntie Annie with me, and Leonora. Moss cannot come because he is required to stay here with the government."

After some discussion, they agreed to this.

Barney and Tanya

When we got back to Moscow, we said goodbye to one another. I didn't know what Tanya was going to do. She always had at the back of her mind her worries about Barney. What if she went somewhere safer and then Barney came home to find her gone? It was a terrible problem and I know how she felt, but on the other hand, something good can come out of something bad. At least he wouldn't be fighting, because he was somewhere in Siberia. By the way, I should mention that, not long after Barney disappeared, Tanya found out where he was. She even managed to go and see him a few times.

Luckily enough for Barney, he played the violin, so they spared him the hard labour. The official who ran the camp had his family with him, and when he learn that Barney played the violin, he thought he would like his little boy to learn to play it, so that helped Barney a great deal. And over the years, wherever I travelled, I used to send parcels to him.

I must mention at this point something else connected with Tanya. At Malakava, in the same building where Tanya had her flat, there was a flat that had been let to a couple. This couple were determined to be friends, with me particularly. Her name was Maria; I think she came from the Donbas, the industrial region in the south. This couple seemed to me so odd, because they were ill-matched: she was beautiful, whereas her husband was not very tall and certainly not handsome. But that I will explain later. I mention it now because it came to matter soon afterwards.

Evacuation

When war is declared, normal life is put on hold; everything stops for war. It is so insidious – it gets into everything. That was what I found so dreadful. When I got home from Ashkhabad, Moss had taken no action yet: the situation was very confused and he wouldn't decide anything without me.

At first Moss couldn't understand why I wanted to leave Moscow. I told him it was going to be very dangerous. The authorities kept pressing the point that women should get away with their children while there was an opportunity, because no one could be sure what would happen. Eventually the bombing started, though not very regularly. Just sometimes the siren would go and we would go down to the basement of the block where we lived. The bombers managed to hit a building opposite us, and did some damage, but – so far, so good – our building still stood unscathed.

When we got back with Leonora, and Moss had reluctantly agreed to our evacuation, he then wanted to know how it was I had made up my mind so quickly.

"What made me decide was when I saw all those people fleeing – it was just a sea of people. I couldn't believe my eyes, how far and how quickly the war had spread, and what had happened to the Baltic countries because of Hitler. But, knowing Hitler, the one thing I felt sure of was this: if he did get anywhere near Moscow, the first people he would be sure to destroy were us, the Jewish people. So there is no option: we have to go. And even though you have to stay, you will be easier in your mind, because you will be by yourself. You won't have to worry about anyone else.''

Then I had to go back to the country, to Malakava where Tanya's flat was, because I had left a lot of things there. When she saw me, this young Maria, who rented the flat next to Tanya's, asked me if I was going to evacuate. I said yes, I was.

"Can I join you?"

"Yes. Why not?"

So she came with us. I think she came back to Moscow straightaway with me, since otherwise she wouldn't know when or how we were going to go. I don't know where she stayed, but Moss arranged everything for our evacuation, though not before he had tried to put a spanner in the works.

I started at once to prepare for my journey. I packed so many things, and not just in suitcases; even things like sacks, whatever I had, I filled them up. When my preparations were nearly complete, I went out to get some food. When I came back, everything was unpacked. I was astonished and I turned round to find Moss there.

"Moss, what on earth have you done that for?"

"Look, it's bad enough that you have your family with you. You can't travel with all that stuff as well.''

"Now, Moss. Don't you worry about me. I've worked out what we need and those things are coming with me. One never knows what the future may bring.''

And how far-sighted I was! I think now it was extraordinary to have thought of so many things that turned out to be essential later on. I tried to explain to Moss.

"Please, we are not going to argue about this matter. You just leave it to me. If I say I can manage, I can manage. I understand these things and I know what war is. I have read a great deal. I know what people go through, especially when I read *War and Peace*. I know what I am talking about.''

He didn't argue after that. I packed everything up again and left very little. I left very little to chance either. I didn't know what might happen to Moss – and I was so right.

Journey east, autumn 1941

Moss took us to the station and we boarded the train. The trains had been converted so that, instead of having compartments with seats, there were bunks everywhere; people being evacuated needed somewhere to sleep on the train. We managed to get a big compartment with several bunks and made ourselves comfortable with our luggage.

Maria was with us, which was very comforting. She was young, which made her useful and also it was nice to have a young person with me, since I had two grandmas and my little girl. Maria was always welcome, and she was pleased to be coming with me. Her husband was delighted because he knew me: he had met us at Tanya's place in the country and he was glad to know that she was going somewhere safer with such nice people as us.

In contrast, Moss was very worried. When the train was ready to leave, we said goodbye to each other and he got off. As he stood on the platform, waving to us as the train moved away, I could see he was very sad.

We travelled for quite a bit until, during the night, our train stopped. Aircraft started bombing us. Well, one never knows how one will cope, but when you are young you don't take things as hard as when you get older. Things happen, you have to face them and you are in the hands of Providence. So I gathered us all together and I said we should all stick together; then, if anything happens, we all go together, it's as simple as that. They couldn't get over my bravery, and afterwards neither could I. I didn't blink an eye. We were stranded for about three-quarters of an hour; then the bombing stopped and we managed to get going again. Now that was luck.

We travelled like that for three days. There were stops for various reasons and, at one particular stop on the third day, I thought: I have had enough. We had stopped in a village and it was so pretty, full of trees. Everything was lovely; even the station looked good. I told them the others we would stop here for a breather; we couldn't just keep travelling, God knows where, every hour of every day. This is far enough for the moment. We will stay here for a little while. To myself I thought, *Three days from Moscow, that is quite a good journey we have done*. And we got off.

The train went on and we stayed there. We got to the station building with all our luggage, with help from various people from the village who had come to meet the train. Then we went to the stationmaster and I placed the others and the luggage under his care, while I took Maria with me to look for lodgings.

Chardaevka

The place was called Chardaevka and we soon saw it was very nice. Everything was in order; everything looked cared for. You could tell straightaway that the roads were properly maintained. People had nice homes; they were quite rustic homes, but nevertheless they were neat. The peasants were very well dressed; they were a kind of half-peasantry, because the village was very large and prosperous.

I found a splendid, big room and the owner was pleased to let it to us. It was big enough for me, my little girl (who always slept with me), my mother and Auntie Annie. We all settled there. I had brought a lot of provisions from Moscow with me, so I wasn't short of food. Maria went looking for a place then, and she found a nice little room for herself.

After that, she used to come every day to see me: we used to walk together and we really enjoyed our time. We found there were many other evacuees there, including some very intelligent people. I met a professor from Poland. There were many Polish people, in fact.

The local people understood why we had come and they soon got used to us. They knew the war had started and in fact they were quite pleased to have us. Well, we brought cash with us. We had to live, so we had to pay for food. Maria was useful in negotiating to buy food, because she understood everything about village life. Where she came from, it wasn't a big town; it was a rather countrified place.

Gradually she told me her life history. She had been married before and they had a little child. Her first husband was a very handsome man, but he never took any notice of Maria. He had a high opinion of himself; he thought he was one to be taken notice of, not his wife. Yet she was an intelligent, beautiful woman.

In the office where she worked, there was an engineer. He was quite a big noise in the sense that he was a first-class engineer and well-known by reputation. When he met Maria, he didn't know much about her background, but he couldn't get over her beauty. Maria told me that every day, when she came to work, he would come with something: he would bring her flowers, he would bring her chocolates.

"You know, Lilya, I never had such attention."

He fell deeply in love with her, and she liked him too. She left her husband with their child, and went off with her new husband. Usa, his name was.

She told me all this, a bit at a time, over a period of several weeks, because we stayed in Chardaevka for about two and a half months, I should say, and we were together all the time. One day she told me, "You know, Lilya, this is very rich, lovely countryside here. They are all prosperous." How on earth did she know that?

Well, her landlady had told her where she kept food. She had a place down a few steps – you couldn't call it a basement, but it was partly below ground level, because that kept the food cool – and she said Maria could help herself to cream or whatever she fancied. She had preservatives there, among other things. So Maria invited me to come and see.

"Lilya, come and I am going to treat you."

"How can you? It isn't yours to give."

"It's all right. She told me I could have whatever I wanted."

We spent a nice time together in Chardaevka, and I was pleased to have Maria with me.

Besides that, we made friends with other people. There were some lovely families there, most of them from the Ukraine. I had been to the Ukraine, because we gave concerts there. We performed in Kiev, a beautiful city, and from there we went to Odessa, where we had probably the biggest success we ever had for our group.

I remember that visit to Odessa especially. In fact, I always preferred Ukraine to Russia itself. The people are so friendly, very kind and very open. They have the best soil in the world, too: it is called 'black soil' (I am translating it from the Russian).

One evening, as we were about to part, Maria asked me to come and sleep with her; she felt lonely. So I agreed and I told my mum and Auntie Annie that I was going to sleep with Maria, so they would know where I was. But Maria wouldn't let me sleep. She kept telling me how much she missed her husband and how he knew that she couldn't be long without him. I thought that was so funny, honestly. In these times when everybody was trying desperately to save their lives and salvage what they could, here was Maria still full of thoughts of love.

Finally we did fall asleep, only to be woken a little later by a knock on the window, and who was it, in the middle of the night? Her husband. So I had to get out of bed and I walked home to my place. Still, that didn't matter.

The following day we found that he had come to take Maria to Siberia, to Sverdlovsk, I think. He was taking her there because he had been appointed to run a big factory. So they packed their belongings and we said goodbye. We never knew if we would meet again. But circumstances always create something, and often something unexpected, because we did meet later on.

Talk about coincidence

When the war reached Russia, all the girls from our group and all our friends quickly made their own decisions and went off. There was usually no time to tell us where they were going, and no time for us to find out. Tanya disappeared somewhere, with her mother; everybody went wherever they chose to go. But I must confess that I had already decided to go to Alma-ata. I had never been to Alma-ata and I didn't know anyone there, though I knew it was a long way, but there was a reason for choosing it, which I will tell you afterwards.

We were able to correspond with Moss, and he wrote to say he was very pleased that we had found somewhere safe to stop, to have a breather. As time went on and Maria went away, our friends that we had made there met and talked about the situation, and I kept reviewing our position. Then I got a letter from Moss, in which he wrote, "Don't be surprised if you don't hear from me" – and that was all he wrote. I thought, *Well, this doesn't sound very good.*

I decided we ought to make a move. Because Moss had said that I wouldn't hear from him, I didn't trouble to tell him what I was up to; I knew he wouldn't get the letter. Perhaps I should have written; I never considered it. I intended to leave a message with our landlady to say where we were going, because Moss knew her address. He could go there if anything happened. I started talking to a family, a woman with two children.

"You know, I am thinking of moving on."

"So am I."

"Shall we combine our forces and travel together?"

"That would be a splendid idea. The more people you know, the better."

"Fine. Well, the first thing we have to do is prepare food for the journey."

We began preparing the food and that took us over two weeks. I had to get biscuits, bread and a big leg of ham. I bought meat and made loads of loads of cutlets. I knew they would last – the weather was changing and going east it would be rather cold. I had two big wooden crates full of food, besides our luggage.

The day came to say goodbye to our landlady, and I left a message with her that our destination was to be Alma-ata. We went to the station, where the stationmaster knew us from before. He asked where were we going? And I said we had decided to go to Alma-ata. There was a group of us.

We asked when would there be a train, and he said they came once a day. We would have to sit and wait, because he couldn't tell us what time the train would arrive. It might be hours before it came. So we went to the waiting-room. There we were, patiently waiting, sitting on our luggage. I can never forget what happened next.

We were sitting very quietly, when the door opened and Moss walked in. Well, talk about coincidence, strange events – they always happened to me. I could not believe it. He looked dreadful. Haggard, but then the weather was cold. At least he was wearing a very warm coat, and he had a rucksack on his back. I ran to him.

"This is a bit of luck!"

"You can say that again."

It turned out that he had arrived earlier, when we were already at the station, but he hadn't come through the station entrance. He had gone straight out of the station to the village, to our lodgings, where the landlady told him that we had left that morning.

"Where were they going?"

"Your wife told me she was going to Alma-ata."

He thought, *Well, there is no point staying here by myself.*

He had been planning to come and join us in Chardaevka, and then he would be able to tell me what had been happening to him. I hadn't written to him because he told me there wouldn't be any more letters. Otherwise, he would have been prepared for us moving on. So he went to the station to ask about trains to Alma-ata, and he was told that the train might be hours yet and he could wait in the waiting-room. And then imagine his joy when he saw us there. He couldn't believe it.

A slight change of plan

Moss looked slightly dazed and I hastened to reassure him.

"Don't worry Moss, I will arrange everything. We leave the two grannies here – I will make up a kind of a bed and they can sleep on that, on top of our luggage. Just wait while I do that, and then I will take you back to our lodgings. You can have a bath there. The landlady will have some supper for you; I know the woman. She is nice and kind, and she is married with children, so she will certainly have food prepared, and we will have somewhere to sleep the night."

And that is what we did. I took Moss and little Leonora to the lodgings where we had been staying, and left the two old ladies to look after the luggage. The people who had joined us also stayed at the station, because they had nowhere else to go. When we got to the place where I had rented the room, the woman was amazed.

"Well, that is absolutely extraordinary, that you hadn't left by the time your husband got there."

I asked her if she could give us some supper, and she willingly did. Then I asked very nicely if my husband could have a bath; because they had no bathroom – that was out of the question in those parts – so it meant boiling a lot of water and gradually filling a very big container, a big tub. I helped him to wash and we went to bed. He was worn out. Even though he had found us and he was safe, he looked worried. I thought he needed to relax a bit.

I wasn't sure what was bothering him. He had taken some food. He had collected a lot of food, but he left in such a hurry that he had to leave most of it at home. Apparently his office phoned and told him to be ready in ten minutes. Well, how can one be ready in ten minutes? Of course he might have known that sooner or later something would happen without warning, and that he had to be ready, but Moss didn't prepare. I found that strange, because I would have had everything ready for any emergency; but I wasn't there, so of course half of the things he wanted to take he didn't.

Maybe that worried him. On the journey, I know he didn't eat for three days. The other people on the train had practically nothing to eat, except there was a stove in the carriage and they used it to make baked potatoes. I don't know what type of train it was; he never told me any details and I wouldn't ask him, because it was bad enough when he told me he hadn't eaten anything. Yet he had brought chocolate, cheese and all sorts of things, and he had never touched any of it.

He said it was for Leonora. I said, "You know, Moss, darling, you should have eaten something, because you know I am very capable of looking after Leonora." I had everything that was necessary – eggs, milk and so on. So I wasn't worried about that. We had food and I knew where we were going, but Moss was with the government. If they were leaving Moscow, that was really frightening.

When Moss learn what I was planning to do, and I got cracking to get it organised, he didn't object. He didn't say Alma-ata was too far or anything. I said we were going to Alma-ata, but I never told him the reason and he never asked. I kept that to myself. I knew it was on the Chinese border and I thought, *When we get there, I shall see*.

On the cattle train

The train did come next morning. We didn't wait very long, we boarded the train and started our journey. It was awful. The train was made up of cattle trucks, which they used to take the cows or horses from place to place, though they had been cleaned out and they had made bunks for us. I had brought sheets, blankets and pillows with me, because I was very far-sighted.

I had travelled a great deal and I had a good idea what to expect, and especially the sort of facilities we might have. In this case we were lucky because our carriage had a little compartment with tap water and a toilet. So this was a great help and cheered us up a little at the start of our long trip. It seemed endless and it was boring.

Moss seemed broken; he had lost his spark. I said to him, "Moss, cheer up! After all, you found us." I was a bit concerned about him. I noticed his behaviour was without any life. And I felt so hurt, because he should have been so happy to have caught us, yet it seemed the reverse. Perhaps he was still stunned at being ordered to abandon his job and flee Moscow. I don't know.

The village where we had been staying was full of food and it was really lucky for us that we had stopped there. Now the bad weather was approaching, though it was still not full winter, and that was a blessing too. The journey was long and tedious, but one had to put up with it. I think Moss didn't object to going so far from Moscow because nobody really knew what the outcome of the war would be. We all knew it was going to be a prolonged business because Russia is vast, and the Germans had plenty of manoeuvring to do, plenty of places to bomb and occupy. They were going to be very busy, and we had to keep out of the way.

I noticed that, when I took a biscuit, he would be watching – I suppose, because I had so many of them. I thought I was just having one now and then.

"Lili, you are not hungry, are you?"

"No, not really. You are quite right."

"Well, don't nibble. One never knows what the food situation is going to be when we arrive wherever we are going."

And I took notice of him; I never liked to upset him over anything. He was right, too, because we had food enough; and the people who joined us, the little family, there was only the woman. Nobody had husbands with them then. The husbands were away fighting. I was lucky that I had a husband with me.

This woman had two lovely children, and they were no trouble. We had stops, and that gave them the chance to run and stretch their legs. We usually managed to make a fire out of logs because the stop would be for a good hour or so. The other person who came with us – she wasn't a neighbour, but she piled in with us because she had heard we were going; I don't remember her name – she was so nice. She managed to make some soup, I remember, and gave us a little each. I had plenty of meat and other things, and bread galore.

I always kept a watch out, because there were people from all parts of the Balkans, entering our carriage, getting off or getting on. I was terrified they would bring some disease, and when we had stops I was always asking the people in the next carriage what happened. They would say, "Yes, yes, children do get ill, some of them very ill; some died even." I was terrified, honestly; that was the only thing that really worried me, that my little girl shouldn't catch anything.

I wasn't concerned at all for myself, nor for Moss and the two elderly ladies; they were fine. We were altogether very happy, except for Moss. I couldn't understand it, and he wouldn't com-municate with me. I thought, *I had better leave him alone until we*

242

get there. And eventually we did get there, of course, because I am here to tell you the story.

Alma-ata, at last

When we arrived at Alma-ata, we were met. There were people preparing for us: they knew a train was coming loaded with immigrants and they had a huge big room ready for us. I don't know what building it was, I have no idea. All I knew was there were beds there prepared for us, so we could relax a bit. Our luggage was safe, too. I know many people lost their luggage, but everything went well with us. Well, everything had gone well so far – except that I watched my little girl and she seemed to me a bit lifeless, only a little, not much. She still ate whatever I gave her.

Now the name of Alma-ata, its name in the local language, translates as 'Cradle of Apples', and indeed I have never seen so many apples on the trees in season. Moss perked up, perhaps because he now saw a role for himself.

"You stay here, Lili. I am going to look for lodgings, to find us a place to go."

When Moss tried to go out, they told him not to bother.

"Don't go to Alma-ata – it is full. You won't be able to find a place to stay there. We will take you to a village called Uzun-argach."

So they took us to this place called Uzun-argach, not far from Alma-ata.

12

Beyond the Steppes of Central Asia, 1941–5

Uzun-argach is very different

The last two thousand kilometres of our journey from Moscow to Alma-ata had been across the steppes; at first it was grassland as far as you could see, but the grass got drier and drier until the landscape was more like desert. By contrast, Alma-ata, when we got there in late summer, was full of apple trees and other greenery, but it was also full of evacuees, so they gave us a little cart for my family and our luggage, and along with other evacuees we set off for Uzun-argach, a small place about 25 miles from Alma-ata.

It took us a little time to get there. The name translates as 'Tall Trees', so I knew this was going to be a pleasant place, perhaps with many trees. And I wasn't wrong. When we arrived, we found that the local people had prepared for us, just as in Chardaevka. What surprised us was that many of the people we saw were clearly not native to the place; in fact, there were many Russians. Now this was a strange phenomenon, the background to which I learnt only later.

Apparently, in the tsars' time and even after the revolution, when people in some way behaved badly, the government used to send them into internal exile, to this corner of Kazakhstan around Alma-ata. They had spread out from there into villages like Uzun-argach, where many of them had settled. These Russians were not peasants; nor were they unintelligent. But neither were they exactly from the intelligentsia: when I got to know them, I found they included some of the cream of the professional classes – lawyers, doctors and the like.

Of course, there were many of the local people there too, with very high cheekbones and slitty eyes, looking to us very much like Mongolians. There didn't seem to be many of them there for our arrival; I think that was because they didn't mix much with the Russians. They had their own places, partly because their diet was so different. They never ate meat from cows or bulls; they ate horse meat. They used to drive a horse and also eat the flesh. We found this very odd.

They were a bit concerned about what they were going to find, we found out afterwards, because they had never seen Jews before. They had often heard about them, but they had no idea what we might look like. They were surprised when they first met us, because we didn't look as strange as they expected. We had to laugh at that. When we got there, they showed us to a big place they had prepared for us. When everyone had arrived, we all had to gather in the square, to get acquainted with the people who lived there. There was a vet, and he was in charge. People came round to greet us and talk to us. They said, "Don't worry, we will make you as comfortable as we can." That was rather reassuring.

After that, we went back to where we had waited first. Moss said I should stay there while he went to look for lodgings. He went off, and now I could see that my little girl was ailing. What it was, I had no idea, but it didn't seem too bad. She was just a bit lifeless. Moss soon came back, because Uzun-argach was not very big.

It's hard to say what sort of place it was. It seemed like a kind of village – to Moss and me, at least – but really I suppose it was more like a very small town. It wasn't just a countrified place, and it had quite a lot of facilities. It had plenty of houses – some a bit nicer than the usual, some not so nice – a central square and proper streets, not just muddy lanes.

We meet the Gauchins

When Moss came back, he explained what he had arranged.

"Somebody recommended me to this chap, and we got talking. He is a librarian – at least, there is a library with some books and he looks after it. I don't know who owns it, but he's in charge. They are willing to let us have a room, but he says he would like to meet you, Lili, because if he is going to take people he needs to see them first."

What he had actually said to Moss was a little different.

"I would like to meet your wife before I agree to take you."

So I went with Moss - Auntie Annie and my mother stayed with little Leonora - and this librarian met us, took a look at me and agreed to rent us a room.

We went back to collect our belongings and Leonora, and told the two ladies. Moss found a place for them as well, because we had to separate. This librarian - Gauchin, his surname was - had a wife and two boys. His wife - I think her name was Natasha - said, "You are going to have dinner with us: I am cooking everything." She was so kind; in fact, the whole family were. They said they would give us the best room, which I thought was very generous of them, but they could not make it ready for us until the following day. For that first night they gave us a bed in a bedroom.

While dinner was being prepared, I made a bed on the stove. I don't know if you have seen those Russian stoves, the kind they have in the villages. They are tiled containers and the top is flat like a floor and big enough to lie on. Even when the stove is burnt out, the warmth just stays, so we made a bed on top of the stove for Leonora and laid her down, and she fell fast asleep. Then we all had dinner at the big table, in the best room, the one they were going to give us the following day.

We were quite taken by their hospitality and of course there was plenty to talk about. Moss even made a joke, and this was the first time he had come to, somehow. He had been in something of a state the whole journey. Instead of him cheering me up, I had been trying to cheer him up, which was odd. Moss and I settled for the night - the two of us in a single bed, and a small bed at that, but we didn't care because we were just pleased to put our heads down - and we fell asleep.

Leonora falls ill

During the night I awoke when I heard Leonora calling.

"Mummy, Mummy!"

"Yes, darling? What is wrong?"

"My ears are hurting."

At that I got very alarmed. I had already had to see to her hair, because it was infested by the little vermin we had picked up on our travels. That was awful. Now I began to wonder what else she might have picked up. Anyway, I put some kerosene on her scalp, rubbed it in gently and then covered her hair up, and she fell asleep.

In the morning she had a fever. In her little ears there was something like pus, boiling over and running down, so there had to be something in there. We didn't know what she might have got during the journey - nothing would have surprised us, since we had been travelling for three weeks with only the most basic facilities - but the infected matter ran right down to her neck and made a kind of ribbon round it.

She had a very high temperature, but luckily they had a hospital there, and Moss - seeing how worried I was - told me to take her straight in. I nearly died of anxiety, but I never lose my head. Moss and I went straight there and it turned out to be quite a clean, pleasant little hospital. We saw the doctor in charge and she had a look at Leonora.

"This little girl has to have some M&B" - that was the name of a tablet in those days, like an antibiotic - "but we haven't any here. However, don't worry. A little later on tonight, I am going to Alma-ata to fetch some."

Meanwhile, she took us to the children's ward and we put Leonora to bed. She had a very high temperature, and I sat there beside her all night. There were three or four other children on the ward, with their parents. One mother came over and spoke to me. She said, "Nobody ever died in this little ward of ours." Well, that did comfort me.

Next morning, Moss was ringing every quarter of an hour, and what could I say?

"Moss, we don't know. She is burning hot, and we haven't got that M&B yet."

"What do you think, Lili? Is she going to pull through?"

"Look, one has to prepare for the worst. If it happens, there is nothing one can do."

Things can happen very quickly with small children, and in this situation they might soon go from bad to worse.

Later that day, the senior doctor came back with the M&B and we started giving it to Leonora. Over the following night, everything cleared and her temperature fell back towards normal. The doctor felt, as I did, that we had been very lucky.

"How on earth did you manage to bring such a tiny flower with you such a long, long way, without her going down with something on the way? Really, it is a miracle she got so far. Now that her temperature has gone down, I think you had better take her away with you, take her home, because you never know what infections she could get from the other children here.''

So I wrapped her up and took her home. When I got there and showed him Leonora, Moss was clearly relieved, so much so that this was the first time I had ever seen him show emotion since we first met. He was absolutely delighted.

After I had brought Leonora back from the hospital, our landlady, Natasha, prepared a Turkish bath for us. She and her husband had to prepare the hot water and the steam, but everything was arranged and we all had this marvellous wash, in steam and plenty of hot water. I really enjoyed that very much, and so did Moss and our little girl. That is one thing that is very important, to be able to have a good wash.

What else can happen?

The Gauchins were very concerned about Leonora, Natasha especially. She was so nice and I liked her, but to be honest I was a bit frightened of her husband. Now, he wasn't a boor. He behaved very well and tried to be as friendly as he could – I also noticed that he read and was rather intelligent in the way that he read. He kept the library of course, and he knew authors too, but nevertheless there was something not quite right there, something I couldn't put into words.

Meanwhile, they prepared the main room for us, the room where they used to eat. It had that big stove, to do your cooking on, and there was a fair-sized bed where Moss and I could sleep together. Everything was fine really, except that I wasn't used to doing hard work, but I had to manage. Keeping the stove supplied with fuel was so difficult, because you couldn't get wood. There was hardly any to be had in that part of the Soviet Union. As the name Uzun-argach implied, there were indeed some very tall trees, but not many, so people wouldn't cut them down for firewood.

What they did have was a strange plant with something like a prickly flower on top. They called it coreye. Towards the end of the year, this flower used to turn in on itself and dry out, and then people collected it. Well, it was easy to collect, but very difficult to bring back. My poor mum tried to help, but she didn't live with us then and anyway she found carrying it even harder than I did.

Natasha – our landlady, I suppose I should call her, since the place belonged to her – used to get enough coreye for all of us, but when it came to putting it in the stove I had no gloves, nothing. And of course I caught my thumb on one of those prickly flowers – it had thorns like a rose – and my thumb became infected and swelled up quite badly. I had terrible pain and I couldn't do anything. Natasha knew what to do though, to get rid of it. You had to bake an onion, put it on the swelling and wrap it up, which I did. That helped and in two days the swelling went down. So that was lucky too.

This place where we stayed was not bad. You couldn't call it primitive, because they had a very nice little Turkish bath, which they had built for themselves, with all the facilities. Among other features, the house had a balcony all the way round the back. We ate well too. I discovered there was a regular market where you could buy food, and I began to do some cooking. We began to settle in, but I could see that Moss wasn't very happy. He missed his work and his colleagues. Still, we were all together now and Leonora was getting better day by day.

As she became livelier again, I noticed something else. If I spoke to her and she wasn't facing me, she didn't respond. I told Moss.

"You know, I don't think Leonora can hear anything."

I took her back to the hospital and the doctor looked in Leonora's ears. There was an infection there. It seemed that, whatever the illness she had had, it had affected her eardrums. The doctor gave me some drops to clear out the ears, and they did help a bit, but Leonora was still in pain. The doctor was not a specialist and she didn't really know what the infection was or how to cure it. What we needed was a specialist in ears, nose and throat, and I thought I should take Leonora to Alma-ata to see one. Moss began to worry again.

I had noticed he was getting a bit restless and not himself. He couldn't find any work to do in Uzun-argach and he needed to be kept occupied, I knew. What I didn't know, because Moss hadn't told me, was that his department had been in touch with him. His colleagues had been looking for him, because they needed him at work. Now he told me that he had written back, to say he would come and join them. When I heard this, I thought, *Never mind, Lili, you'll get over it. If he has decided, don't try to talk him out of it. If he wants to go, let him go.*

"Yes, you go."

"Will you manage?"

"Look, dear, of course I'll manage. I always manage."

By now we had been in Uzun-argach a little while and we had made friends among the evacuees. There were people from Poland, from various parts of the Baltic states and a lot from the Ukraine, who were lovely people. I wasn't going to be friendless.

People thrown together

There were neighbours on each side of us. Our landlady, Natasha, had a brother and he lived to the right of us in an enormous lodge, a sort of *dacha*, a beautiful place with a huge open fire. I had never seen anything so lovely. Not long after Leonora came back from hospital, our landlord killed a pig, and he and his wife had a party for their family to celebrate the whole pig. As his wife's brother had this big place, they decided to have the party there; we were invited too, as their lodgers.

The brother also had lodgers, a husband and wife. At least, I thought they were a married couple, but I found out afterwards – I met them quite often from then on – that they both came from Kiev, in the Ukraine, but they had simply been friends there. They had run away, but I don't know the circumstances. She was blonde, a beautiful-looking woman. He was married, but I don't know what happened to his wife. I knew he was Jewish, and that was about all I knew. They were very nice, so it didn't matter. You know, people were thrown together because the whole country – the whole of Europe – was upside down. When you got talking to people you didn't know, they would say, 'We are lucky to be alive'. That was what you heard all the time.

Anyway, they had this big party, Natasha's brother and his wife, and they made their main room just like a big hall, with tables all the way round the walls, and benches. The cooking was based on their national dishes. When they killed an animal, especially a pig, they used to make these *pillamainy*, as they called them. The English don't eat that sort of thing; at least they never used to, but now they sell them, sometimes stuffed. They made pastry, very thin, and cut it out; then they stuffed it with that fresh meat, minced. But you can't imagine how good it tasted, what with the way the mince was

250

prepared and it being so fresh! It wasn't just the *pillamainy* that were stuffed with good food. We had a very good time.

We all sat down and I thought Moss would liven up a bit, but at least he was pleased; I can't say he wasn't. They were serving this wonderful dish, hot, steaming – the smell was delicious, I remember – and we had a little drink they had prepared for us. That drink seemed to do Moss a power of good. We spent a very lovely time there. I thought they were such nice people. It was funny to us that up till then they had no idea what Jews were like, and they thought we were absolutely wonderful. But that is how it is when people meet one another: they often get a pleasant surprise.

To our left there was another nice family, from Poland, I think. Not long after we had arrived, I needed something – a grate or some-thing, for cooking – and Moss said he thought these people seemed *sympatiya* and the wife would be willing to help. And of course she did, and we became friendly. I know they had suffered some mis-fortune. The husband had found a job as a secretary. They had a daughter – about 16, a very nice girl. They had a cousin with them – a pleasant young man, I remember. I don't know what happened to the whole family: I never asked, and it takes time before people tell you about themselves.

They did tell me how they had been robbed of a lot of their luggage. They were very well-to-do people and their winter coats, beautiful fur coats, had been stolen; I felt very sorry for them. Their journey had been longer and more difficult than ours. We had fol-lowed one straightforward route from Moscow, whereas they had had to leave their country, cross the border and get through a battle zone, to reach Alma-ata.

Next day, I went to see the doctor and told her that Moss might have to go away. She said, "You know what? Be happy, Mrs Muscat! We have the leading ear, nose and throat specialist coming from Kiev, and he will be here any day." I felt a lot better when I heard that. I told Moss, so he would be relieved of the worry. He had been given a date for his return to duty, so now he packed his things, ready to go.

I felt rather empty at the idea of being without him, so far from home. As we said goodbye, Moss promised to be in touch and said not to worry. He went to Ekaterinaburg – I think that was its name – but afterwards they called it Sverdlovsk. It is in Siberia and that was where the government went.

Not for all the tea in China

But now I must tell you something that I forgot to mention, which happened earlier. We had come to know many people, lawyers and professional people, and a group of them wanted to go to China. They were talking about this and they asked me if I would be interested. I said, "Yes, I would." When I got home, I put this idea to Moss.

"Don't you think it's a good idea? They say crossing the border is nothing to worry about, because nobody's there. The Russians aren't guarding that border; the Chinese might be, but not the Russians because they are fighting a war in the west. This is an opportunity. There's a big group of Polish people who want to go to China and from there they are planning to make their way to America or wherever. Look, if you're worried about our two grandmas, that's not a difficulty. We can take them with us."

"But what would I do?"

"You will throw your passport away, and the first big place we come to in China, you will go to the embassy – wherever we end up, there is bound to be an English embassy – you will ask for a copy of your birth certificate and then get an English passport. After that, we can go wherever we like."

"And what about Leonora? She might not survive the journey. We cannot take the chance. No."

Moss flatly refused. Maybe he was sorry later; I don't know. But it was no good. I couldn't do it without him, and in any case I wouldn't. It was after that episode that he got in touch with his colleagues, found out they were looking for him and agreed to go back. In the meantime, Leonora had this calamity.

He perhaps thought that, if we had decided to go to China, I would just pack and go, but I wouldn't. First of all I would have seen to Leonora, because there was no hurry. We had nobody to pester us – the government were far away – and they had their own rules in Kazakhstan. It wasn't Russia. So I would have taken her to Alma-ata to see to her ears. Then, Moss had a lot of money, so we could do something about getting foreign currency, I knew that. If you try in your life, you succeed; it is only when you don't try that you don't succeed. But he refused. It was no good me explaining how we would manage. He was adamant that Leonora might not survive. Well, on that ground I would not argue, because one can never be certain of anything.

The hospital porter

It is very strange how people meet. For instance, a man appeared at the hospital, God knows where from, a nice, intelligent man. He wasn't young, he wasn't that old, and he picked up the job of hospital porter. You might wonder why I took notice of him. It was simply that, when I came to the hospital with Leonora, he happened to enter the building at the same time. For some reason or other – one cannot tell how people pile up together – but in some way he liked me and my little girl, and we became friendly.

His first name was Lazar and his surname was Sobel. It is the Russian word for a little animal – mink, I think. Anyway, I was often at the hospital with Leonora, and one day I asked him where he had come from: "From a prison camp." "Goodness! What were you doing there?" Well, he had been taken away during one of Stalin's purges in the 1930s, when they used to arrest people for nothing. You can imagine what people went through. I know what it was like when we lost Barney, and he was still in the camp.

Lazar was willing to help us get to China. Moss met him too and liked him, but he turned this offer down. He was very frightened that Leonora might not cope. I think he found the whole idea of trying to leave the Soviet Union too worrying even to think about. Yet I would have managed with Leonora, and he would have been able to get his birth certificate, because I have a copy now; I had to get it when my daughter was getting married.

Still, we became very friendly with this Lazar Sobel, who was a very intelligent man, though he was doing the job of handyman, really. I asked him how he managed the work he was doing. "Well, after what I went through in the prison camp, now there is nothing I can't do. Whatever it is, I am helping people who need help. I do various things, whatever is needed."

Meanwhile, with all these visits, I had also become very friendly with the doctor, the head of the hospital. The day came when she told me that this eminent specialist was coming the next day. I couldn't wait for tomorrow, to see him. Well, he did arrive and I took my little girl to see him. He had a look at her ears and asked what I had been giving her; I showed him the drops. He soon told me what to do with them.

"No, no, throw those drops out: they are eating at her eardrums. I am going to give you some of these yellow pills. Dissolve one in boiling water, dip some cotton wool in it and then dab it inside the ear, and that will gradually clear it.''

I started treating Leonora that same day. It might seem simple, that treatment, but it was just like anything else in the world: when you know what to do, it's easy. Within about two weeks, her hearing came back and she was well again. Things were getting better, and we had lovely new neighbours where we lived. Yes, now I must tell you what else I did.

On my own

Mr Gauchin was getting a little too friendly towards me, and I didn't like that. His wife, Natasha, was lovely. But I didn't care for my landlord; I didn't feel comfortable with him around. Not that I was frightened of him, but I was concerned that he would start pestering me. I had met men like him before.

I decided to move out. Besides, I wanted my mother to be with me. I missed her. So I went looking, and in the centre of the village I found a room in the house of a little old lady. Mind you, she wasn't that old: she still went out to work. When I asked whether she would be willing to rent me the room, she said she would, with pleasure; but she would have to sleep in the corner. It was quite a spacious room, so I told her not to worry about that.

I set to work to make it comfortable, but I had to improvise. I got hold of some planks and I used four of them to make a bed; for a mattress, I found a container and put some hay in it to make it firm enough to sleep on; I had sheets and pillows and a blanket, but nothing else. Now that I had a bed for myself, I began to look round for something for my mother and I managed to get a settee that she could sleep on. We had a little table and there was a big stove in the room, the usual kind of stove.

Our little landlady, this elderly woman, worked at the *kolkhoz*, the collective farm, and she worked very hard. I forget what we used to call her, but I know we gave her a name of some sort. Her teeth were half gone and she looked old to me then, but nevertheless she was so tough, that woman.

She had a son and a daughter, but they were away from home. Her daughter had gone to stay with her aunt in Alma-ata, because she wanted to study. They were not dull, these village people; they knew

254

exactly what they were doing. Her son was away in the army, fighting. He was married and normally lived at home, so she had given him and his wife half of her house – or rather 'hut', I would say. I don't know if it was made of clay, but it wasn't wood.

In the other half of her home lived the daughter-in-law, and she had brought her sister to live with her. There was also her son's little girl, her grand-daughter. These three occupied just one room, and they had their own facilities there, though very sparse of course. They lived in a strange way. You couldn't call them Gypsies, but they slept on the floor. I know her mother-in-law, our grand little lady, used to complain to me how awful they were and how they would take liberties with her. And I would say, 'Well, you can't help it: that's life.'

She had a cow and chickens, so we had fresh eggs every day for my daughter – and we wouldn't have had those in Moscow. She used to bake delicious bread, in that big stove of hers. The best thing was she used to share everything with us. Of course I paid her for whatever we used. She had a pig as well. I remember that because the pig had a litter and she brought one of the piglets inside, into our room. It didn't matter really; we understood how it felt. We wrapped it up to keep it warm, to help it survive, just as we had wrapped up when we first came to Russia in 1921. It was a struggle for that piglet, just as it had been for us.

So we settled in, my mum and I. Auntie Annie stayed where she was in the village and of course I didn't neglect her. I used to go to see her periodically and she seemed to be managing all right, but she used to get depressed, like her son. I think she and Moss had something in common there. I know he was very fond of her, and so was I, but when we returned home from this evacuation, I found out that she was not so nice as I had thought she was. But that is nothing to do with this part of my story.

Leonora got well again, and we all got on well with the woman too. I contacted Moss and told him what I had done. He was pleased I had settled, and he sent me money. Of course it wasn't enough. More than ever, I was glad I had packed so many things when I left home – that time when Moss unpacked everything and I had to pack it all up again. Now it all came in useful, because I had to start selling things – well, not selling exactly. What I did, I bartered them for food.

I had some wonderful embroidered tablecloths with me, and that was the reason I took them: to have something to barter, that many people might want. I had travelled from an early age, so I knew that when you arrive in a strange place, somewhere you know nothing about, you won't always have money – or not the sort of money that people in that place will accept. So to me this wasn't something unexpected, a thing I wasn't prepared for. I knew exactly what was needed in such a situation, and I proved to be so right in my preparations and the way I managed things.

More about Lazar Sobel

I told Lazar where we had moved, and as time went by he used to come to see us. He liked my mother too, and he was so nice. When he had free time, he used to tell me all the details of what went on in the Kremlin, the bickering and the terrible schemes that the apparatchiks were working on, before he was arrested. He told me how they used to go to Paris – things like that, all the details.

One day I asked him something of more immediate importance. Physically, he had begun to pick up a bit, but he still looked rather thin from the camp.

"How are you managing with food?"

"Not very well, really, because they don't cook in the hospital. They only nurse the children, and the parents or whoever brings the child supplies the child with food."

"Look, Lazar, you need a bit of fattening up, and my mother is a marvellous cook. Why don't you come and eat with us sometimes? Even if it's just soup, it will soon build you up."

My mother cooked once a day, and often it was soup; but, when I say 'soup', I am talking about real soup, a thick broth with beef and vegetables. She used to go every morning to the market and get everything she needed for a really rich soup.

Each day we had one good meal, a good dinner. I don't know what we managed on in between, but mum would make an omelette or some pancakes when the stove was on. Our diet now was superb, and I invited Lazar to join us for dinner. Before long, he used to come every day and have a bowl of that wonderful soup that my mum cooked. He used to say, "How can I thank you?" and I said "Don't talk about that. We all have to help one another."

We had good water too. I had a little pail, which I had brought

256

from home. I had tried to think of everything. I thought I would be glad of this pail, especially for my little daughter's needs, and I was right. I used to go and fetch water from a spring. There was a little stream coming down the mountainside. That was pure water, really clear, sweet running water and I used to fill my pail there.

The scenery pleased me too. I used to like that little walk up the mountain road, even when it was winter. I had brought plenty of warm clothes from home, because I took everything I could lay my hands on. I used to walk to the spring each day, and on my way there and back I used to turn over my memories and talk to myself in my head: *Yes, I will get there. I will get to London. I will manage. I don't know how, but I will.* I used to like thinking about pleasant things, and Uzun-argach wasn't bad either.

In fact, I really got to like the place. It had beauty as well, because it was on the border with China, near the beautiful mountains of Tibet. It was fantastic, especially when spring came: then, it was absolutely glorious. Even my mother noticed the scenery, because she commented on it. "Lili, isn't it beautiful?"

By then, spring was approaching. I got a letter from Moss, saying that he had settled in fine and sending me some money, and of course he sent his mother money too. He had plenty of it; there was no problem there. The problem was that he never sent me enough, because we had to buy everything on the black market, even bread. You just couldn't get decent bread from ordinary shops. They seemed to sell nothing at all, but you could buy things if you asked the right people and paid their price.

You had to adapt yourself to their way of life, and I found that most interesting – in fact, I rather enjoyed it. The whole village was like that, an extraordinary mixture of shortages in the midst of plenty. That was the funny part. There we were crammed into one room, yet there was that marvellous freedom, because there was so much space: they had these plains, the steppes as the Russians call them, plains where they grew wheat. I mean, they could have supplied the whole world with wheat, whereas all I wanted was enough flour to make some bread, but you just couldn't buy flour. I wondered how I could get at that wheat. So I talked to my friend Lazar, and he said, "Don't worry, I will arrange something."

Usa's family

There was another family who became very friendly towards me. This husband and wife came from Kiev. He was an official of some sort. I don't remember his surname, but I think his first name was Usa; I am fairly sure it was. Her name I can't recall, but their daughter's name was Clara. I knew her better, because whenever she could be in my company she would always be there. She actually just fell in love with me. Well, I was young then, I was not even 28, and she was a lovely girl. Her mother too was very fond of me.

Usa used to help us a great deal. If I needed extra potatoes, he used to get them for me, and I used to help him in other ways. I used to help Lazar, and he did odd jobs in return, so he too became friendly with them. In addition, he was free to go wherever he wanted – but that was later on. I will return to that. We were all very good friends indeed. It was extraordinary. I would say our mutual help and friendship lasted nearly five years before the war stopped.

I had said to Lazar that I would like to get hold of some wheat, because my mother could bake wonderful bread. So he talked to our new friends, this family, and Usa he said he knew a village where we could get grain, a place where the people native to that area lived, but they wouldn't take money: you had to have something to barter. And I had. I had still a lot of lovely cloth that Moss had brought from London. He had never had it made into a suit, because he couldn't find anyone who could do that expertly enough. Well, I wouldn't say they can't sew, but there were certain things the Russians couldn't handle. They never really had much private enterprise of their own. You could get a good dressmaker, but never a good tailor.

Now I knew where you could get wheat and I had something to barter with. So I asked Lazar how we would get there, and he told me not to worry: he could arrange for us to use a little horse and cart from the hospital. So we fixed a date.

Journey through Kazakhstan

He got this little cart with a horse, and Usa came too, and the three of us set off. I took my cloth to barter, but I don't know whether the other two had anything to barter nor, if so, what they were trying to get. I think perhaps they went just so that I wouldn't be by myself; and of course Usa knew that place, and acted as go-between.

It was quite a journey, because Kazakhstan is rather vast, I would say. It was coming towards evening when we reached this place – it wasn't a village, but anyway some kind of settlement – near the Chinese border, where these Kazakhs lived. They were what we called then 'slitty-eyed people'. When we arrived, they had just finished their dinner. They met us with great hospitality and said they still had some food left over, and would we like to sit down and eat?

The meal they were eating was called *bishbarmak* – I remember those strange names. Their food was extraordinary and so was the way they ate. They didn't have spoons or forks, and they didn't use sticks as the Chinese do. They ate it with their five fingers, and that was why it was called *bishbarmak*, meaning 'five fingers'. They all dipped their fingers in the bowl and picked out whatever they found, but their basic food was always made from wheat. They also made dough, and they put it in hot water with meat to make us a kind of stew or something. They thought we would sit down to eat that as well, but Usa discovered that the meat was horsemeat, so we thanked them very much, but explained that we were not hungry any more.

So we got to know one another. They asked what brought us there and we explained that we wanted wheat. "Oh, we have plenty of wheat," they said. Then I told them that I had a wonderful exchange for their wheat, some really fine cloth, all the way from London. I showed them, and their eyes nearly popped out. After that, a deal was quickly arranged. I was to get two big sacks full of wheat, huge sacks – and, if I say huge, I mean it. On top of that, they gave me a little piglet. It was a little honey, that piglet, and in any case they insisted we were not to refuse it: they had plenty of pigs, and horseflesh too.

They made us a bed on the floor in a spare room and we all slept there. We had a very good night's sleep because we were tired out. The following morning, we set off back with all our goods. It was quite a long journey, but we had so much to talk about and think back over. That visit had been a strange event, and the people themselves, their food and how they lived, their primitive life, which they loved so much, everything was new, strange and different to us. They loved their freedom and they lived on land that had never been occupied by anybody else, near China.

"The most wonderful time we had"

Well, on the way back home, I couldn't help talking to Lazar, because he was my very good friend, though I was fond of Usa too. He was so kind to me, because he thought I needed help, and we got on very well. They had given up two days and gone on that long journey, just so that I could get wheat. These were my best friends after the ones I had in Moscow.

When we got home and I brought in the two sacks, my mother couldn't get over it. She was so happy, even though the sacks took up so much room. Leonora was happy too, now that I was back. Next my mother had to find out where to get it turned into flour, but our little old lady, she knew – she knew everything – well, I call her 'old' because she had white hair, but she had energy galore. She also had some wheat that needed grinding into flour, because that was her diet. She liked anything made with flour. So she took my mother to the mill, and they came home with sacks full of flour.

We stood it near the stove, so it would stay dry. When the first batch of bread came out of the oven, with that lovely smell, then Leonora was really happy. And that bread wasn't the only good thing that came to Leonora with the flour, but she only told me this later.

"Mummy, you don't know, because I never told you. Whenever you put me to bed, to sleep, when you went away I noticed that some little mice came out and they were so sweet. I used to lie as still as I could, so they wouldn't hide."

"You naughty little thing, why didn't you tell me?"

"No, mummy, I didn't want them to go away. I liked watching them."

I thought that was so sweet. Actually, my little girl was very happy the whole time we were there. She still remembers it. If I ask her now, she always says "They were the most wonderful time, those years we had there". We were nearly there for four years, you know; it was a long stretch.

Our landlady's daughter-in-law had a little girl, a nice girl, but rough and always full of dust. That was what my daughter loved and that was a pleasure I would never deny her. If you can't play in the dust when you're a child, when can you do it? They were so friendly and I could be sure, if I went anywhere, that when I came back they would be wallowing in the dust. I would pick up my little girl, go inside, wash her down and change her clothes; but the other girl didn't mind, and it didn't matter to her mother. She was brought up in that dirt – well, it wasn't really dirt, just dust. The place they lived in, however bare it was, they kept clean.

Leonora liked her little friend next door. That little girl looked so scruffy, but she was very sweet in her own way. She adored my little girl and they played so well together. They never once had any differences; they never fell out. Leonora had other friends nearby too. She loved the friendliness of the place and she loved the place itself, not just the dust, but the scenery, the tulips in springtime and the good food.

When harvest time came, we had an abundance of fruit, especially apples. But the tomatoes! I have never seen anything like the way tomatoes grew there. They grew all over the place, even in the street outside our place. You could buy them for very little money. I remember I bought an awful lot of tomatoes, and they showed me how to dry them, because they knew how to preserve fruit for winter. I managed to dry sacks and sacks of tomatoes.

Then the melons came and oh, they were fantastic! These melons were quite long, very different from the round cantaloupes that are sold in England, but very sweet. We dried the melons too. I learnt how to put them on sheets on the roof, where there was plenty of sun, and let them dry in the sun. Then my little old lady showed me how to treat the melons in order to preserve them. When they had dried, you had to cut them in slices, as if you were going to eat them, and they would dry up even more. When the slices are fully dry, they become very soft, and you make a big plait out of them. That was how we preserved them. Then, through the winter, if you wanted to eat some, you just sliced a piece off. I can't explain the taste, but it was delicious.

They had extraordinary soil there so, when the harvest came, everything was in abundance. But of course wintertime could be harsh, so they had learnt how to preserve not just fruit, but cabbage and various vegetables. That was very attractive.

Things to do in Uzun-argach

No matter that the war was on somewhere, and we were far from home, I see now that we had rather pleasant times there. Not only was it a beautiful place, but the village itself – or little town,

261

whichever it was – had many good facilities. Where we lived, it was quite a busy street, right in the centre of this village of ours. Just down the road was a chemist and the young Russian woman there was very friendly and took a liking to me. She said if I wanted anything, I was to let her know and she would get it – and she did. For instance, I wanted some material, some voile, to make a partition round the corner of the room where the little old lady slept, so she could have a little privacy, and she got me that. Whatever I wanted, she would get it for me if she could.

She was an excellent rider; she went long distances on horseback, taking medicine to various places, like that little settlement where we went to buy wheat, which was quite a journey. We used to go out together and she decided to teach me to ride.

"You can't live here unless you can ride a horse. Otherwise, you can't go from one place to another."

The horses were extraordinarily tall, with no saddle. It looked alarming to me.

"How on earth do you manage?"

"Simple. I just get on it, that is all. You try."

I plucked up courage and I tried.

"Good gracious, I feel as if I am going up to heaven. No dear, this is not for me. I am not made for horse riding. Could you try and help me get down again?"

I came down, I scratched myself a bit, and I thought: Never again will I try that. All the same, I found her very *sympatiya*, as I would call it, so friendly and nice. We enjoyed ourselves together.

There were other amusements too. Uzun-argach had a kind of club theatre and sometimes they showed films there. If I were to tell you one of the films we went to see, you perhaps wouldn't believe it, but once they showed *Lady Hamilton*, with Vivienne Leigh and Laurence Olivier. Churchill used to say it was his favourite film starring her. That was the first time I had seen her, and I thought: *Good gracious, what a most gorgeous creature she is!* There was something about her that drew me. As Lady Hamilton, she showed grace and beauty, and I liked her acting too. No matter what they showed, all the old films, like *Gone with the wind*, I would never miss Vivienne Leigh. I liked her always. I know she was very much criticised her in England, but I found they were wrong. She had great talent, unknown to an average person. She was beautiful but also charming, and that is a very rare thing.

The audience was a mixed crowd, but an appreciative one. All the evacuees used to go and they were such intelligent, decent people. I had so many friends there that it would be impossible to tell you about them all. The very first day I went into hospital with Leonora, there was a woman from Kiev there with her little girl. She came up to me and said "Don't worry, nobody here ever died from this war". She and I became very friendly, and her family too. I used to go to see them, and we kept the friendship up all the years we were there. I met such marvellous people; I still think about them.

Then they asked me if I could do something to help.

"Yes, I could teach ballroom dancing, if people would like me to."

"Oh yes, they would."

As a professional dancer, I danced very well, I had taught people and I liked ballroom, so I danced whenever there was an opportunity – the tango, foxtrot, waltz, slow waltz. People came and I showed them how to dance all these. They liked to move about.

They put a show on and asked me to join in. I said, if they wanted me to act, I didn't think I could manage it. "Oh, just try." They had a play written by God knows whom – I vaguely remember the story – and for one part they needed a young woman. Now, I would never say that I could act; in any case, acting never interested me – I only liked dancing – but they talked me into it, saying I had the right appearance, looked smart and would just fit the part. Well, I did it. I acted. I learnt my lines, something I never knew I could do.

I will try anything, if I am talked into it and if it amuses somebody. We had an audience and they liked it very much. The second time they asked, though, I declined. "No, you find somebody else to do it. I can't." It was strange; I just didn't like acting.

A meeting in Alma-ata

It was amazing the transformation when spring came, and summer too, but especially spring. The mountains would be covered with tulips. I don't think they had daffodils, but they had wild tulips, and they were quite a sight. Even my mother noticed them. She used to correspond with her younger brother, Peter, and in one letter she wrote about the beauty of the place where we were staying. He wrote back, "How can you write about these beautiful things, when there is a war on?" Well, when you are far away from the war, you don't think of it. I don't know where Peter was staying, but he was obviously nearer the action. We were about as far away as you could get.

Then there were times when I fancied going somewhere with one of my friends. One day Clara had a suggestion.

"Let's go to Alma-ata, Lilya. Do come."

"All right, I will go."

There was always something I needed to get there. I used to make arrangements for our parcels from Alma-ata to be picked up by the lorry that delivered goods each day to our village. I don't know what the lorry brought, but nevertheless it came every day. So now I spoke to the driver.

"Would you take us with you, when you are ready to go back to Alma-ata?"

"With pleasure!"

"And would you bring us back?"

"Yes, yes. Definitely."

Clara was so pleased when I told her what I had arranged. I knew Leonora would be fine, with my mother looking after her.

It worked out very well. We got to Alma-ata safely, and this was the first time I had been there since we first came. The day we arrived, we were too distressed to notice anything. Now we had picked up. It was interesting and quite pleasant. Like Uzun-argach, it was full of Russian exiles and evacuees.

As I was walking along the street, who did I bump into? Schneider's sister. I knew the whole family, and this was Sarah Lynechna, the eldest. She was a very smart woman, married to a manager of some sort; he had a very funny face, but she was rather attractive. She looked astonished.

"Lilya, what on earth are you doing here?"

"What are *you* doing here? We evacuated."

"So did we."

Well, there you are, the world is not that big anyway, so one does meet God knows where, somebody one would never dream of. We spent some time, my Clara and I, with them. It was nice to know somebody in a place like Alma-ata. I always knew it would come in very handy one day. I had that premonition. And it always works out as I think because I thought: *I am not going to stay here for ever, and these are very competent people and they know their way about.*

So we spent the day in Alma-ata and bought whatever we wanted. In the evening we went back the same way. The same lorry picked us up, but – unhappily for us, or even unluckily I would say – the lorry broke down during the night. So Clara and I, and the driver, we had to abandon the lorry and walk all the way home. I took my shoes off and walked barefoot. I couldn't walk in the shoes, but barefoot I could. Clara did the same; she didn't mind, and neither did I. It was nearly 20 km (12 miles).

Finally we got home. Clara went to her place and I had to knock on the window. My mother was surprised I was so late; she had started to wonder when I was coming. I told her what the calamity was. She said, "Don't worry. I will make you some hot water to wash your feet." So it worked out not too bad. I got whatever I wanted, I don't remember, it might have been soap. There were many such things that you could get in town, but not in the village where I was.

The village

I must tell you more about the village and give a little insight into the extraordinary people who lived there. They were extraordinary, quite unlike the Russian peasantry. They were settlers, in many cases from hundreds of years ago, from Russia – entirely different from the local people. I would compare them with the Australians, in the way they formed their country and the fact that they hadn't originally chosen to go there. And it wasn't their country, in the sense that there was a scattering of people living there already. Although the two groups didn't mix much, they seemed to get on very well. Nobody ever interfered with the native peoples; they lived their own lives, as they had done for thousands of years. It worked: that was the beauty of the place.

Once I had settled in, I began to recognise the various types of people. First of all we had the evacuees. They weren't poor people, because they had lovely belongings, yet nobody was ever robbed there. They were honest. You could even leave your door wide open and nobody would come in and take anything. That was a phenomenon to me. They had proper streets there, not just dirt tracks, and their way of living was so organised. There were other things to notice too.

That first day, when we had just arrived and we gathered in the square, I noticed the type of people who came to meet us. One man in particular – he was a vet – stood out from the others. He was tall, wearing one of those Russian *parpaha*, hats made of Persian lamb. Well, it was winter, but he was dressed in all the gear. He had very good clothes; I would say he was wearing sheepskin, but there were plenty of cattle there too. He caught my eye, so I remembered him.

I caught his eye too. He looked round at all the evacuees and he stopped looking when he saw me. I remember that. He looked very intensely at me, then he looked all round and came back to me again. Well, at the time we had just arrived and I never took much notice, except to remember that I had seen him there.

I knew he was a vet and a kind of *starosta*, as they called it, the headman of the village, because he looked after all the cattle and the surrounding collective farm; that was his duty. I learnt afterwards that he had a young wife, a typical Russian blonde, and a little child. They had a very nice house too because, even in Uzun-argach, there were some better off than others – just like anywhere else in the world.

Meanwhile my social life too was improving. People used to meet at that theatre club, and sometimes they would invite us all to come and meet one another. They would have some music playing and make an evening of it. I made a bit of an effort to make myself look nice, and I did my hair. I had very good hair, adaptable – in that climate it never frizzed, it just nicely curled – and I managed to give myself a bit of a hairstyle. I wasn't really dressed up – after all, I wasn't going to the opera and I would never try to show off or look extra-smart – I just wanted to look nice. I had a pretty blouse and a skirt on, and a nice little wrap. My mother stayed with my little girl, and I went off to this gathering.

Everything was fine. There were many people there, evacuees especially. There was a young woman there, with a coarse, but very pleasant face. I know she came from the Ukraine, but I don't know if she was ever married or not – I knew her only vaguely. There were crowds of people, and she was trying to get through them to say hello to me. Eventually she managed, and why I remember that is because she made all that effort and then she said such an extra-ordinary thing. I couldn't believe it.

"You look so beautiful."

"Thank you. That is kind of you."

"I can't take my eyes off you."

When a man pays a woman a compliment, that is one thing, but when a young woman comes up to you and says such a thing – well, that was something extraordinary. Still, it soon flew out of my mind and didn't come in again until recently.

There was a young man there, one of those natives of the place, with oriental eyes, a very young, handsome man. He came across to dance with me, and I could see he wanted to make friends, but I was very cautious. After this little party was over, we all stayed on and chatted. We had a splendid time. Eventually it was time we went home; he was determined to escort me, and I didn't mind. I said I hadn't far to go because our little place was in the middle of the village, though not in a prominent street, and he walked me home. It's a funny thing, whenever I think of that village, nearly all my memories of it are pleasant. Somehow, people showed extraordinary friendship, the families there were wonderful and my little girl was so happy. Even now, when I ask her "Do you remember Uzun-argach?" she answers "Oh yes, I never will forget it."

One thing leads to another

Before long, I heard from Moss that things were getting more settled. The war was going well, they had prevented Hitler from taking Moscow and pushed him back, and now the government was thinking of moving back to the capital city. It seemed things were looking brighter.

Life went on and we had to occupy ourselves, so the library that Gauchin ran was a wonderful thing. It had some very good books. I read one of Stendhal's books in French, the one that brought him overnight fame, *The Charterhouse of Parma*, based on a true story about a family. It made him so important in French culture.

My visits to the library and my reading also helped to widen my social contacts, and that was very nice indeed. There were families I became really friendly with. Many of them were delightful people, and I found the Ukrainians particularly warm and lovely. Although I had plenty of time, I was always occupied, if not with one thing then another.

We got to know some Polish people who lived not far from us. There were seven boys in the family. When the war came, they got separated and then their parents had been killed. I never asked any details about the parents because I thought it would be very hurtful, but I was very taken by their attitude. The boys were wonderful and the eldest looked after the others.

This eldest brother became friendly with us. He was telling me about Tel Aviv, about the Jewish settlements there.

"That is our dream. I want to bring my family there, my six brothers."

I felt so sorry for those young boys. How on earth would they manage to get to Tel Aviv? But I have learnt that if you make up your mind to do something, it will work, with just a little knowledge and good sense, so I listened to him when he talked about this place in the Middle East.

"Have you heard of Tel Aviv?"

"No, I haven't."

"Well, they say it is absolutely wonderful. It's a place where all the Jews live together and they live in harmony."

They were such good, friendly people; they deserved to realise their dream.

Rosa

You remember, when I took my little Leonora to the hospital, to the children's ward, and that young woman came across to speak to me? It was so friendly and kind of her.

"This ward is lucky: nobody has ever died here, so you have good reason to hope."

I was there two days with Leonora, this young woman was there with her little girl and we got talking. She told me about how she got married, how she felt when her husband-to-be proposed to her and she thought how fortunate she was, that the man who was offering marriage to her had such a good position and was such a nice man. He was a blond too and I thought, *Well, I remember that feeling, it is very pleasant. I feel very pleased for you.*

Strangely I don't remember her name, but her little girl's name was Rosaline. They called her 'little Rosa'. She was blonde, with a dark complexion and grey-blue eyes I remember, because I always observe and remember images.

From that time on, we became close friends. Her husband was with them at the time, and she introduced me to her sister-in-law, her husband's sister. The sister had a son, about 16, a very lovely, handsome boy. They lived quite a distance away, but we met nearly every day because they had very big houses, and they insisted I should come. They liked my presence and I used to bring my little girl with me, because she and little Rosa could play together.

But every time I went there I found Rosa's mother doing the ironing. One day I saw her ironing again and I couldn't understand how she never seemed to finish it.

"Good gracious, how on earth do you manage with so much ironing?"

"Oh, I have to do that, because I was told it kills the germs."

That seemed so funny and yet it was so right; it was just that I had never thought of it. Now that we were settled ourselves, I suppose my mother and I never thought about germs very much. We thought of infections as a hazard of homelessness and long journeys without proper facilities.

Besides, the village was very well organised for evacuees. I must mention that they used to arrange a Turkish bath for us every week. The women went there separately from the men, and we used to have a very good wash down. There were all the facilities you needed. That was fantastic, in this out-of-the-way place. I can't get over the way they organised all the things that are so important for people to exist, to look after themselves and to be clean, as well as they can. That was marvellous.

The vet

It was wonderful to have a hot bath, but unfortunately I couldn't get soap for love or money. What I had brought with me was soon used up, and even when I went to Alma-ata I couldn't get any, it was so short. Now every so often I used to see this vet, the one who had caught my eye on that first day, and he used to stop and talk to me. He was very friendly and he said that if ever I needed anything, he would try to help.

The next time I met him, I asked if he might be able to get me some soap. I thought as a vet he would have access to it. He said he was going to town that day and he would do his best to get me some soap. If I came over that evening, he would give me whatever he had managed to get.

I knew where he lived, just outside the village, not very far. That was fine; I wasn't afraid. I just never thought of any danger. I didn't realise that one has to be very cautious with such a man, young, tall, handsome, and a big man at that. That evening I told my mother I was going to this vet's house, because he had promised to get me some soap. My mother said "Do – it will be a great help". She had tried to barter with people to get soap when she went to the market, but she found they never had any to sell. It was a terrible dilemma. So off I went.

I did wonder whether to tell you of this unpleasant episode. And then I thought, why not? One can only speak from experience, and this was something I had never foreseen. After it was over, I thought to myself, *How careful one has to be*. I was at that age when men would be tempted. I was then 28, a good, ripe age, and I looked fit and well, because my life was so leisurely and the air there was wonderfully pure.

When I got there, he met me at the door, showed me in and sat me down.

"By the way, my wife had to go to her parents and she took the little girl with her."

I thought, *What on earth did he tell me that for?* I didn't say anything. He was very hospitable. We had a little drink and something to eat that he had prepared for me. I was surprised. It all seemed at odds with the reason for my call. I decided to ask.

"Did you have any luck with my request?"

"I'm so sorry, but I really couldn't get any."

I thought: *Why didn't he call round and tell me that it hadn't been possible? Why did I have to come to him?* But he was a cunning man, which I had never foreseen.

I could see his eyes were sparkling and, before I could do anything, he got hold of me and threw me on the bed. Well, I don't have to tell you what I went through. It was awful, because I had thought he was such a lovely man. I won't say that I wasn't frightened of him, as a male, but much more than that I was outraged, that he would try to do something without my consent. I was absolutely incensed. I managed to free myself and I ran out of the front door. He tried to follow me and I said "Please don't. I will find the way myself; I can find my own way home," because by then it was getting dark: autumn was coming.

Of course, after that incident, whenever I was out walking out and he came towards me, I used to turn my head aside. He would stop and I would pass him by. He looked surprised, because clearly he thought he was irresistible. Well, that experience was unpleasant, but it didn't matter; there was no harm done. I was just disappointed, that's all. It wasn't pleasant to trick me and then try to seduce me without my consent. But then, for one man like that, I met many others like Usa and Lazar.

Letters from Moss

Time went by and I heard some good news from Moss. He thought the government – or at least his department – might be moving back to Moscow. I don't know just when they did move back, but I imagine it was about this time.

After that, I stopped getting letters from my husband, and I thought this was very odd. A month or two passed and nothing came. I felt sure he would be back in Moscow by now, so I decided to write to my neighbour, who had stayed put. I know she never left Moscow, because when we returned she told me that she and others like her were not afraid of Hitler, since they were not Jewish. On the contrary, they were rather looking forward to freeing themselves from Stalin, one way or another, so they were disappointed that Hitler never took Moscow. However, that is a different thing entirely. It shows that every person in this world has to think of themselves and their own interests, but they must still be very careful what they wish for.

My neighbour was called Olga Yakanova and I knew she would tell me what was happening, because I had been very friendly with her. I wrote to ask: 'Can you tell me if there is anything wrong with my husband? I feel sure he is at home.' Quite soon I got a letter from her. She always addressed me by my full name, Lilya Josefna, Joseph being my father's first name. That is how Russians speak to one another – by your first name and your patronymic – but only if you are very friendly or related.

She wrote: 'You know, I was worried. I have been thinking about you, Lilya Josefna. My heart was thinking, should I tell you or not? I must tell you that your husband is going through a second summer.' I didn't understand that phrase, but then she went on to explain: 'I think he is having a very good time, because there is a young woman coming to him.' Fine. I didn't answer her, but I decided I must write to Moss, to tell him that I had found out.

To be honest, I wasn't surprised because four years is a long time, nearly four years not seeing one another. Having said that, I knew that other families of evacuees in Uzun-argach had had visits from their menfolk, even those who were fighting at the front – and Moss was never fighting. Of course, I knew it wouldn't be easy for him to come and see us.

So I wasn't all that surprised, but I just wanted to know how serious it was. I wrote to Moss and told him that I had found out about it, but only because he had stopped writing to me. And I went on: 'Look, Moss, you are free: you decide. If you feel you want to break away from me, do so. You are welcome. I would never try to keep a man who didn't want to be with me. It is your choice, but if we broke up I would be really very disappointed.'

I sent off that letter and I got a reply very quickly, I must say. After all, it was a long way to send a letter. From where we were, it took about a week and a half to get a reply. At the end of that time, a very thick letter came and I opened it. Eight pages he had written, saying how he was devoted to me and his little girl, blah, blah, blah, and this little affair had never been anything serious. He explained everything in detail, how he felt about me and much more.

I thought, *Well, that remains to be seen. I wasn't born yesterday.* I realised I was very disappointed and upset. All that long period, I had missed him, I had seen all the other families having visits from their husbands, and I had understood that he couldn't leave his post. Having such a special skill and working for the government, it wasn't easy: he couldn't just ask for leave – or perhaps he could? I don't know.

13

Leaving for Good, 1945-6

Arranging to leave Uzun-argach

The time came when we were told we were allowed to go home. Moss wrote to say that he was arranging everything for our return. He sent documents, but there were things that he couldn't do from Moscow. We still had to buy tickets and how could we arrange that? After all, we were not in Alma-ata; we were in this village.

Meanwhile, a new person appeared in our village. I don't know what connection she had there; in fact, she was a bit of a mystery. However, she looked rather nice and she made a point of wanting to meet me. When we met, I quickly realised that this woman was rather intelligent, very knowledgeable and shrewd. I told her my plans and she explained why she was there.

"I know many of you are going back home, and I thought I could aid you."

"That would be a great help."

"I have people in Alma-ata who can help you arrange things."

She gave me their address and told me what sort of assistance they could give me, and in fact this contact proved very useful. Funnily enough, about a year later I came across her again, but in Moscow, and she remembered me.

Some other people in the village, who were already in touch with her, told me that she was a very knowledgeable person and trust-worthy. So I decided to take her advice and go to Alma-ata. I thought I would see Schneider's sister too, because she would still be there.

It was not easy, but I got to Alma-ata. I had to rent a place there while I made arrangements. I had been given a private address where I could get a room, and when I went there the owner had a surprise for me.

273

"You know who I have here, Lilya?"

"Who?"

It was my friend Maria, who had asked to come with me when I left Moscow, the one who lived next door to Tanya.

Then I went to see this strange family. They greeted me kindly, and I told them who had recommended them to me. They did know her and they were very pleased to meet me and help. They had just two rooms – nobody had a room to themselves – and in the best room the mother was ill in bed, with some kind of instrument or apparatus alongside.

"What is wrong with your mother?"

"Oh, she has problems with her stomach, or something."

"Anything serious?"

"Not very, but nevertheless she has to undergo this treatment."

"I see. Fine."

They had a son, a young man, who used to organise things. How all this came about, I have no idea, but I met his family. One of his sisters had a beautiful voice, because she used to sing in opera at the theatre in Alma-ata. That was sister number one. Then he had a younger sister, and she was rather beautiful. He himself wasn't anything striking, but he was a very good organiser. He agreed – at a price, of course; everything has to be paid for – to get us tickets and fix the date when we were to come. We arranged all that, I went back home – by 'home' I mean Uzun-argach, of course – and I told my mother and Auntie Annie.

Saying goodbye

I began to get ready to leave the village. This period was rather sad, I have to say. I have spoken of the many good friends I made there, especially Lazar Sobel – I did say that his surname, if I translated it into English, would be 'mink', except that now I remember that *sobel* is that little animal the sable, so I am excusing myself – but the time had come to say goodbye to all my friends.

There were two families that I was particularly attached to. One was the family that I first met when my Leonora and their little Rosa were in hospital. It was Rosa's mother who, whenever I visited them, was always doing the ironing because, she said, it killed the germs. Her husband was with them some of the time, I think, though I am not certain. Her husband's elder sister lived with them and she had a son, who was getting on for 17. There was also a younger sister, who didn't live with them, and her name was Shelley. They were all planning to go to Moscow. I know that, because I recall giving them my address in Moscow.

The other family had the lovely daughter who was so attached to me, Clara. I don't know what her father was; to me, Usa seemed like some kind of official because he always wore army uniform, but I never really asked him what he did. He was usually to be found in the village, where he helped many people and especially me, because I was very friendly with his wife and daughter.

I had to sell a few of my beautiful things and she bought them. She seemed to have a lot of money, but I don't know where it came from. I never went into details of how people arranged their lives. I knew it was useless leaving an address with Clara's family: they would never travel to Moscow. Lazar Sobel was very friendly with this family too, so he would not be alone, but he and I were sorry to part.

In between saying goodbye to all my good friends, I started to pack our goods. There was quite a bit to pack, because I took plenty of food. Among other things, I had some dried tomatoes and dried, plaited melons. It was a lot of work, but eventually everything was ready. We had a van, and we went.

The journey back

I had arranged to be met in Alma-ata, because there were some things I didn't know – where to stay the night, where the railway station was, when to be there – and there were bound to be some things I hadn't thought of. When we arrived, the woman that I mentioned, who got in touch with me in Uzun-argach, was there to meet us and she was helpful in several ways. She was Jewish herself, she understood the plight that Jews were often in, and therefore she offered her help.

When I went to collect the tickets and make the necessary arrangements, it was that young chap again who came and organised them. First of all we had to stay in a hotel overnight. This was the first time in years that we had slept in beds, and that was wonderful. It was a lovely hotel too.

Our train journey started the next day. When we got to the station, that woman was there again and she warned me that we would have quite a long journey – which I knew, because I had made that journey before, more than once. But she did tell me that on the way we could do something to help ourselves if we had our wits about us.

She explained that when we came to the Aral Sea, which was on our way – and we would know when we were near, because the land would look very dry – we should look out and buy salt, as much as we could, a big bag of it, because elsewhere salt supplies were difficult to obtain. In the villages they were short of salt, she said, so along the way we could exchange the salt for butter, or whatever we wanted to get. And that advice came in very useful.

The next morning, that young chap came down to the station and arranged everything. We had a compartment to ourselves with comfortable beds; there were four bunks, with soft mattresses and beds already made up. My mother and I slept on the bottom ones, Auntie Annie slept on one of the top ones, and the other one, well, we left it. Leonora sometimes would sleep there, but often she wanted to sleep with me.

The journey went smoothly and we were very comfortable. *En route* there were many stops where you could buy supplies. Peasants usually brought smoked fish, which we liked, and fresh bread. They knew what was needed and we managed our journey very well.

When we came to the place where they were selling salt, I told Auntie Annie – at that time she was still able to do things for herself – and advised her to get some salt. I knew she had money because Moss used to send her some. I was very pleased when she bought some salt, because I had a limited amount of money to spend. I had to sell things to keep us going: me, my mother and Leonora. I had enough money, because Moss did send me a little extra to get home, but I had to be careful.

I bought quite a lot of salt. A few stops further down the line, not very far away, they all came out with containers of loose butter, and that stays longer than fresh, so I exchanged some of the salt for big containers of butter. The weather was becoming a little fresher, so it wasn't difficult to keep the butter. I am not sure, but I think it was coming into autumn when we left. I could see that Auntie Annie too managed to get as much butter as she wanted. She knew she would be going to stay with Tanya when we got to Moscow.

276

Back in Moscow

Well, at last we got home. How long it took us I haven't the faintest idea. All I know is that we got home. I was surprised that Moss wasn't there, but then in another way it wasn't surprising. He couldn't know when we were arriving, because I didn't know how to get in touch with him. You couldn't telephone, not that distance, in those days, and I didn't want to send a telegram. I didn't know myself, even, when we would arrive. So I left it at that.

We got out at the station and I hired a *gyp*. We managed to put all our things in it and I told the driver where to take us. He brought us home to my place and we got all our luggage upstairs. We lived on the third storey, so I left Auntie Annie downstairs with her belongings and reassured her that she would soon be home.

"You stay put until somebody comes to escort you home."

Next I phoned Moss and told him we had arrived. I didn't try to make any jokes and I didn't make any fuss, because I didn't really know what I was coming home to. He came straight home and he was pleased to see us, and I was very pleased to see him. He was happy and yet I could see traces of not being happy too. I told him that Auntie Annie was downstairs, and he immediately stood up.

"Well, she needs taking home. I'll go now."

"Do you think you should? You look so tired."

He hesitated, and one of our neighbours, a young man, stepped in. He called her 'Auntie Annie' too, because he was on friendly terms with our family.

"I will go with Auntie Annie."

"Are you sure you can manage?"

"Yes, yes, definitely. There is nothing to worry about."

So Moss relaxed again and this young man, Vova, went off downstairs to take Auntie Annie home. In any case, Moss naturally wanted to talk to us. He was delighted to see little Leonora, who had grown since he had last seen her. She was 6 by then, a delightful age – quite a big girl for her age, and lovely to look at.

We put away all our things, and I set to and made a meal. I had brought plenty of food with me; in fact, Moss couldn't get over it, we had so much food. That passed a little time pleasantly, and in a way he was pleased to see us. Then Vova came back and he was very disturbed. The problem, which I had never foreseen, was that Auntie Annie had forgotten where she lived. Of course Moss knew where she lived, so it was my mistake. I should have let him go with her, but I hadn't seen him for such a long time – three and a half years is a long time – and you can't always think of everything logically. It never occurred to me she would forget her own address.

What had happened was this. When she got to her place, she sent Vova to look at the number; she thought he would know which was hers. But then she told the driver to wait while she went to see if she could help. As soon as she did that, the cabman drove off with all her luggage. If Moss had been there, he would never have let that happen. He would have made the driver take the cab into the yard and unload it there.

Auntie Annie found her flat and got in; Vova went down to get her belongings only to find they had gone. That was such a misfortune and a shame, and I felt sorry. Well, that was a bit of a blunder on my side, and Moss went for me.

"Now look what you have done."

"I am sorry, I didn't mean to. I thought you were so tired and wanted to see us so."

"Well, now you will have to share all the food we have."

"Of course I will give some to Auntie Annie; I won't keep it all for us. Anything I can do, I will."

Somehow he never forgave me for that, because his mother mattered more than I did to him. I was rather hurt and he was irritable, which I didn't like. We sat down to eat and I gathered there would be problems, but I didn't say anything much. After we had eaten, we unpacked the food and I still had plenty. Besides, I am so resourceful that I would always get food one way or another, and Moscow was coming to life again, now that people were returning.

Back to not-normal

We spent the night together and he seemed to be all right, quite contented even. The following day he had to go to work, and I started getting the flat straight. I had already given some thought to what I would do, and I had decided I wouldn't rejoin the dance group. I thought I would do better to concentrate on putting our lives back together.

I couldn't do it, because the government had announced that all women who had somebody at home to look after their children would have to go out to work. They would have to take whatever job they were given, and that meant heavy work. When Moss came home that evening, I told him that we had a problem and we hadn't any choice: I had to work, because I had my mother to help me. The government wouldn't allow two women to stay at home, and if the government had made up their minds to do something, they would do it, no two ways about it. Unless I didn't mind working in a factory or a steelworks, I had to start dancing again.

Somehow he couldn't take it, and I knew why. It was because he didn't like me going away. Of course he missed me, that was reason number one; but reason number two was that my mother wasn't able to look after things the way I did. She was a lovely cook, but the rest was rather vague. He liked order, as I do, and everything was just so when I was at home. Straightaway I saw that he was getting irritable. The thought that I might go off somewhere, even though I hadn't started dancing again yet, was gnawing at him.

The following day, I gave him his breakfast separately and then I fed my little girl. When we sat down together for lunch, Leonora was very playful. She was sitting next to him and she was getting a bit naughty. So what? She was happy. Then she went to take something and he smacked her hand. I was taken by surprise.

"Moss, why did you have to do that?"

"Well, she should be obedient."

"Good gracious, she is only a child, and if sometimes she is playful and wants to be a little bit naughty, so what? After all, she didn't do anything very terrible."

I let it go at that, but I didn't like it.

In fact I didn't like his attitude generally. I could see he was torn, and I knew why. The woman he had teamed up with was his secretary, and they are the worst enemies to wives. I learnt that the hard way, but of course if I had been with him all the time, there wouldn't have been a choice. In any case, I was much better-looking.

When Tanya got back and we met up, she expressed her disgust.

"Lilya, I can't stand that woman."

"Well, what can we do?"

Shortly after that, even before I started dancing again, they gave Barney leave to come home from the camp. They were going to release him completely, but at that point he was just home on leave. Well, we were all very happy, Tanya especially.

On his return, he came to see me. That was the first time he had

279

seen my daughter. I could see he was charmed with her: he couldn't take his eyes off her. She was shy, though; until then, she never knew she had an uncle.

Barney knew there was a bit of a rift between Moss and me, but – I suppose because he was Moss's brother – he saw it differently.

"Lili, you are going to have to put your pride away."

"That is nothing to do with it. It is not my pride; it is the situation. I have to go back to work, whether I want to or not, and Moss has to make an effort to cope with it."

What I said was true and fair, but, even as I was saying it, I knew Moss would never do it. If anyone was going to make an effort, it would have to be me. But I wouldn't: I didn't want to, and why should I? I had done nothing wrong. *He* had; I hadn't.

I could see Barney was very disappointed. But somehow he didn't see things in proportion: we had all gone through such terrible years of anxiety, deprivation and God knows what. Awful things had happened to people, we had nearly lost our little girl, and none of that seemed to count. All that mattered, apparently, was that Moss wasn't happy. I didn't like that. I don't like people who don't give any real thought to what is fair and right, and what isn't, who just see things on the surface and follow their own emotions.

Isadora's dancers together again

Since the government insisted I should be employed, I had to contact our manager, Schneider. The other girls who had come back to Moscow did the same and we all gathered at Schneider's place. We were naturally glad to see one another after all that time: it was a sort of reunion. There was Mooshya – I was very pleased to see her – and Doda, who was Marsha's neighbour.

Doda came with us to China, but she had a weak heart and that was why Irma never took her to America. Doda was fond of me, I remember, and now she came up and spoke to me.

"Lilya, you look as if you've just come back from a holiday."

"To be honest, I suppose I have. The place where we stayed was very healthy: the air was wonderful and so was the food, and the whole way we lived in the village."

"I can see. You look absolutely wonderful."

"You look well, too. Tell me, have you seen Marsha? Where is she?"

And then Doda told me that sadly we would not see Marsha again. What had happened to her was something just extraordinary, and that was one reason that Doda had come to see us all, to tell us this terrible news.

I missed Marsha; I loved her very much. She had that flighty streak in her, and I was always telling her, 'Marsha, think before you do anything.' But she never did, of course. Then, when the war started, everybody concentrated on doing whatever they could for themselves. Society disintegrated into families.

I learnt from Doda that Marsha had married. Her husband was a lovely man, but she didn't have long to enjoy being with him, because he was killed in the war. At some occasion - perhaps at the funeral, I don't know - she met a pilot, and he offered to take her away with him. Later I found out more of the details, though I never discovered the whole story.

Marsha had a close friend that she often talked about, whose name was Lukya. What I didn't know was that Marsha had decided to go with this pilot, and Lukya said she would go with her. I don't know even where they were planning to go. Not long before they were due to set off, the two girls began to notice that this pilot was not completely right in the head. They thought maybe he had become a little unhinged by the war, or by what he had had to do. I don't know the truth of that.

Anyway, the two girls made up their minds they would have to get away somehow, without him knowing. But he smelt a rat and then did something dreadful and almost unbelievable, I would say. He killed them both, set fire to the place where their bodies were and then allowed himself to be burnt to death there. To think of what the war did to people. Even now I think about those events; I still can't get over that tragedy, it is so distressing. However, I can't keep dwelling on that misfortune.

The frozen north, winter 1944–5

Schneider, our director, said he would arrange bookings for us, but we would have to be prepared to go away. The first place we were to give concerts was Murmansk. He said he couldn't arrange train tickets for all of us at one go, because it was very difficult. The reason we went was to entertain the crews of the English ships that used to come to Murmansk and Archangel, to deliver supplies and know-how to help the Russians, and their naval escorts. The war was coming to an end, but it was not yet over.

I told Moss that I would be going with the dance group to Murmansk and Archangel, but I couldn't tell him for how long, because we didn't yet know. Somehow he didn't object or say anything much, but the relationship between us wasn't the same. Looking back, I saw that it had really started when he joined us in Chardaevka, after nearly missing us. I don't know what had happened to him, because he wasn't a man to speak out, as I would. To me, if you are troubled, it is nice to talk to the person who is closest to you. But he didn't seem to want to talk; he just watched me, and I didn't know why. I know he was frightened we would be short of food, but we never were.

So it had all started a long while back. I had become used to this change in him, but I still didn't know what the outcome would be; I felt that was up to him. Whatever he decided to do, so be it. I would never fight to keep a man – I can assure you of that – no matter how much I liked him and loved him deep down, because that is a different feeling from being infatuated with a person. But whatever happened, I wouldn't go under – it is not in my make-up.

Schneider told us that he couldn't get tickets for us all on one day. Three girls would have to go first, and the rest would be able to travel the following day; our concerts were due to start the day after that. I was one of the first three, along with Shura and Vera. So we went to Murmansk, found our hotel and settled in, and then we wondered what to do, because the others would not arrive until the next day. At the theatre where we were to perform, they had a production of an operetta that evening, and we decided to get tickets and go to see that. We did and we enjoyed it.

Victor Frobel

As we left the theatre, in the dark somebody came up to us. All I could see was that it was a man in naval uniform. He said he would like to escort us to our hotel and he asked us in English if we minded.

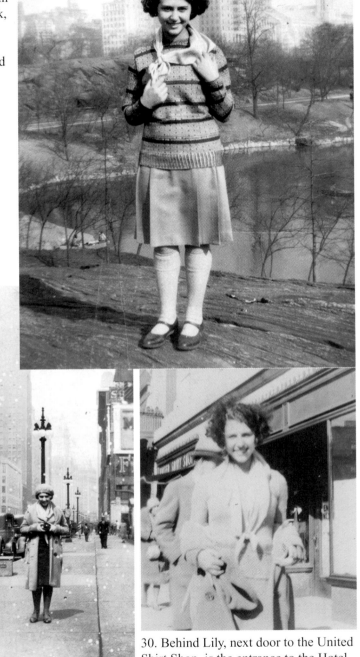

28. A very happy Lily in Central Park, New York, on the second North American tour, still wearing clothes she had brought with her from Russia.

29. Another week, another city: Lily in Pittsburgh, ready to go shopping. The joys of retail therapy were something new.

30. Behind Lily, next door to the United Shirt Shop, is the entrance to the Hotel A La Marque, which was still not quite finished when they first stayed there at New Year 1928.

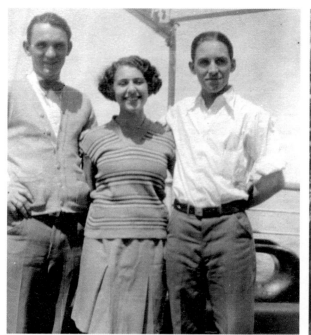

31. Sailing to France on board the liner *Carinthia*, summer 1929. Lily was amused because Frederick (left) and his brother were both pulling on her: each of them wanted her all to himself.

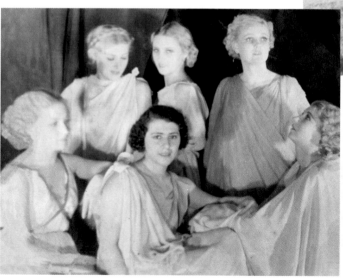

32. A fly in sour cream! The blondes are (from left, back) Tamara Lobanovskaya, Elena Fedorovskaya and Shura Aksimova, with (front) Maria Mysovskaya and Valentina Boye. The only one with dark hair is Lily Dikovsky. This was probably taken in 1936, just before the trip to Polyarniy in the far north.

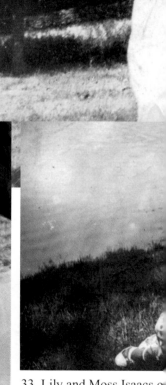

33. Lily and Moss Isaacs o their honeymoon in spring 1933, by a little lake not fa from Moscow. They had known each other since the were children,

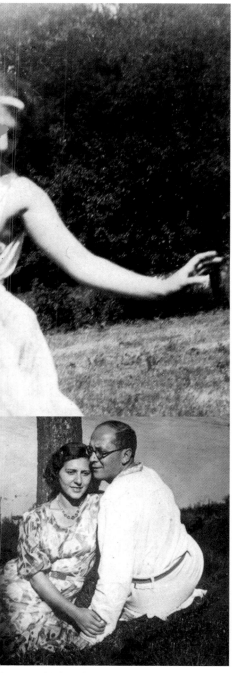

34. Left: Lily dancing for sheer pleasure one morning in the garden of the *pension* at Pontchartrain, aged 16. Manya came out and took the picture.

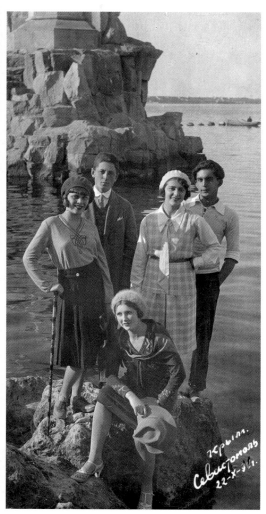

but saw little of each other as they were growing up. After they married, Lily felt that Moss completed her education, telling her about world affairs and everything from stars to atoms. At work he was called 'The Walking Encyclopaedia'.

35. After the Isadora Duncan Dancers' return from America, they went on tour to the Crimea. Here are Tamara Semenova, Lily and Shura in October 1930, having some time off by the Black Sea, at Sebastopol. The two young men were silent admirers, who followed them around.

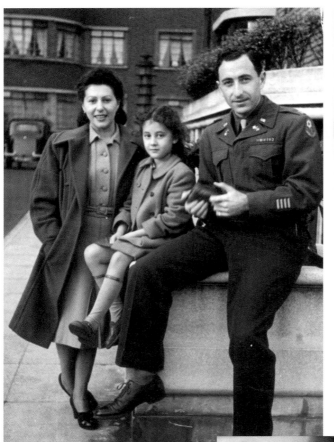

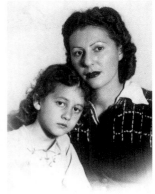

36. In 1941, the Nazi advance threatened Moscow and Lily fled to Kazakhstan with her daughter Leonora. Moss could not go, and they were separated for three years. Back in Moscow in 1945, Lily found things had changed. She had this photograph with Leonora taken, to accompany her application for her British passport.

37. Above: In 1921, as a girl of 7, Lily had set off from London to go to Russia. In 1946, Lily finally arrived back in London with her own 7-year-old daughter. They are seen here with George, the American husband of her cousin Eva, in front of Regency Lodge – their first London address.

38. Right: Lily's mother chose to stay in Moscow. Her husband Moss had no choice: he had given up British citizenship to take a post in the Kremlin, which meant Lily herself could go only if they divorced. It was the only thing Moss could now do to help her, and he did it. Nonetheless, he was there to see her off at the station. Lily never saw him again.

Shura and Vera didn't speak English as fluently as I did, so I told the girls in Russian

"Do you mind? He would like to escort us home."

"No, not at all. Tell him we don't mind at all."

"They say yes, you can, of course. Thank you."

It turned out he was from the convoy that had just arrived from England, the one we had come to entertain.

So we walked together, but we couldn't talk much because he was restricted in a way. He couldn't talk freely, because I was the only one who could really speak English, but next to him was Shura, then came Vera, and I was next to Vera. So I had to talk for the other two, and also across them, which wasn't easy at that distance. Anyway, our hotel wasn't very far.

When we reached our hotel, the three of us said goodnight and thanked him for the escort. At that point he spoke just to me.

"May I speak to you for a moment?"

"Yes, of course. What is it?"

"I would like to show you my boat, where it is moored."

"Yes, if you like."

Our hotel wasn't very far from the shore; he pointed out his ship, then said goodnight.

"Could I come to see you tomorrow?"

"Fine, of course you can. We will be very pleased to see you."

I was so surprised that he chose me, and not Shura or Vera. Still, he chose me.

The next day he came as he had said, and in the daylight I had a good look at him. He was very handsome, a lovely Scotsman, and he told me his name.

"I am Victor Frobel, from Dundee. Please will you accept this? Your name is Lily, isn't it?"

And he gave me a huge parcel. I thought: Good gracious, I must have made quite an impression on this man, because he remembered my name - though I suppose Lily is simple and it is an English name.

"Lily, you don't mind accepting this present?"

"Well, it is very generous of you -"

"Look, just accept it. Don't ask questions."

The weather was getting a bit cold, I remember, and I wasn't really dressed for it. He could see my clothes were not warm enough and he was afraid I would catch cold, so he had brought me a big hand-knitted scarf.

"I am the youngest, I'm the baby of the family, and my mother knitted this scarf for me before I left Dundee. Now, you wear it and keep yourself warm."

It was a beautiful navy colour and it wasn't so much a scarf - it was a shawl really, it was so wide, and he put it on me. He was so nice. I had to laugh with pleasure at the generosity of a man I didn't know, had never even seen before in my life.

He took such a fancy to me, yet I couldn't understand it because we had never been introduced or anything. He had only seen me in the theatre foyer with the other two girls, but he said he was walking by and he noticed me.

"Why?"

"Your long black hair - and you shouldn't ask so many questions."

That was really funny, so I accepted. I wouldn't refuse such a lovely man, when he had been so kind to me and shown his affection straightaway.

Later in the day, he had to go back to his ship.

"Can I come and see you dance?"

"Of course. The rest of the company, all our girls, will soon arrive and tomorrow we have the concert."

He said he would be only too pleased to come, and he didn't come just to our first concert, either. After each concert he came backstage to see me and said, "I enjoyed that very, very much."

We became very friendly. I introduced him to the rest of the group and to Schneider, who liked him too. We became very close to this Victor, and he got very attached to us. This was a strange phenomenon. He arranged for the sailors from his ship to come to our hotel, which had a large restaurant, to meet us there. He pointed out that one of us was an English girl. The sailors were pleased and came up to ask me questions.

"Oh, Lily, how nice: you were born in London?"

"And you still speak English?"

These young chaps were delighted. Later on, they were singing, 'It's a long way to Tipperary'. They enjoyed themselves and so did we.

One day I asked Victor when his ship was sailing. He said it was up to him, but he thought they would wait a little longer. He wasn't in a hurry to go. We had concerts in towns round about, and he asked if he could come with us. Schneider said, "Yes, of course - he is such a nice man." He travelled nearly everywhere with us, and we liked that.

This went on for over three weeks, while we had engagements in Archangel and various places, though in between we came back to Murmansk. He was just charming, and our attachment of course grew. Even though our director hadn't enough English for a conversation with him, he said what a lovely man Victor was.

This romance just came to me. And it came so unexpectedly that it was extraordinary. At the time I was in a peculiar situation and an unsettled state of mind. I wasn't angry – the anger had gone – but I was disappointed.

Victor begged me to have a photo taken with him, but I told him I was terrified of the KGB. He then begged me to come back with him to England, but I couldn't.

"Victor, I can't. I have a child, and at the moment I have a husband. I don't think that will last, the way things are. The war did damage to all of us. Nevertheless, I have a child. But I promise you one thing: if I ever get to England, I will certainly get in touch with you."

He gave me his address, and I still have it with me, in his handwriting.

One of his sailors, his First Mate, said to me, "You know, Lily, you are beautiful." I couldn't take notice every time someone said that – I had got used to it by then – so that wasn't important. Victor never said anything like that to me. I asked him once what attracted him: "Your lovely, long hair." We left it like that, but his attachment went beyond that. The time came to say goodbye, and we did so with sadness. I promised to send him a photo of mine, which I did when I got home. I still don't know if he got it or not, but his memory lingered on.

Moss moves a little further away

When I got home, my mother told me that Moss was out.

"You know, Lili, the last three nights he hasn't come home."

"Well, in that case he can stay there."

I wasn't going to make any attempt to get him back. I would never consider it. I knew he was torn, and I felt there were many reasons for that. It was mainly that he didn't want me to travel, but I had no option: the government insisted I work. In any case, I couldn't give up a well-paid job, because everything was so uncertain: I thought about what had happened to Barney, and the war was still on. But he came to me.

Victor had loaded me with cigarettes, among other gifts, and I knew Moss had started to smoke. Only one or two of the girls smoked; Shura and Vera, that I shared a room with, they never smoked. I didn't smoke. I had no inclination to smoke, even before I had Leonora. The advice to pregnant mothers was, 'Even if you smoke just four cigarettes a day, give it up.' I gave it up. I didn't miss it. But I didn't throw them out. We never realised then how dangerous smoking was – there was no publicity in Russia then, as there is in Britain now, that tobacco is a killer.

Moss came to me. I didn't make any fuss. I only said that I had some cigarettes and, if he wanted them, he could have them. He thanked me and he took them. We never mentioned ourselves or our future. From that time on, we never spoke about how things were going to be. He decided to move out. He didn't completely do so, because some things that belonged to him were still there.

I got used to it, but I felt empty without a doubt. Although I was invited out and I had many friends, that didn't compensate. When I took my little girl to the park or anywhere, there were just two of us. I so wanted her to have a father, and it just didn't happen.

Why does history repeat itself? It was very much like what had happened to me, with two differences: my mother felt it was better that I never knew my father, and so I never did; whereas I really wanted Leonora to have a father, and Leonora did know him and understood what had happened. She was a very bright girl, but now she was very quiet. I never made any fuss, though.

One day Moss called round and asked if he could take her out. I said 'yes' straightaway. He took her out, and when Leonora came back she had wet feet, because her shoes had leaked. I got really angry that Moss had never noticed that; he should have bought her a pair of shoes. I suppose he simply didn't notice, but his attention was divided. Leonora was unhappy about that.

"Mummy, there was a kind of woman with him. I didn't like her."

"Don't take any notice, darling – something happened. I'll tell you about it when you are bigger."

The idea of returning to England

Our group continued to give concerts here and there, and it was after one of these that I met a girl I had been at school with, May Peters. Her father was English without a doubt because, though he signed his name as Petersen, I knew he was called Patterson. He had taken Russian citizenship when he became a Soviet official. He was a commandant in the Kremlin, and people feared him.

On my way home, I bumped into May near the Grand Theatre, the Bolshoi, because I had to pass that if I was coming from that part of Moscow.

"Oh, Lily, you are just the person I wanted to meet."

"Yes? What is it?"

"Well, I have decided to apply for my birth certificate and get a passport. I want to go back to England. Do you want to join me? You can – after all, you are British. You were born there."

I also knew that my father wasn't Russian, and never had been, but May was now considered to share her father's Russian citizenship; in the same way, until my marriage, the authorities considered me to be Austrian, and my mother too. I wasn't sure how May would be treated. I started to say that, but she misunderstood.

"Mind you, May –"

"It's all right, I've heard about your personal affairs."

Somehow, in our circle, people who had some connection with the school or knew any of us were always well informed.

"Yes, it is very sad. But really and truly I haven't anything here to stay for."

"You know, Lily, I will tell you something I've been thinking about."

Now, May being English and living not far away from me, we used to bump into each other every so often and keep in touch that way; and she had been quite a while at our school before she left, so I knew she could do exercise and things like that.

"So we can go to England and start a group or whatever – not a school, we couldn't do that – and I will help you with the project."

She knew I was a good dancer and a good teacher. I knew she was very efficient and also she understood how to move.

"May, it is a good idea!"

287

A visit to the embassy

We decided I should apply straightaway for my birth certificate and passport. May had already done this.

"Don't waste your time with the Russian authorities. Go straight to the embassy. That is what I did."

I went to the embassy and spoke to the First Secretary to the Ambassador. I remember his name: Mr Boston. He interviewed me, and I explained what I wanted. He looked at me dubiously.

"Mrs Muscat, are you sure you want to do this? You have a good position here."

"Yes, I am sure. My husband and I, we have had serious differences."

"But you have everything here. I have seen you dance: I never miss your programme when your group dances in Moscow. I like tremendously what you do."

"Nevertheless, I want to go to England."

"What are you going to do there?"

I explained our idea and he listened. He didn't comment, but he told me that England was not very nice: it was dull and grey, the weather was bad, there were shortages. If only he had mentioned that they weren't interested in the arts, I might have had second thoughts. But I was determined to get my English passport.

"Whatever I decide, Mr Boston, please get me my passport and my birth certificate."

"Very well, Mrs Muscat, I will."

He took down all the particulars and we parted as good friends. From that time on, he kept in touch and was very kind to me.

He always invited me to the embassy if they had a film show or any event there. I remember once I went to see a beautiful film, starring Ronald Colman. He was so handsome, I liked him so much. At this film show I met a defector, a girl from the big theatre, the Bolshoi, who was there with her husband. Her name was Valya Prohorava; she was very lovely and she made a name for herself. One of the rising stars in the embassy had proposed to her, and they married. She was a very good-looking girl. Was she a very good dancer? Only medium, I would say. I knew them all in the Bolshoi, who was good and who not so good, and I saw Valya Prohorava dance several times. She was not an especially good dancer.

Whenever I used to go to the embassy, Mr Boston always kept me in the picture. On my next visit, he pointed out something I hadn't considered.

"You know it will take time."

"That doesn't matter: I have plenty of time."

"Have you begun divorce proceedings?"

"No. I wasn't planning to divorce my husband. Should I?"

"You have to have a divorce. Otherwise the Russians will reject your application. If you are still married, they will say you are a Soviet citizen. So you have to make up your mind which you want, your husband or your passport."

"In that case, yes, I will divorce him."

Are you sure?

I arranged to see Moss. We sat down and talked, and I told him what I intended to do.

"I have decided to go to England."

"Are you sure?"

"Yes, I am. I don't want to stand in your way and I want to make a life for myself."

He didn't say anything, but I could see he was perturbed.

"Before I can get my passport, we have to get a divorce. Do you agree?"

"If you want to, yes. But what are you going to do there in England?"

"What am I going to do? Whatever happens, I won't sink. Besides, your brother Fred is there and he will definitely help me. We were always good friends, and I don't think he will forget me just like that."

He didn't say anything, but deep down he was clearly really worried.

"What are you going to do there? How are you going to manage?"

"Just what are you worrying about? Were you going to offer me something? Did you say you were coming back to me?"

"No."

"There you are, then. We will leave it at that."

And that was how we left it. I knew deep down he wanted me to stay at home. He might have come back to me if I had said I would give up dancing. But I was nervous of doing that, because you never knew what the Russian Government might do. They were devious really and capable of all sorts of mischief. Besides, I don't think it would have helped, because Moss was torn.

I thought, *He is weak; let him get on with his weakness*. By that time he had come to take away his belongings. I think I was away when he came. He took whatever he had bought and the things he wanted to have. That didn't worry me. I had made up my mind, and we had a divorce. That was easy: you simply went to the registrar and said, 'We are separating.' We did that; then I went to the embassy and I told Mr Boston exactly what I had done. I thought, *Now I have to face things on my own - but I am definitely not going down on my knees to anyone*.

Alma-ata, of all places

Meanwhile, our group gave concerts wherever we were asked to go, and one of our bookings was in Alma-ata. Now isn't that strange? Even more remarkable was that, when I got there, my friends from Uzun-argach came along - not the family with little Rosa, because I knew they had moved back to Moscow, but Usa and his family, with Clara, that girl who was so lovely, that I liked so much, and Lazar Sobel as well. They all came to see me dance, they really liked it and of course they invited me round to their place.

That was quite a reunion. They were all asking me how I was, and I had to tell them that there was a rift between me and my husband. I don't think they were surprised, because the same thing had happened to many people - especially those, like us, who had been separated for years by the war - but they were very kind and delighted to see me. Little Clara by then was not so little: she was 17. She said, "Lilya, you are going to stay with us overnight. You are going to sleep with me." And I did. That is how generous they were.

Of course, the next day I had to say goodbye, and Clara was sorry to lose me, but I felt sure she would do well without my help. Her disposition was so caring, she was a loving daughter and she was beautiful.

"No, darling, you will have your own life. You will make your way, don't worry."

We had had a delightful relationship, but nothing in the world lasts: there is always an end, even to the loveliest things. We parted, and I travelled back to Moscow with the rest of the girls.

May Peters

When I got back, I met May again.

"Lily, come over to my place. I am having a little get-together this evening and I want to introduce you to somebody."

So I went. And I thought, *Perhaps my social life is picking up.* I used to go quite often to see May, since we were both waiting for our British passports. Mr Boston, at the embassy, never forgot about us, and he used to invite us there.

When May invited me round to her place for a little party, she wanted me to meet a young Englishman from the embassy. I think she had been going to their parties for some while, and that may be where she got the idea of going back to England. Her parents were no longer alive, as far as I know, and she felt anxious about her future. She had some English friends at the embassy, so we used to meet there sometimes and had quite a nice time. And that is how the time went.

Moss is torn between three women

Although I filled my life with activities, the emptiness was there. I was really hurt. I had so wanted Moss to be there to meet me when I came back after those years of enforced separation. I had so wanted him to be happy, and it didn't happen. I could never forget that disappointment, though I tried. I didn't know how to win him back.

He was in a difficult position, I think, because in my absence he had become attached to this other woman. That was the result of circumstances; what didn't help was his mother's intervention. Until then I had never known the real Auntie Annie. Gradually I came to see that deep down she was a very cunning person. Moss of course was her favourite, because he loved her very much. I didn't mind that; it didn't worry me in the least. I had always been very fond of Auntie Annie myself.

We all tend to think that other people will do the thing we would do. Moss and his mother thought like that, I soon saw. I had been away for nearly four years: what had I been doing? Moss was still carrying on his affair: why wasn't I making any fuss?

I had never met his secretary. I wasn't inquisitive; I wasn't interested in her. I don't know what her father did, either; all I know is that he was high up in something or other, and that attracted Auntie Annie. Moss must have said to his mother, "I don't know what to do." She evidently said, "You stay with this new woman; after all, she has a good position and you will be better off." Moss was torn two ways, but his mother was on his side and he took her advice. How ill she advised him, how very ill.

Her son was having an affair, but what her son was doing didn't matter. Perhaps she thought it was all right for a man, but it was different where a woman was concerned, though she was the last person to be able to talk about that. Nevertheless, whenever Auntie Annie and I went anywhere together, she always watched me. I didn't know why she was watching me, but it seems she was afraid I might have a little affair with somebody. She told Moss and his secretary of her suspicions, and they too turned against me. They made up all sorts of stories about me, which I discovered only much later.

A meeting in Poland

Anyway, my social life was good and I had many loyal friends. I used to go to parties downstairs, where Mahmet and Sonya always saw to it that I wouldn't feel lonely. But I would feel empty whenever I went out with my little girl, because there weren't three of us. When her father visited us, he would try to buy her interesting toys, but that wasn't what my daughter was interested in.

Sonya was one of my best friends and she was very good to me. Mahmet, too, was fond of me and very kind indeed. He always said, "Lilya, if you are ever short of anything, let me know." I was also kept busy with rehearsals for our group's second visit to Poland. This time we gave concerts in Lvov. It was quite a nice place and strangely enough there were very many Jewish people there. Our performances were a big success, I have to say.

At the hotel in Lvov, I got a message that there was somebody asking for me. I went down to the foyer, and there was Mahmet. I was so surprised, and he had been too, when he saw the posters for our show.

"Oh, Lilya, I never knew you were coming here."

"And I didn't know *you* were coming here! Otherwise I would have let you know. So, why did *you* come here?"

"I will let you into my secret. I came here to buy furniture."

"No. Really?"

"Yes, really."

"Well, good for you, Mahmet: get whatever you can."

"I am trying to."

He bought a complete set of dining-room and bedroom furniture made of bird's-eye maple. I remember that well, because I saw it when it arrived. He had a beautiful apartment, but you couldn't get anything so lovely in Moscow as you could get then in Poland, which had not yet been dragged down by the tyranny of our lovely Stalin – the good uncle that everybody thought he was, especially the American working class.

I also bought a few things in Lvov. We had a very pleasant time mixing with society there. I did especially, mixing with the Jewish people, dancing and being made much of. That is where I picked up that lovely Jewish song, 'Bei mir bist du schön'. Oh, I liked it so much, but I could never get the record. In any case, by that time I had lost my Pet-o-phone, which was stolen from Tanya's place in the country, where I had left it. Tanya always kept in touch with me and so did Barney. Eventually, as I mentioned, Barney returned to Moscow and that was when Auntie Annie behaved very badly towards him, and there was a rift between them. That was even before I left Moscow.

Return to Murmansk

Our group had to go back to Murmansk: an American fleet was there and they asked us to dance for them. I had such lovely memories of the British fleet. A few American chaps became friendly with me because I spoke English, and I asked them how they were bearing up. They said, "We are all homesick."

Now the British sailors never mentioned that. They were such brave lads and they stuck to reality, but the Americans weren't used to war. They took it very badly because they were not used to these terrible discomforts. I understood that, and we did our best to entertain them. We didn't stay there long and then we came back to Moscow.

On my return, again the English Embassy got in touch with me, to tell me how things were progressing. Meanwhile, we were preparing for another tour. At this point I must mention my mother's sister, Auntie Clara. They lived in Moscow, but I was only occasionally in touch with them even before the war, though I recall they invited Moss and me once, and we had such a lovely evening. All their girls were there, the whole of my cousin's family.

A tour in Siberia

Our next tour was to Siberia: we went to Sverdlovsk, and there I met Rosa, one of my cousins. She came to see me and we became friends. She had a husband and two children. He wasn't a Jewish man. She invited me to come round and stay the night with them, which I did. Her two girls were blonde, with long plaits. I had never seen the children before, but I thought they were lovely. As for her husband, well – as long as she liked him, that's all I can say. We used to spend time together, Rosa and I, and we got on very well.

One day, when I went back to the hotel in Sverdlovsk, the girls told me I had a visitor, and there was Maria. She was still beautiful. I hadn't seen her since the time we were leaving Moscow, when we went away together. Really, I was so surprised that she turned up here.

"Didn't you know, Lilya, that we work here? We learnt that you were coming here to give some concerts, and of course I had to get in touch with you."

We talked and I must have asked about her family.

"You know, Lilya, I am so trying to have a child."

"Well, how is your little husband?"

"Oh, he is still adorable. I love him just the same."

I thought that was lovely – but she could not have a child. I felt sorry for her.

"Do you ever get in touch with your son from your previous marriage?"

"No."

And that was it. I was very pleased to see Maria, very pleased indeed. She promised to be in touch and asked me where I was living. I gave her my address and she said she might come to Moscow.

"Lovely! And now you know where I live."

"Yes."

That is how we parted.

The other girls took notice of her, with her beautiful blue eyes and dark hair. She was lovely. Ulya commented on her.

"Isn't she beautiful?"

"Yes, I know. I like beautiful women."

I went to see my cousin Rosa and told her we would soon be going away. I think she was only in Sverdlovsk because they sent her husband there: he was a party member. She had to go where he went. Her youngest brother had been killed in the war, I did know that, though the rest of her family were alive. She was very pleased to see me, but naturally she was a little sad when I had to go. I tried to cheer her.

"Look, don't worry: they may send him back to Moscow before long, and you won't be so alone."

It was just circumstances: my life was entirely different from theirs.

We said goodbye and I went back to the hotel. We began to pack, because our tour had finished. It was quite nice – we went there in summertime – it was not bad at all, because wintertime in Siberia is very severe. However, if you live there permanently, you get used to the severe winters, and there are two good things about them: there is never wind, it is always still, and the air is so pure.

When we were ready to return to Moscow, we found we couldn't get tickets. All we could find were five seats on an Army jet plane. It wasn't a passenger plane, but five of us decided to fly back that way, and the others eventually went by train. It is a long, long way.

So we flew back. As we were getting off the aeroplane in Moscow, the pilot said he had never experienced such luck. It was a three-engined plane and two had conked out. We had been flying on one engine, but the pilot got us home and we never knew. I don't think it would have made any difference if we had known, because when you are young you take things in a quite different way from when you are older.

The war ends

Very shortly after we got back, the war was declared at an end. I had a phone call from Moss to celebrate the fact that the war was over. He seemed to be so very happy, and I was pleased he phoned, but that was it. Nothing followed, though, and after that I went on my way. I was quite occupied with friends and meeting other people.

Moss used to come now and then to see Leonora and - I think - to see me as well. But I never stayed in when he came. In any case, I was always being invited out. One day, I was out walking in the centre of Moscow and I bumped into Lazar Sobel. Oh, he was so pleased to see me!

"How are you, Lilya?"

"I'm well. Actually, I am trying to go to England."

"Splendid idea! Don't waver: just go. Get out of this country, if it is at all possible."

He had done his time in internal exile, and now he was back in Moscow. He had met up with his wife and daughter. The reunion with them had made him extraordinarily happy. I felt happy for him, too. We parted and each went on our way. I don't now remember where I was going, but I was always meeting somebody at that time.

We all make mistakes

The embassy had told me that my documents would be ready soon, so I was starting to pack and the news got around my circle of friends - some of them people I hadn't seen for years. I met Lucy Flaxman, who wanted me to get in touch with her husband, Jack Chen. He was in London, apparently, writing for the *Daily Worker*. Lucy was still regretting that she hadn't stayed in America with her father. She had left her father because she felt something he had done was wrong.

"I shall never forgive myself for making such a dreadful blunder."

"Lucy, everybody makes blunders. You can only look back and wonder what made you do it. I know it myself; I know it very well."

"But why did I ever come back?"

She asked herself that again and again. I could only say I would try to find Jack, but I could not promise anything.

A young chap also got in touch with me, someone I'd never seen before, short and very funny; his name was William, I think. His father was Harry Pollitt, a prominent Labour politician, who had strongly advised him against going to Moscow. William had gone anyway, now could not get out and was pining for his family. He was something in the theatrical world.

"What made you come to Moscow?"

"I just fancied it. But please would you get in touch with my father, and beg him to get me back to England?"

I don't know what he had done with his passport. Anyway, I said I would try my best when I got to London.

My passport, at last

Just after that I got a phone call from the embassy.

"We have your passport. You can come and collect it whenever it suits you."

I could hardly believe it. I felt really happy. The bad news was, May Peters hadn't got a passport. This was a blow: I needed someone with me. May met me and explained.

"Lily, it's so unfortunate. The authorities won't let me go, because of my father."

"I'm very disappointed. You know, May, you gave me the idea of going – I might never have thought of it, but for you – however, I'm still going to go through with it."

Moss came round for something. I told him my passport was ready, and he wasn't happy. Then he started thinking.

"What are you going to do when you get there?"

"Don't worry about that. The only thing is, a friend was going to come with me. It was through her that I decided to go, but the authorities refused to let her leave. All the same, that won't put me off. I am going to the embassy to get my passport."

Of course the reason he wasn't happy was because of what he himself had done, when he gave his passport away. Why had he done it? That perturbed him terribly. Had it not been for that, perhaps he might have come with me; who knows? Up to then he had still thought I might change my mind, but I didn't. I was determined to go through with what I wanted, but there was one more thing I had to ask him.

"Of course I have to have your permission to take our daughter."

297

"I will let you know about that."

That didn't sound promising, and I was afraid there would be problems there, but I knew Moss would never go against my wishes in that. He just couldn't do it.

From that time on, I started my real preparations. It wasn't a case of just making a list and ticking things off – a 'one, two, three' job. For one thing, I had to have a certain amount of money. For another, I had to get rid of lots of things that I didn't need to take. So began a busy, busy time for me.

Mooshya and a man

I liked Mooshya, one of the girls in our dance group – she was so gentle and kind. We had become quite attached to each other, ever since the time a few years earlier when I told her not to marry the first time. Eventually the truth of the matter dawned on her.

"Lilya, how far-sighted you were. If only I'd listened..."

"Well, I knew just what to expect even then, because I had seen that man of yours and he was so unreliable, he would never be any good for a husband."

After that she took notice of everything I said – I was young, like her, but I knew what was what.

We used to meet up and go out together. We often went to orchestral concerts at the Tchaikovsky Hall. It was a lovely hall for music, rather than anything staged, such as ballet. Mooshya and I booked tickets for a concert that included Tchaikovsky's 1st Piano Concerto.

Although I was preparing to leave, there were still plenty of chores to do at home. We had a very nice home, with all the facilities to look after ourselves. I also had to help with shopping for food. My mother had to buy most things on the black market, because there was hardly anything to buy in the shops. Often you could only get bread, so I had to go to the market for meat, vegetables and various groceries – even milk wasn't always to be had in the shops.

On the day of this concert, I had to go out to buy milk. We had a special can for it, so I took the can and went to the market. On my way back, I got off the tram near home to walk down the little side road to where we lived. As I stepped off the tram, a young chap came up to me.

"May I stop you a moment and ask you something?"

"Yes. What is it?"

"Well, I have just come back from the army."

"Yes?"

"I wonder if you could come with me tonight to a concert."

"I am so sorry, but I can't. I would have helped you out there if I could, but I can't: I have arranged to meet a friend tonight."

I wanted to be kind; he seemed such a nice chap.

"What a shame."

"Well, goodbye."

We left it at that. I never asked where he was going to take me. I couldn't go and, after all, a concert could be anywhere.

That evening I met Mooshya, and we sat down to listen. Next to her there were two empty seats, and who should take them but that chap I met on my way back from the market. He had brought a friend with him. He didn't see me at first, so I leaned across Mooshya and spoke to him.

"Ah, there you are. I don't know if you remember me."

"Of course I do."

"This is quite a coincidence, meeting you twice in one day."

This was the first time I had heard the Tchaikovsky No. 1, and Mooshya and I fell in love with it. At the interval, the four of us had a good time together, walking and talking, and we parted after the concert. But I thought how strange this incident was.

Grigori again

In the middle of my preparations to leave, who should turn up? Grigori! I was astonished.

"What made you get in touch with me?"

"Well, I heard that you had split with your husband, and I thought I would try my luck again. I have a very good position now - I have been made a director, and they are sending me to Tallinn as director of a fur factory."

"Grigori, I am really flattered in a way. After all these years, I thought you would have forgotten about me."

"No, never. Can't you at least spend an evening with me? We could go out somewhere."

"Where?"

"Wherever you wish."

"Well, I would like to go to a concert."

I knew already what was going to happen, but he agreed and I kept my word.

For half of the concert he was asleep. That was nothing new to me, though. As we were coming back home, he stopped on the pavement.

"Lilya, decide."

"I decided years ago, Grigori. It could never happen. I am going to London – that is settled – and I have a daughter, so it is out of the question. Look, Grigori, as time goes by, you are sure to meet somebody else. Just say goodbye."

"Can I do anything for you before you go?"

"There is one thing you can do for me, if you are able. You can get me a fur coat –"

"With pleasure."

"– but on one condition: that I pay for it."

He agreed and he kept his word. He got me a lambskin coat – it wasn't Persian Lamb, it was from a young lamb – I think it was called Broad Lamb. I didn't care for the way it was made, but I thought, *It will do*. I thanked him and paid whatever it cost.

"Thank you very much; that was very good of you. Goodbye."

"Goodbye, Lilya."

He didn't trouble me any more. That was a blessing.

Rosa and Shelley

Some friends from Uzun-argach turned up. You remember that lovely family with the girl called little Rosa, that I met at the hospital? It was her father's sister who called, the mother of that boy of 17. She came to visit, but she missed me. I had had to go out; she waited for me, but I was detained and of course I never knew she was going to come. When I got home, my mother told me about it.

The following week, the youngest sister of Rosa's mother appeared – it's funny, but I remember her name, Shelley – and she brought with her the boy I mentioned. He was now a very nice young man. They came several times, and I liked Shelley very much, but I thought it was not right bringing that young chap with her.

"Shelley, dear, you know I like you very much. The trouble is that

I feel I am so busy now that I cannot give you my attention; so we will have to call a halt."

I could see she was disappointed and a little surprised, so I spelt out the problem.

"It is because you are so much younger than me and your nephew is becoming a little too interested in me, so I think it would be better to stop there."

I had to laugh, really, at the idea, but even so I knew from other people that such things do happen. It was a pity, but nevertheless it had to be so. And I really was busy. I had to prepare everything, I had to sell many things and these things take time.

Preparing to leave: buying and selling

Although my wardrobe was marvellous, I couldn't take half of it with me. There was too much. However, many people wanted to buy various garments. A neighbour I was friendly with bought many things, saying, "Your clothes were always so wonderful." I sold them, even to far relations, and that money was useful.

I began to think, *How will I manage when I arrive in London?* When the embassy got me the passport, I asked about getting some sterling currency from them.

"Well, the best we can do for you, the most we can allow you to change, is £150."

I had to pay for that, but they didn't charge me a lot; they needed Russian money to pay for things in Russia.

That was settled, but that money was to pay for the journey itself. I knew it was quite a distance and how would I travel? All that had to be arranged. As well as money, I felt I ought to have some other valuables with me, some jewels at least. I had never thought of them before, but now they seemed a good idea. The staff at the embassy were very good: when they look after you, they really do look after you. I spoke to a woman there who was in charge of finance and organisation, and asked her.

"Do you think I would be able to take some jewels with me?"

"Certainly, if you wish."

Funnily enough, Moss had never taken any interest in buying me jewels. It wasn't the fashion in Moscow then, but now in some way

301

my preparations got him interested. He thought I should have something from him and he bought me a beautiful set all made in platinum: a necklace with a real aquamarine, set with little diamonds, and matching earrings. He also bought me a beautiful sapphire ring, which I have to this day.

I also started buying things, first of all from Tanya. She said she would miss us. I said, "Look, Tanya, I know, but nevertheless I have to sort out my life." Tanya understood. She was a very good friend to me, and she put me in touch with a friend of hers who had quite a number of things to sell. I managed to get various bits of jewellery, though nothing spectacular.

Moss asked me if I needed anything else and I said yes, because there was a place in Moscow where they bought jewels and other valuables from private individuals. Whatever they bought was then sold in another shop, which they had recently opened, where you had to pay for things with gold.

Moss said we should go and see what we could get. As we waited, we spoke to the other people in the queue and asked them what they had to sell. The lady in front of us showed us a brooch with three diamonds, but of course I didn't understand jewels and neither did Moss. We didn't know the value of it. They did offer her a price, but we had warned her beforehand what to expect. We told her that, whatever they offered her, we would pay more if she sold it to us privately. And that is what happened.

I found out afterwards that there was a slight flaw in one of the diamonds, but it wouldn't have stopped me from buying it. They were a fair size, about three-quarters of a carat each. I thought it would come in very useful on my journey. I knew the consul at the British embassy would do whatever he could to pay for my hotel and meals, but if I wanted to buy anything, I would not have any local currency. Jewels are always acceptable.

In the end I had gathered quite a few bits, but one thing happened that I regret to this day, and why? Because I was still indecisive. I wasn't sure how things would turn out when I got to London; I might not be happy, I might want to come back again.

A person I knew called Laritza, who was related to Tanya, got in contact with me.

"Lilya, I have something to offer you, a beautiful thing."

It was a very clear diamond, one carat in weight.

"Laritza, dear, I have run out of cash and I can't ask Moss to pay."

"What a shame, Lilya, because it is a lovely buy and a reasonable price."

However, I had decided that I now had enough to carry me through. So I had to refuse that. It was a shame really that I never bought it. I could have squeezed myself and found the money to get it, but sometimes you feel you have reached the limit. In any event, I thought, *How am I going to carry it through customs? There is bound to be somebody who wants to know what valuables you have.*

What would my mother do?

I mentioned the efficient person who arranged our tickets when we were still in that village near Alma-ata. She also helped me to get in touch with various people. I don't know how – probably through friends of friends – but she got to know I was going to London.

So she got in touch with me, found out my address and just turned up one day. I was surprised. It's funny I don't remember her name, but I do remember her.

"I hear you're going to London. What will you do with your place in Moscow?"

"Well, I don't know yet how well I will settle in London. It is difficult to tell, going by yourself, but for me it's going to be a strange place. I was brought up in Russia from the age of 7."

"Look, I would buy your flat."

She knew my mother owned it, because all the flats in our block were built for sale.

"Money you don't need, but I can give you diamonds or whatever you want. I have plenty."

I suppose she assumed my mother would be going with me and we would rather sell the flat for jewels than for roubles, which would be no use to us in London. If she bought our flat in Moscow and we bought one in London, then, if we found we didn't like England, she could offer to exchange the flat in Moscow for the one in London.

She had her own reasons for making this offer. Her daughter, who was very beautiful, had been having an affair with a journalist called Ruddock. I remember him: he often visited Paris, where he was well known, and he wrote for a magazine of Russian literature. He was very much taken with her, and she with him.

"Really I would love my daughter to have a place of her own in central London. Well, anyway, think about it."

"To be honest with you, I am definitely going – I have made up my mind – but my mother really doesn't want to come, and I don't want to insist."

And we left it at that.

The embassy told me not to ask permission for my mother to come with me, because in 1920 she had signed an agreement that she would never return to England. I was an only daughter and we only had each other, so I could have insisted on my mother coming with me and they could never have refused us.

But my mother was reluctant. She probably thought, *Let her try England, if she is so keen*. I think she had got a little tired of me and Leonora, and the whole situation. I sensed my mother's doubts.

"Look, if I don't like it there and I can't settle, I will come back."

I told Moss the same. I could see he was a bit concerned, so I tried to reassure him.

"Moss, let's make a deal, you and I."

"Yes? What is it?"

"Look, if I don't like it there, I will come back to you. In that event, would you come back to me?"

"Yes, Lily, I would."

We said no more about it.

In those last few days, paradoxically, I was enjoying my life, going to say goodbye to various friends. I heard that Barney was coming home for good. When I next saw Tanya, she was very excited. By this time she had moved to the house of a very old friend of her mother's. Tanya was now really comfortable, because she had a very nice apartment with good facilities. When Barney did come back, she would have somewhere decent to welcome him and big enough for both of them. She was really looking forward to it.

Tanya's mother used to call me 'Lilikin'. She liked me and was sorry I was going, saying it was a shame, but nevertheless she could see that I wanted to make a new life. All she was concerned about was that her daughter was still there in Moscow and her son-in-law was going to be released completely. So she was contented.

I sold whatever I could. I knew my mother wouldn't want the mahogany double bed, so I sold it to a neighbour, who was delighted to have such a beautiful bed. My mother still had a bed-settee and I left the whole place full of nice things, including plenty of crockery and a lovely dinner service. My mother wasn't destitute.

However, she was used to me getting everything for her. I always supplied whatever she needed and made sure she was never in want. Now that I wasn't going to be there, I made arrangements with Moss.

"Look, I am going away. I know you will be worried about me, but there's no need. But I'd like you to look after my mother and see that she is never in want."

"Don't worry, Lily. I will do that, I promise you."

Leaving Russia for good

Very soon the day came when we had to go. My mother came to see us off, and so did Moss. Leonora and I got on board the train. We were sitting there, Moss was standing next to me and he was stroking my hair. I felt sad, and so did he.

"You know what, Moss? I am going to try and get you back."

If it had been possible, I would have done it too; but deep down I knew there was no hope of it.

I suppose I could have said, 'Come with me now: don't go home. You are on the train already. I will hide you somewhere,' but I never considered it. Of course I didn't know then that the bunk in my compartment had a lid and you could put your things inside. Probably it would have been dangerous to hide him from the border guards, but I didn't think of that either.

He had to get off because the train was ready to depart, and I could see he was so very sorry that he was not coming with us. My mother said goodbye, Moss promised me he would look after her, I said I would be in touch and he said he would too. And the last thing he said was, "Have a kipper for me."

You know, afterwards that played on my mind: it was so poignant. That man, he was so English. He was more English than I was. I had always admired England from my childhood, and I always took notice of what was going on there, but I knew that Moss was much more English. Very English. He never could fit in, in Russia.

It was a disaster when his department made him change his nationality. I don't know what made him do that. Maybe it was just that he loved his work, was scared of losing his job and didn't feel

305

secure enough to turn down promotion. He was very close to his brother Barney, who had done the same, but that didn't make Moss any less English. He didn't tell me until he had done it, or I would have stopped him, and that was why he never told me. He didn't want to be talked out of his decision; but before long he too began to grieve over this misjudgement of his.

We said goodbye, he embraced me and then Leonora, and she was delighted. She thought this was going to be a very big adventure, and she was right. She was 7 years old and so grown-up by then, a lovely child. I don't know how Moss could ever bear to part with her, and with me too. And I was so right in the decisions I made. Later on I found out how right I was.

14

A Passage to England, 1946

The train started. As it began to move out of the station, I settled my luggage, keeping the things to hand that we needed on the journey. I had organised all that when I was packing, and everything I took came in very useful. I glanced at my daughter and she looked so happy.

"So, Leonora, how do you feel?"

"Well, I am sorry to leave Grandma, but this is interesting, all the same. What is the journey going to be like?"

She never mentioned her father.

As our train rattled through the outskirts of Moscow, we settled down for the long journey to Helsinki, which took a day and night even when everything was running smoothly. We had the compartment to ourselves, just the two of us. One of the people travelling in the next compartment was a young Russian. I was always very fortunate with young men, and we got talking. He wanted to know where we were going.

"Well, really we are going to England."

"Are you really? And where is your first stop?"

"Helsinki."

"Have you any Finnish currency on you?"

"No."

"But how are you going to manage?"

"We will be met at the station."

"But say, for instance, they miss you and you have no money: then you would be stranded. How on earth would you manage?"

"I don't know."

"Then I will tell you something. I go very often to Helsinki, so I know what I'm talking about. And I will give you a packet of cigarettes. You can buy the whole of Helsinki for a packet of cigarettes!"

"What do I want with a packet of cigarettes? I don't even smoke."

"Don't refuse it. Take it."

"No, no, I couldn't possibly."

"Yes, yes, take it. You'll be glad of it."

I did and I was.

I forgot to mention that, before we left, my aunt – my mother's sister, Clara – sent her eldest daughter, Luba, to help me get ready to go. Luba was a great help in arranging things and doing jobs, but then she was my first cousin after all. Aunt Clara had given Luba a 20-dollar note. It was a very old one, but she told her daughter, "Give it to Lilya. It will come in useful to her." It was kind of her and I was grateful – it was a nice gesture. I stitched it up in the lining of my coat, in case any official tried to take it away from me.

I must mention here another thing that happened before I left Moscow. My Maria told me she would come to see me before I left. When she turned up, it dawned on me: *Of course – there will be a reason why she has come*. It soon came out.

"Lilya, I have come to say goodbye, but there was also another reason why I came. I want to buy your watch. Sell it to me, Lilya: you are going abroad, where you can always get yourself another one. Here I could never get such a beautiful thing."

She meant the beautiful watch, made of white gold and adorned with real sapphires, that I had bought in New York. Maria had always admired it, I knew that. So I sold it to her, and that was another bit of money that helped to buy other things I needed.

Helsinki

We slept on the train, though there were no bunks, just the seats. Not long after St Petersburg we reached the frontier between Russia and Finland. At the customs, they asked me if I had anything of value to declare, and I said, "No, not really." They didn't even open my cases and luckily they didn't search me, since I had a little container on me with the few jewels I was carrying. So we got through customs, and the train set off again, leaving Russia behind.

It carried on for several more hours until at last we reached

Helsinki. We got off the train, Leonora and I, and my little girl suddenly became very efficient.

"Mummy, I am going to watch the luggage. You go and see if there is anybody there to meet us."

I did that, but I couldn't see anybody, so I took a cab and told the driver to wait. I went back to get Leonora and all our belongings, and the cab driver helped us. I asked him to take us to the English embassy, which he did.

At the embassy, I told them there had been no one at the station to meet us. They said they were sorry; they must have missed me. I asked where I was meant to go now. They were all apologies, saying of course someone would take us to a hotel. This person escorted us there and said the embassy would get in touch with me within a few days. We thought the hotel was quite decent, Leonora and I. We had a nice room, but there was no bathroom. I was very disappointed and I told the proprietor.

"There seems to be no bathroom. What facilities are there?"

"Well, we have no bathrooms, but there is a Turkish bath, which you could use. You can have a good wash there and sweat out all the dirt."

"Right, yes, I would like that very much, whatever it is. Can you arrange that for us? We have just come from the station after a long journey – we travelled on the train overnight – so we want to wash first."

They prepared this sweat bath for us, and Leonora and I went in. But after a while we were in despair; we couldn't find how to get out of it. We had to get down on the floor to get away from the steam, it was so awful. In the end somebody came for us. I said to them, "Good gracious, we are not used to such steam and heat!" So we finished up laughing. We were given towels and we went to our room.

I only vaguely remember Helsinki. We didn't stay there long, just two or three days, and I was glad of that because I wanted to get on my way. In any case, there was nothing very exciting about it. Leonora and I went out in the evening, and we felt quite lost – as you do, in a place where you don't know anybody. I stood by a shop window because there were a few people there, and I noticed they were speaking Russian, so I approached them.

"Hello, good evening. I have just come from Moscow."

They just looked at me and said "Sorry" in Russian before walking away. I thought, *Fine*. I could tell they were frightened, because everybody there was terrified of anybody who spoke Russian, in case they were from the KGB.

Before we went any further, and knowing we would be in Helsinki for a few days, I decided to write home. I still thought of the flat in Moscow as home. In reality, it was just my mother's flat; Leonora and I had no home now. I thought, *I must tell them everything that happened on the journey, with all the details*. I used to write very well, and I liked a little laugh, so I told them all about the chap who gave me the packet of cigarettes that would buy Helsinki, and the Turkish bath where we nearly died, and the people in the street who spoke Russian but were terrified to speak to us. I wrote a really long and interesting letter. I knew they would enjoy that.

Crossing the Baltic

After a day or two, a message came for us from the embassy to say they had arranged our passage and now we could set off for Stockholm, on the next stage of our journey. Oh, I was very pleased! We went down to the harbour with our belongings and boarded the boat.

We were a couple of days on the boat, and there were many other passengers. Among them was a family that I noticed, since they seemed to take great interest in Leonora and me, because we spoke Russian or perhaps because of my appearance. I looked nice, I have to say, because I was wearing a fur wrapper. I knew the weather would be a bit fresh in the Baltic. Now I had a fur coat, but I didn't like it, so I bought myself this wrapper made of mole trimmed with ermine. It not only looked very nice, but it hid everything else; by now I hadn't many clothes to wear, because I had sold everything. After a short while, the woman – of this family I mentioned – approached and spoke to me in Russian.

"Can I ask you something?"

"Yes."

"Where are you going?"

"To Stockholm, and from there we are going to London."

"Oh. I hope you don't mind, but we noticed that you and your daughter were speaking Russian. That is why I asked."

"That's all right. And who are you?"

310

"Well, we were at the embassy in Helsinki and now we are going to Stockholm."

"Oh, that's interesting."

So we became a little friendly and that made the journey pass more quickly.

Our first night in Stockholm

Eventually we docked in Stockholm, where I was met and taken to the hotel, which turned out to be extraordinary. It was a lovely hotel. We settled in, but Leonora couldn't get over it: the people, the shops, the lights. To her, it was like Fairyland.

"Mummy, look how beautiful it is."

"Yes, isn't it? Absolutely splendid!"

We were both charmed. We walked about the city for an hour or so and came back to the hotel for our supper, as we called it. The dining room was packed with people. The waiters were very kind. I suppose they guessed that, when the war was on, we must have been short of everything. Sweden hadn't been to war, so they had everything intact, just as it was before the war. They even had fruit. There was a bit of a shortage, because at the end of the year it is not easy to get citrus fruit, but they had managed to get some oranges, and these they gave only to children. Leonora had never seen an orange before; she had seen mandarins, but never an orange. I peeled it for her.

"Mummy, what will it taste like?"

"You try, darling; you may like it."

"Oh, Mummy, it's very nice."

I was surprised to see a big trolley being wheeled up to every table. This carried the hors d'oeuvres, and there were all sorts of savoury foods and various salads. My favourite was those wonderful herrings, especially smoked herrings. But all the food there was just wonderful: they were very good cooks. It took my breath away, because I was always fond of very good food.

And then we thought we would have an early night. We felt a bit tired. Leonora and I found we had a splendid room, but we hadn't yet had time to look around, even to see what our windows looked out on. We had a big double bed - lovely, very comfortable - and Leonora liked sleeping with me, so we had a good night's sleep.

Making good use of our assets

The next morning, after breakfast, I told Leonora we were going out now to do some shopping. Oh, she did get excited! I had a good idea what I was going to get, because we needed clothes, coats and various things, but first I had to sell the brooch.

I found a jewellery shop, we went inside – just the two of us, because I was always very competent in such dealings – and I went straight up to the proprietor.

"Do you buy jewels?"

"Yes, what have you brought?"

I showed him my brooch, and he had a good look at it.

"Yes. Did you realise one stone is a bit flawed?"

"Yes, I know."

He named a price, and I couldn't argue. I remember it was £35. Well, even £1 was quite a lot of money then, so I agreed. Then I asked him if he knew a good shop for clothes, and he gave me directions.

We found the shop and went in. Leonora needed clothes, and this was my chance to dress her up beautifully. I bought her dresses – pretty, but warm – and a beautiful camel coat, lovely warm boots and woollen stockings. She needed to dress up because the weather was getting cold there in Stockholm. When I had finished buying clothes for her, we went to another shop where I could buy things for myself.

I remembered that when I went to the British embassy in Moscow to see the woman who took charge of arranging my money, she wore nice things, and I had taken particular notice of one dress I liked, a dark blue dress. I would call the colour peacock blue; anyway, I really liked it.

The proprietor of this shop and his woman assistant showed me what they thought might suit. It was a kind of pinafore, in that colour blue, and I bought a white blouse to go with it. I liked brown, I remember, so I chose a camel coat that would match my daughter's and a nice brown beret that I liked. I clothed myself very well. We went back to the hotel and I was very pleased with my purchases.

Before we left Russia, my aunt Clara had also brought me a crocheted angora shawl as a present; ironically, it was traditional to give this kind of shawl to a bride. They were hand-made and famously so fine that you could push one through a wedding ring. I used it to cover my shoulders when I went out in the evening, whatever dress I was wearing, because the weather was turning chilly by then. I know we looked rather nice, because people started to take notice of Leonora and me. We heard them asking, "Who are these people?" And we heard other people saying, "They are a mother and daughter, and I think they are going to London." It was interesting to hear yourself being discussed like that.

We found out that amongst the people who were talking about us was an American. A few days elapsed, then he got talking and we became very friendly. So I asked him about Aunt Clara's bank note.

"I wonder would it be possible to change a 20-dollar note? It is an old one, but perhaps it can be changed into Swedish currency. What do you think?"

"Of course it would. I will go to the bank and get it changed."

He went to his own bank, and they told him the note was so old it was outdated, but this was of no consequence. It was still real American money, after all. They changed it into new dollar bills for him, and he gave them to me. I knew you could buy things with American dollars, wherever you went, and now I had some.

Swedish interlude

This young man was very kind and friendly; he used to tell me that, if I wanted to go out in the evening, his room was not far from mine, so he could keep an eye on my daughter. That was nice of him because I did get invited out.

There was no British embassy in Stockholm, but there was a consulate. A young girl from the consulate, well a youngish woman, came to visit me and we soon became friendly. Her name was Margaret and she used to invite me to the consulate or whatever function she was going to, and take me with her. The first time this happened, this young American encouraged me to accept.

"You go; don't worry, your daughter will be looked after."

"Darling, you don't mind if I go, do you?"

"No, Mummy, you go. I am a big girl now."

So the time there passed like that. It was very enjoyable, and I wrote home again, this time to tell them how much Stockholm had impressed me. Before long, we had been in the hotel two weeks, quite a while. Margaret from the consulate came to see me, to explain the delay.

"The trouble is, they can't get a passage. There are not enough berths and it isn't easy to get a passage to London. So we will just have to wait until one is available."

Meanwhile, the hotel proprietor was getting a little windy. I suppose he was worried the bill might not be paid.

I must say something about the hotel. It was so unusual and beautifully kept. We were not on the ground floor; I think we were on the first floor – the second storey – because I remember our room looked out over the garden and we were only a little way above it. It was a kind of half-garden, like a rose garden. But it was beautiful. I took photographs of that hotel and kept them, because I admired it so much. Leonora used to go to play in the garden and I went out with her. It was full of flowers, but so was the interior.

The whole place was charming; indeed, the whole of Stockholm was delightful – in fact Sweden was lovely altogether. The Swedish people were handsome, even beautiful, and the city of Stockholm was so attractive, not just the buildings, but the streets, the parks, the water – everything. I quickly notice whatever is lovely; my eyes have always been attracted to beauty.

In the course of the third week, the proprietor asked me how long we were planning to stay there. I explained we were waiting for a passage and as soon as they found us a berth on a boat to England, we would go. I said I didn't think it would be long. Because I had waited so long, the consulate had tried to get me a seat on an aeroplane, but they couldn't. Maybe that was just as well, because I preferred to travel by boat.

Margaret had said I could expect to get a passage shortly, and I hurried to finish my shopping. I needed to get shoes and of course I still had no watch, but otherwise I was well equipped. The place where I had bought most of my clothes gave me a very smart umbrella for nothing, because they were so pleased to have my custom. Perhaps they thought that was essential for anyone going to London. The money I had from selling the brooch, together with the 20 dollars, was just sufficient to pay for my stay there and to see that Leonora and I were well dressed, with decent shoes and everything we would need when we arrived in London.

The day came to say goodbye. The time in Stockholm seemed to have flown, because it was so beautiful there; the walks I had with

Leonora, she so enjoyed them. It was a delightful place: neat and very orderly – just the way I like things – with beautiful Gothic buildings. We had such a pleasant time there.

But I felt sad, because somehow I felt that – even if some day I returned to Stockholm – it would never be like that again. Whenever I looked back, even then, I could catch in my mind the impression that places first made on me: when we first went to Riga as youngsters, when we first saw Paris, and then New York. It was exactly the same feeling each time, that it was a lovely place the first time I saw it, but somehow it was never the same again in years to come. The exception was when I went to Austria, to Salzburg and a beautiful lakeside resort, Zell am See – they impressed me deeply. I loved Austria.

Crossing the North Sea

The boat was ready to sail from Stockholm, so we said goodbye to the people we had got to know at the hotel, and to the proprietor, who was so nice to us, and we went to board the ship. It was a Swedish cargo boat.

They took us to our cabin, which was quite pleasant. We had our own facilities, with a bathroom attached to our cabin, so we had some comforts there. We sailed out of the harbour and out to sea. I must say the journey was a bit rocky to start with, and during the night sometimes I heard a siren go, but I never really took much notice. We spent a comfortable night.

The following morning we got ready and then went to find breakfast. Leonora and I entered the dining area, and met our fellow-passengers. I found out it was a cargo boat that carried a few passengers as well. There were no other women on the boat, only me; there were five other people, but only one of them was English. The rest were going to England, but somehow I never got round to finding out who they were.

I don't even remember the Englishman's name, but I know he was a doctor. He and the others used to chat among themselves. Many times, when Leonora and I came into the dining room for breakfast, I heard them saying, "My! Doesn't she look fresh? Fresh as a daisy." Well, I had nothing else to do but keep myself in good shape.

The weather was turning cold, very cold. Even as we left

Stockholm, flakes of snow started coming down. I wouldn't say we had a wonderful passage either – the boat rocked and plunged quite badly at times – but the nearer we got to England, the further south we steamed and the milder the weather became. Our passage was uneventful.

Whenever we went down to dinner, they would lift their glasses and say 'Skol' to one another and to me. They made me very comfortable, the men, especially the captain. He was Swedish, but he spoke English very well, so we managed to talk quite easily to one another; he personally became very friendly towards me. It was very pleasant to have good company like that; it might have been very different.

Our days of doing nothing were drawing to an end. There were big seas now, and it was not very pleasant. It was colder too. I remember once sitting on deck and I had to get out my fur coat – whether I liked the coat or not – just to keep myself warm, because you couldn't sit anywhere without a coat. Leonora, though, was running about: she didn't seem unhappy.

The night before we reached England, I heard a knock on the door during the night, and I said, "Yes?" In came the doctor, and he said I had better keep my door open. I didn't ask why. I supposed it must be something to do with the boat rolling so much, so I kept it open. The doctor coming in must have woken Leonora.

"What is it, Mummy? The boat is rocking so much – can I climb in with you?"

"Yes, darling, of course."

So I picked her up and we lay together, and we both fell asleep with the sirens going and the boat pitching and rolling. It was so stormy that night, but nothing was going to disturb my sleep. Isn't that extraordinary? Now, when I look back, I think, *Good gracious! How plucky I was!* But it wasn't that. It was simply the age I was. Things don't disturb you at that age in the way they do when you get older.

Back in England

The following morning, my door was still open. I never bothered to close the cabin door because there was nobody else there. At breakfast I discovered we were coming into Middlesbrough. After breakfast, we went back to our cabins to start packing. Everyone came along to say goodbye to me, including the doctor who was so attentive to me.

"Where are you going?"

"To London."

"Have you got a ticket?"

"No."

"Have you any money?"

"No."

"Well, how on earth are you going to get there? Now, you take this £5 note."

"Thank you, but you must give me your address. I have to return it to you."

He wrote down his address for me. It was good of him to think of a stranger like that.

By now we had docked, but we still weren't able to go on shore. The formalities took a little time. Meanwhile I was packing my things, and all this time the cabin door remained open, as the doctor had advised. Now, this wouldn't have mattered except that I had hung my fur coat on it. Since I had left the door open, I never noticed the coat. So I didn't pack it and I forgot all about it.

Although the captain was Swedish, like his ship, the other officers were all British. While we were waiting to land, one of them walked up and down with me, and we talked.

"Where are you going to settle in London? What is your address?"

"Regency Lodge in Swiss Cottage."

"That is a very good address."

It was nice to hear that, of course, but at the time I had no idea what he meant. That was never a problem in Russia: whether it was a good address or not, you just had to take what you were given.

Then the captain made his appearance and started walking with me and chatting.

"Are you in a hurry?"

"What on earth do you mean by that?"

"Well, why don't you stay on the boat, stay for two or three days more? It would be nice to have you."

"It is very kind of you to offer me such hospitality, but I am going to London."

I had to laugh, really. You never know where you are with men. Honestly!

Our trains came and we all said goodbye to one another. The captain was rather sad to see me go, I discovered, and said he would miss me. Well, I never even knew that he liked me, never mind liking me enough to invite me to stay on for three days more; but of course I never could accept such an offer.

We all departed, and I set off. It was quite a journey from Middlesbrough to London, and we had to change trains on the way. But there were always chaps that would help me with my luggage, which was nice. They would make sure Leonora and I got on the right train and then put all my belongings in the carriage – well, all my belongings except for the fur coat, which I forgot about completely. Freddy was able to go later and get it back for me.

And at last we reached London, 25 years after I had left. Freddy was there to meet me, with a car. It was his cousins' car, but none of them could drive; so Fred drove. In any event, he would never have let me arrive without being there to meet me.

I talked about Freddy earlier in the book, how close we were as children and how well we always got on. I knew that he had a mixture of feelings seeing me now, because he was so disappointed that I had married his brother and not him; and the fact that things had gone wrong and here I was on my own, with Leonora, made it harder to bear. But these were facts – they couldn't be changed – and these sort of things do happen to people.

When he caught sight of me at Kings Cross, I could see that he couldn't believe his eyes. He hadn't seen me for a long while and he was clearly stunned by what he saw. Leonora he had never seen at all, and he was delighted with her too.

Then Freddy introduced me to his first cousins, my relations by marriage, whom I had never met before. They were a middle-aged couple, very kind. We got talking, because of course I spoke English, though Leonora couldn't yet, but that didn't matter really. Then Freddy put our luggage in their car and they took me to Regency Lodge, to begin life all over again, almost – but not quite – a stranger in my own country.

15

Epilogue, 1946–2006

After 25 years, I was back in England, the country where I was born, where I had such wonderful memories of my childhood. I had left behind my mother, who did not want to leave Russia; I had left behind my English husband, who was no longer free to leave and no longer my husband.

I also left behind May Peters, the friend who really started me thinking about moving to England. She was refused permission to travel because her father now held Russian citizenship and a sensitive job in the Kremlin. So in the end I had to travel by myself – with my daughter Leonora, of course.

Two years earlier, when I got back to Moscow from Central Asia, I had been warned to get hold of my birth certificate and a British passport. I must confess I had also been warned that England had changed since 1921, but how it had changed one could never understand until one saw it.

Popular movement

In 1945, I felt I couldn't afford to go to America – I was very short of cash at that time – so I decided to come to England. Not only was it my homeland, but May and I thought we could teach the movement of Isadora. We assumed that Isadora Duncan's name was well-known all over the world; we thought the English would be pleased to have somebody who had been taught by Isadora and could carry on her ideas.

I danced very well and I just wanted to pass on these graceful movements of Isadora's to ordinary people. I knew from experience that I had abilities in teaching, but I had very little experience in organising things. May Peters would have been better at that, and we could have helped each other. I was very green. But then, until I was 30, I'd had everything done for me: by my mother, by Isadora, by the school, by Moss.

Nevertheless, I had arrived. I didn't know anyone in London apart from Fred, my husband's brother. He and his family tried to help me, but they also had no idea how to organise such things.

After some time, I got permission to teach in one of the Maccabi clubs in the East End. I was pleased when I first entered that club, even though I had only three pupils. Imagine how I felt when, after three weeks, I had 36 pupils!

Now that was encouraging, especially since the girls came from factories and other tiring jobs with long hours. Wherever they came from, they loved the movements, they loved what I was showing them, and this was exactly what I had hoped for. Although my pay wasn't much and certainly not enough to support me – they paid me only 10 shillings an hour and I did two one-hour sessions a week – yet I enjoyed it.

Diploma in Bicycle Movements

But then officialdom stepped in. I thought that was only a problem in Russia – people always used to say 'England is a free country' – but then I never understood politics. In any case, politics had changed: the Labour government had come to power. The people at the top now came from very different backgrounds and some of them didn't know much.

Well, of course, the person who was in charge of physical training in the area heard what was going on at this club and she came to see me while I was taking a class. She watched the lesson and then came to talk to me when I had finished. I pointed out how enthusiastic my pupils were, how well they were doing and how many there were.

"Yes, it is very interesting, but I see you haven't got the English diploma."

"But surely I don't need one? I have all the documents to show that I was a pupil of Isadora Duncan and that I was a very good teacher at her school in Moscow, because I gave the examination to many children who applied there."

320

"That may be so, but nevertheless we cannot allow you to carry on teaching like this, until you get a diploma."

"Surely you don't think I am going to study for some Diploma in Bicycle Movements? I would never do that."

"Then I am very sorry, but you will have to go."

She didn't look very sorry. The girls were in uproar when they heard about it. They all crowded round me and said, "We are going to fight for you!" but I had no heart for it.

"I am not a fighter. If they don't want me, so be it." And I left.

What now?

That was the biggest disappointment I had ever had, but I was still young and I still had a little money left. Instead of giving up my idea, I should have gone to the American embassy and asked for permission to go to the United States. I know I would have succeeded there very well with Isadora's ideas.

But somehow it never came into my head. I just thought, *Well, that is it. I tried and I failed, and now I have to forget about it*. Still, it was very, very disappointing, and I never really got over it. Yet now I had come to England and I had to make the most of it.

I rented two rooms, for myself and my little girl, and then I looked around for a place where she could learn the language, since she didn't speak English – just as I didn't speak any Russian when I first came to Moscow. I found a little school for her, in Bexhill, on the south coast. Once she was settled there, I started to look around to see what I could do.

This period was very stressful. When I reached England, I was a healthy 31-year-old, yet I lost two stone in weight – that's 28 pounds – within a short time. I never noticed, but other people did. My relations, Moss's family, came to see me. They were kind, but they knew nothing of the arts. They didn't understand what was needed, so none of them could help.

I thought, *I can't rely on other people; I have to find something myself*. I looked around for some work and I succeeded. With my family background, naturally I was very good with a needle, so I found work in a dress shop, a very posh dress shop, in fact. Mrs Davies gave me a job – "I knew you were so capable" – and before long I had a new flat too, in west London.

News of Vanya

One day, while I was still staying with my husband's relations in Swiss Cottage, something extraordinary happened. When I got home, they said, "Guess who rang?" It was Vanya, our friend who used to come and see us in Moscow, the London jeweller who was robbed. I was amazed to find he was back in London.

Anyway, we arranged to meet, and his first question was, "How did you get here?" to which I responded, "Well, how on earth did *you* get here?" He told me that when the war reached Russia, he had gone to Tashkent; we compared dates and it was at the same time that I went to Alma-ata. We were both in Central Asia and we never knew.

I told him how I had begged Moss to cross over into China with us, and he wouldn't do it. Moss said our daughter would not survive: she was too young for such a journey, because we would have to cross mountains and semi-desert. Well, if he didn't go, I wouldn't go, so there you are.

Meanwhile, there was Vanya in Tashkent with the same idea, but his wife died of hunger there before they could travel on. After that he and his young son walked nearly all the way to China, crossing over the border secretly. They may have had some lifts on the way, but nevertheless they did it. So Moss, Leonora and I could also have done it. In all this, he never lost his British passport.

His brother was dead by now, so he was pleased to see a familiar face and so was I; he was a great comfort to me, because I felt very lost in London. About this time, the British Government asked Freddy to go to Germany, as a translator, I think. While he was away, Vanya used to come and see me, and sometimes take me out; I was really pleased to have his company.

What happened to Moss

Not long after this, I discovered that Freddy and the whole family were trying to get Moss out of Russia, over to England. But his family and friends in Moscow wrote to warn us not to try any more and just to forget about him. When I wrote to my mother, I said, "Perhaps I should come back to Moscow, so I can do something to help."

Her answer was, "No: you stay where you are." I understood then that something terrible had happened to Moss. I knew I would never see him again; I had to make a new life for myself. My mother had told me, "Forget about him," so I did. I really tried.

Joseph

It happened one day in the school holidays that one of my daughter's friends from school got in touch with me. Her eldest sister wanted to go out dancing, but she was still young enough to want a chaperone, so she asked me if I would come with her to a club, the Anglo-Palestinian Club.

My landlady, a young woman, encouraged me to go.

"You go, Lily. I will be at home and I shall look after Leonora. She will be fine."

So I went. While she was dancing and I was sitting, after about ten minutes a young man came up and asked me for a dance. He danced like a dream. After a while, we stopped and went to sit down. He wanted to know more about me.

"You dance beautifully. How is it that you dance so well?"

I laughed and said, "Well, you dance very well yourself. As for me, I am a dancer."

Joseph had been to the club the week before, but the club was so full he couldn't get in. What I didn't know was that, on the evening we met, as soon as he came through the door he saw me – he had eyes like a hawk – and he said to himself, *That's the woman I'm going to marry*.

Joseph was determined to see me again, and eventually I agreed. He used to take me out, sometimes we went out for a meal with another couple and one thing led to another. Then he asked me to marry him, and I thought, *Well, I could do worse*. He had a very quick mind, he was a good man, a decent man, and I agreed.

We married and settled down together. He was doing well in his job, but then the directors wanted to cut his earnings, so I encouraged him to set up his own business. He was cautious, but I advised him and the business took off straightaway.

We carried on with our life and I introduced Joseph to Vanya, who approved of him. Vanya and I still kept up our friendship, and Joseph and I got on well, but deep down I was never happy.

Isadora and I

I came to England to teach, and they closed my classes down. I was never really happy after that, because it seemed no one was interested in Isadora Duncan. They seemed unaware that she had created such beauty and movement. It is a pity, because music and movement are important: through them one can learn how to be graceful and how to be composed, whatever happens in life.

This book is for Isadora. I feel I owe her something, because she gave me so much. I was always unhappy that people didn't give Isadora Duncan her due. She was such a marvellous dancer and she created something fresh: she turned the whole idea of ballet upside down.

The best ballet dancers in the world do what they do today because of Isadora Duncan. The Bolshoi production of *Romeo and Juliet*, that was so admired, would never have been born if Galina Ulanova had not studied what Isadora was doing. When the critics saw that production, they were all very taken by the way the dancers moved; what they saw were Isadora's movements. From then on, more and more ballet dancers started to dance properly.

Whatever my abilities may be, I can't just sit around and twiddle my fingers. I tried to teach and I wasn't allowed to, so I went on and did other things. Why I am saying all this is because I still can't get over the loss of what I came to do. But you can't re-do what has passed.

Joseph Lotterbach

Up to now I have said very little about my father, because my mother told me very little. She decided that was the best way, and she was very determined. But then so am I. The main thing that made her different from me, I think, is that she was brought up in a village and I was not.

She said I was a lot like my father, in looks and personality. He was very quick, sharp: he noticed things, and I am the same. Those were things my mother liked about him; she wasn't like that. But I never met him and he never saw me. My mother had walked out and left him, and that seemed to suit him. He seemed to disappear, and then

324

there was no way of finding him again, but I found this wasn't quite true.

When I came back to England, I stayed at Regency Lodge, but I was determined – and of course the family understood – that I wanted my own place. Freddy had a friend who knew somebody in one of the turnings just off Golders Green, where I could rent two rooms, which I did.

Opposite me were a young couple, also with a little girl. When I moved in, the young woman rang the bell and introduced herself. I invited her in and she wanted to know where I was from and how had I come here? We got talking and I explained that I had been born here, but I never knew what had happened to my father and really I would have liked to find out. To my astonishment, she said, "I think I can help you there."

She offered to take me to the East End of London, where she knew somebody who, she thought, would know about my father; and she was right. He told me that, yes, he knew my father. When my mother left him, he tried to find us. He looked for us for a whole year, while she evidently hid from him. It must have caused him terrible anguish, knowing that he had a child that he had never seen. After a year, he gave up and went to Paris, where in time he got married again.

Well, I thought, *it is a shame*. He was in Paris when I was dancing there and he never knew. He would have been very interested to meet me, and I so longed to meet him. But my mother never even told me his name; I discovered that much later. I was known by her maiden name, Dikovskaya – or, when touring abroad, Dikovsky. If I had kept my father's surname, which was Lotterbach, it would perhaps have caught his eye on the theatre programme and he would have wondered, *Who is that girl?*

As far as this man that I met knew, my father was still alive, but that only made it more sad, because apparently he loved children and now had quite a large family. So I couldn't get in touch with him, because how would his children feel? What would his wife think? Did they know of my existence? Did they even know he had been married before? Had my parents ever divorced? What would happen if his family found out that his first wife was still alive? None of this would be welcome and neither would I.

I thought I would be intruding so, though I found my father in the end, I never met him. That's sad, I think. But that's life, and you can't retrace your steps.

Index

Since it has not been possible to identify all the people and places mentioned, some surnames are lacking and some names may be mis-spelt. The publishers will welcome corrections or further information.

327

INDEX